6

D1384574

# Behavioral–Social Aspects of Contraceptive Sterilization

# Behavioral–Social Aspects of Contraceptive Sterilization

Edited by

**Sidney H. Newman**
National Institute of Child Health
and Human Development

**Zanvel E. Klein**
University of Chicago

**Lexington Books**
D.C. Heath and Company
Lexington, Massachusetts
Toronto

*301.321*
*B419*
*C - 1*
*5/80*
*19.00*

**Library of Congress Cataloging in Publication Data**

Main entry under title:

Behavioral-social aspects of contraceptive sterilization.

 Outgrowth of a workshop sponsored by the National Institute of Child Health and Human Development.
  Bibliography: p. 217
  Includes index.
  1. Sterilization (Birth control)—Social aspects—Addresses, essays, lectures. 2. Sterilization (Birth control)—Psychological aspects—Addresses, essays, lectures. I. Newman, Sidney H. II. Klein, Zanvel E. III. United States. National Institute of Child Health and Human Development.

| | | |
|---|---|---|
| HQ767.7.B44 | 301.32'1 | 77-94 |

ISBN 0-669-01442-7

*Copyright ©1978 by D.C. Heath and Company*

All rights reserved. No part of this publication may be reproduced or transmitted in any form or by any means, electronic or mechanical, including photocopy, recording, or any information storage or retrieval system, without permission in writing from the publisher. The material in this book grew out of a workshop sponsored and supported by the National Institute of Child Health and Human Development, of the National Institute of Health.

Published simultaneously in Canada

Printed in the United States of America

International Standard Book Number: 0-669-01442-7

Library of Congress Catalog Card Number: 77-94

# Contents

CAMBRIA COUNTY LIBRARY
JOHNSTOWN, PA. 15901

# Foreword

More and more individuals are using contraceptive sterilization to control their fertility. Indications are that use of this method is spreading rapidly, both in the United States and the rest of the world.

It is heartening, therefore, to see this report of a workshop in which experts discussed the significant behavioral-social facets of contraceptive sterilization—including public health, social-demographic and family planning, psychosocial, economic, and methodological considerations. These experts emphasized the tremendous need for behavioral-social research on contraceptive sterilization. They stressed that there has been and is a high degree of utilization of the method without the complementary behavioral-social research necessary to understand differences in use of the method in various parts of the world, as well as the consequences of such use. Research is also essential to planning, administering, and delivering contraceptive sterilization programs in the United States and other countries.

It is hoped that this book will inspire and encourage behavioral-social scientists to engage in significant, meaningful research on contraceptive sterilization.

*Arthur A. Campbell*

# Acknowledgments

Grateful acknowledgment is made to the following sources for permission to use copyrighted material in this book: Christopher Tietze, "The Current Status of Fertility Control," from a symposium on Population Control appearing in *Law and Contemporary Problems* vol. 25, no. 3, summer 1960, pages 426, 441 published by the Duke University School of Law, Durham, North Carolina, copyright 1960, by Duke University; Commission on Population Growth and the American Future; R. Freedman, P.K. Whelpton and A.A. Campbell, *Family Planning, Sterility and Population Growth*, New York: McGraw-Hill Book Company, Inc., copyright 1959 by McGraw-Hill, Inc.; Charles F. Westoff "Trends in Contraceptive Practice: 1965-1973" in *Family Planning Perspectives*, vol. 8, no. 2, 1976; J.M. Stycos, "Female Sterilization in Puerto Rico," *Social Biology* (Eugenics Quarterly) 1954; M. Woodside, *Sterilization in North Carolina*, Chapel Hill, North Carolina: University of North Carolina Press; Harry Sharp, *Growth of American Families, II (Interview Schedule)*; Worldwatch Institute; Excerpta Medica, Amsterdam; N.B. Ryder and C.F. Westoff, *Reproduction in the United States*, copyright 1971 by Princeton University Press; P.K. Whelpton, A.A. Campbell, and J.E. Patterson, *Fertility and Family Planning in the United States*, copyright 1966, by Princeton University Press.

# 1

## Introduction
### *Sidney H. Newman* and
### *Zanvel E. Klein*

The actual and potential importance of contraceptive sterilization in regulating fertility throughout the world can hardly be overestimated. Essentially a twentieth-century development, contraceptive sterilization has shown tremendous worldwide growth during the 1970s (Ravenholt, 1976; Speidel and McCann, 1976; Potts, 1976; Stokes, 1977).

Research is needed to establish accurate figures on the use of contraceptive sterilization in individual countries or on a worldwide basis. Attempts have been made to estimate how many couples in the world have used contraceptive sterilization and to compare these estimates with the use of other fertility regulating or terminating methods. The results are presented in Table 1-1 (Stokes, 1977). The table indicates that the number of couples using contraceptive sterilization more than tripled between 1970 and 1976, a much greater increase than occurred for any of the other family planning methods. This differential growth has made contraceptive sterilization the method of fertility control most used around the world; in 1950 no more than four million couples were using sterilization as their method of birth control (Stokes, 1977). Although the estimates must be validated by future research, they reflect the magnitude of current and probable future use of contraceptive sterilization throughout the world.

Harder data are available for the United States. As a recent report by Westoff on U. S. couples (Westoff, 1976, pp. 54-55) has pointed out,

Probably the most dramatic change since 1970 has been the acceleration of reliance on surgical sterilization. In less than three years, the proportion of contraceptors sterilized for nonmedical reasons grew from 16.3 percent to 23.5 percent. As of 1973, there were an estimated 4.4 million couples among whom one or the other partner had had a contraceptive sterilization. Both male and female operations have increased since then, with the female procedures still slightly more prevalent than vasectomies.

There has been much greater theoretical and research emphasis on the biomedical and technological aspects of family planning than on its behavioral-social

---

Much of the preliminary editing of the papers included in this volume was the responsibility of Zanvel Klein. Our thanks go to Ms. Micki Stock, Ms. Connie Czarnecki, and Ms. Kathy Kostelny, who worked with Klein, typing and retyping manuscripts. We also express our appreciation to Ms. Dorothy Tengood who worked with Newman in the handling of many details and who did much typing.

1

**Table 1-1**
**Estimated Number of Couples Controlling**
**Their Fertility by Family Planning Method**
(in millions)

|  | 1970 | 1976 |
|---|---|---|
| Sterilization | 20 | 75 |
| Pill | 30 | 55 |
| Condom | 25 | 30 |
| IUD | 12 | 15 |
| Other | 60 | 65 |
| Total | 147 | 240 |
| Abortion | 30-55 | 30-55 |

Source: AID and the Population Council. From
B. Stokes, *Filling the Family Planning Gap.*
Worldwatch Paper 12 (Washington, D.C.: World-
watch Institute, 1977). Reprinted with permission.

features. Older methods of contraception and fertility regulation such as withdrawal, the condom, and the diaphragm received very little behavioral-social
research attention. More modern inventions like the pill and intrauterine devices
fared no better. Although abortion has been studied by the social scientist, it
has not been studied nearly enough.

Unless behavioral-social researchers investigate sterilization—an area that has
so far attracted little study—this method of fertility termination will continue to
be used quite differentially in the various nations of the world without the understanding necessary for adequate planning, administration, and utilization.

Recognition of the rapidly increasing importance of contraceptive sterilization gave impetus to the organization and conduct of a workshop on Behavioral-
Social Aspects of Contraceptive Sterilization in June 1973. The workshop, held
in Bethesda, Maryland, was sponsored and funded by the Center for Population
Research of the National Institute of Child Health and Human Development.
Although some time has now elapsed since the workshop was held, the articles
presented in this volume continue to represent the best and most current thought
in the field. Moreover, all of the workshop participants were given the opportunity to review and update their articles for publication in this book.

The workshop participants were selected because of their special expertise
in the subject they were asked to discuss. Each prepared papers prior to the
meetings and revised them later, following discussions which involved both
participants and commentators. The role of the commentator was of special
significance, since the three commentators who reviewed, analyzed, and discussed
each article were well qualified to express pertinent points of view. The commentators and their backgrounds were: H. Bradley Wells, population statistics;
Barbara Hulka, epidemiology; and Kurt W. Back, social psychology and sociology.

We then edited the articles in their revised forms, and returned them to the authors for review and further revision. The authors' changes were incorporated into the final, sometimes updated, version.

The purpose of the workshop was to review and highlight the status of contraceptive sterilization in terms of behavioral-social theory, methods, and research—to indicate what is known and to identify the gaps in knowledge, the methodological problems, and the needed research.

The workshop was organized into five sections. Section I dealt with the public health aspects of contraceptive sterilization; public health considerations were reviewed by Charles Arnold, who stressed the scarcity of research. The social-demographic and family planning aspects constituted the subject matter of Section II. These were viewed from an international perspective, with major attention given to the countries in which, historically and currently, contraceptive sterilization is of major significance. Sterilization in the United States and Puerto Rico was compared by Harriet Presser in her article; India was analyzed by Moni Nag. To Dorothy Nortman fell the large task of discussing the features of contraceptive sterilization in the other parts of the world.

Section III of the workshop examined the psychosocial aspects of contraceptive sterilization, so important for analyzing and understanding problems basic to the initiation, administration, development, and use of contraceptive sterilization. David Rodgers presented the theoretical-conceptual-methodological framework. Edward Pohlman considered contraceptive sterilization in males, Warren Miller in females. Helen Wolfers discussed the consequences of contraceptive sterilization; Henry David and Herbert Friedman reviewed the factors related to acceptability. Everett Rogers focused on a neglected problem—barriers to the diffusion of contraceptive sterilization—and Duff Gillespie, William Spillane, and Paul Ryser reported on their work on the role of knowledge and attitudes in use of sterilization.

The economic aspects of contraceptive sterilization (Section IV) have received little attention, but the promise of such inquiry is reflected in the article presented to the workshop by George Simmons. The last section of the meeting confronted the methodological problems which have beset and hampered research on contraceptive sterilization. Section V, on survey methodological aspects, is the contribution of Leonard LoSciuto and Nancy Cliff, whose article identifies some of the problems as well as possible approaches to their solutions.

The title of our workshop and of this volume aroused some discussion among the participants. Is the term *sterilization* appropriate to the procedures we are examining? Should the term be changed in scientific parlance or clarified because of the various connotations that it has collected over the years? The questions are not new. It will perhaps not surprise readers that the matter of nomenclature was quickly identified as an empirical issue whose resolution depends on research. The various labels applied to the surgery probably reflect how the procedures are viewed by the scientist, the medical practitioner, and the layman. Nonetheless, we need some usable terminology at the present moment. Among the possible choices, *contraceptive sterilization* was most acceptable to the participants in the workshop. It best describes the procedure and carries the implicit notion that use of the method is voluntary.

## References

Potts, M. "Demand Grows for Sterilization." *People* 3(2), (1976), 33.

Ravenholt, R.T. "World Epidemiology and Potential Fertility Impact of Voluntary Sterilization Services." Unpublished paper presented to the Third International Conference on Voluntary Sterilization, Tunis (February 2, 1976).

Speidel, J.J. and McCann, M.J. "Minilaparotomy—A Fertility Control Technology of Increasing Importance." Unpublished paper presented to the Association of Planned Parenthood Physicians, 14th Annual Meeting, Miami Beach, Florida (November 11-12, 1976).

Stokes, B. *Filling the Family Planning Gap.* Worldwatch Paper 12. Washington, D.C.: Worldwatch Institute, 1977.

Westoff, C.F. "Trends in Contraceptive Practice." *Family Planning Perspectives* 8(2) (March-April 1976): 54-57.

**Part I
Public Health Aspects of
Contraceptive Sterilization**

# 2 Public Health Aspects of Contraceptive Sterilization
### Charles B. Arnold

## Introduction

The public health aspects of surgical contraception intersect a number of disciplines, including obstetrics and gynecology, sociology, psychology, anthropology, demography, statistics, and epidemiology. This article reviews only the issues associated with medical problems arising from contraceptive surgery itself.[a]

### Anatomy

An understanding of the anatomy of the male and female reproductive systems is essential to the discussion of the complexities of the various surgical procedures.[b]

The female organs lie within the pelvis and are covered by peritoneum; to transect or remove them, considerable surgical skill and an effective supporting facility (usually a hospital or major clinic) are required. In women, the surgical interruption of the reproductive process focuses primarily on the oviducts, though among surgeons there is a small, vocal group of hysterectomy advocates as well. Surgery in the pelvis is generally considered as "major" by both the surgeon and the public. Although recent developments in "band-aid surgery" have modified surgical techniques somewhat, these procedures have only reduced, not eliminated, the surgical skills needed and the risks that women encounter.

---

This review and analysis is selective, primarily focusing on the North American health and medical literature since 1960. It has considered only studies in which surgical outcomes have been documented statistically. Sample sizes are at least 100 cases in all instances referred to or cited. In assessing the literature, one is limited by the frequent absence of appropriate information concerning methodology.

The writer wishes to acknowledge the help provided him by the bibliographic and review efforts of Harriet Presser (1970) and the Department of Medical and Public Affairs, George Washington University Medical Center (1973). Any incompleteness in this article of course, is the responsibility of the author.

[a]"Medical" refers to those problems (as consequences of surgery) in which demonstrable organic pathology results, that is, morbidity resulting from pathophysiological processes or physical organic change, mortality, pregnancy, or demonstrable failures of attempted surgical contraception. Excluded as outcomes are those conditions which are behavioral or involve dynamic psychosocial states, the subjects of other chapters, in this volume by Miller, Pohlman, Rodgers, and Wolfers.

[b]Female sequelae are given the major emphasis in this chapter because of the greater procedural complexity of female sterilization and the greater total complication rate.

The site of the male sterilization procedure (*vasectomy*) is the vas deferens, the conducting structure for spermatozoa, which lies immediately beneath the skin on the back side of the scrotum. Because of the relative ease of accessibility, the operation is generally a brief, out-patient procedure, regarded as minor surgery, and poses no particular technical problems to the surgeon. The simplicity of the operation is exemplified, in part, by the use of mass vasectomy camps in India and other parts of the world.

The sequelae to the surgery are directly linked to these anatomical dictates. The old surgical maxim applies: The briefer the surgery and the less tissue handled (surgically), the fewer the postoperative problems. Men may thus resume normal activities, including sex, almost immediately postoperatively, while women, depending on the procedure, may be ten days in hospital. Important as anatomy is to the nature and likelihood of postsurgical problems, however, the issues are much more complex.

## Theoretical Framework

There is relatively limited precedent for the construction of a theory related to social medical problems like the medical/health sequelae of contraceptive sterilization. Even a tentative theoretical framework within which to understand postoperative problems, however, seems important because of its dual relevance for research and maternal care services. In the virtual absence of well-conceived research in the public health aspects of contraceptive sterilization, the theoretical level of the questions posed and the conclusions to be drawn is relatively low.

When a field is relatively underdeveloped theoretically, a large number of the relevant questions are of interest to both researchers and practitioners: basic definitions, incidence rates, prevalence rates, and reporting standards. To plan research or services, furthermore, one needs to know the relative contribution to the outcome variances made by the major independent variables (assuming these variables have been fully identified). Some likely variables currently lacking research definitions include the technical preparation of surgeons, staffing patterns for postoperative care, culturally-based standards of heterosexual activity and beliefs affecting the postoperative period, and the preoperative health of the patient. How much of the variance associated with morbidity, mortality, complications, and failures related to sterilization procedures can be explained by such variables? Currently we cannot answer such questions. In effect, we are near, if not upon, the bottom rung of the ladder of theories of the public health determinants and consequences of contraceptive sterilization.

Figure 2-1 is a paradigm presenting some major factors that are hypothesized to contribute to the outcomes observed in the literature. The figure represents a modification of the traditional epidemiological interaction model ("agent-host-environment"). As a paradigm, it is presented primarily to suggest a theoretical approach to outcome studies.

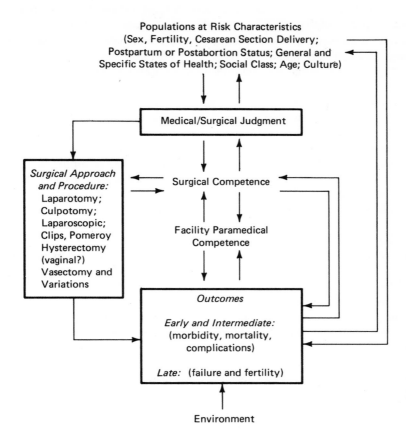

**Figure 2-1.** Paradigm depicting major factors interacting with medical and health outcomes of surgical contraception

The model specifies what seems obvious: that environmental, institutional, and medical factors interact to produce the observed health outcomes of surgery. Some of the implications of the paradigm are listed.

*Sex Differences and Medical Sequelae*

As noted earlier, the anatomy of the reproductive system determines the speed and the amount of tissue damage demanded of the contraceptive surgery. The female's oviducts (tubes) lie anatomically against the broad ligament in the interior part of the pelvis. They are covered by peritoneum. The male's vas deferens is located bilaterally just under the skin in the posterior lateral aspect of the scrotum. In contrast to that of the female, the site of male surgical contraception is surgically easily accessible.

Tubal occlusion may be approached several ways surgically (John, 1972; Johnson, 1972; Laufe, 1972; Roe, 1972). There is little agreement among surgeons about the best approach. Vasectomy uses only one direct surgical approach, although here as well a number of variations are available to the physician (Hulka and Davis, 1972).

Anesthesia for females is nearly always of the general inhalation type (laparoscopy may be an exception). The anesthesia of choice for males is delivered by local infiltration. The necessity of general anesthesia and its duration are definitely associated with morbidity and mortality; local anesthesia carries virtually no comparable bodily or systemic risks (Barnes, 1970).

Surgical risk is greater for women than men. Risk of death for nearly all forms of tubal ligation in the United States is approximately thirty per 100,000 ligations (Presser, 1970). Except for one or two deaths in India, attributed to postsurgical wound sepsis tetanus, there has been no reported mortality from vasectomy, worldwide (Speidel, 1973).

For women many different surgical procedures can be implemented for producing permanent tubal occlusion. Each has its own risk of failure or complication (Yuzpe, 1972), with some risks unique to given procedures. Tubal electrocauterization, for example, carries a risk of accidental cauterization of the bowel or bladder (Hulka, 1972B), clearly a hazard to health. Subcutaneous emphysema, an untoward side effect sometimes associated with laparoscopic surgery, is only temporarily socially disfiguring, at worst. Damage to the bowel or bladder may not be visible, and may or may not be a cause of morbidity. Although not a morbid condition, subcutaneous emphysema's effect on the patient's appearance could result in poor public relations for surgical contraception and decreased popular appeal. Both complications are thus potentially important problems, different in kind; their possible impact on acceptance rates for surgery is, as yet, unknown. With voluntary surgical contraception dependent on popular perceptions to sustain participation, the surgery's cosmetic and other nonmorbid complications are a subject of practical, if not theoretical, interest.

For men, the different procedures for vasectomy involve different failure rates. Other sequelae produced by male procedure are not, however, clarified by the literature.

Postoperative care for females may run seven to ten days; laparoscopy is an exception, necessitating only six to eight hours' observation if uncomplicated (Wheeless, 1972). In men, postoperative care is virtually unnecessary.

High surgical competence, including level of technical skill, is demanded for the female procedures. Considerably less arduous preparation is required for the development of adequate skills in simple vasoresection of the male.

## Cultural-Social Factors

Besides the obvious influence of tradition and reference groups on attitudes, expectations, and beliefs, the simple physical environment of the community regarding public sanitation and personal hygiene practices may increase the risk of postoperative wound infections.

## Surgical Judgment

Probably no issue related to understanding or predicting public health aspects of contraceptive sterilization is more central, yet more difficult to study than is surgical judgment. The decision-making processes of surgeons in selecting technique and candidates for contraceptive sterilization have thus far been inaccessible to research. Universally very much in command, surgeons usually do not subject their judgment to the questioning of others. Even the medical record may contain no hint as to the rationale for a particular timing, procedure, or surgical approach. There have been few, if any, scientific studies of surgical judgment, though objective criteria are now evolving in medicine that may assist research on health problems which include surgical intervention (Payne, 1968).

In judgments about sterilization, some of the surgical reasoning seems based on no more than tradition. The so-called Rule of 120, for instance, despite its obvious inherent inequities, is still cited by surgeons as a guide for decision-making (Claman, 1971). According to this usage, fertility multiplied by age should equal 120 or more to qualify a woman as a candidate for contraceptive sterilization. A 25 year-old woman with three children would not be eligible, whereas a 30 year-old woman with four would be. With no empirical basis, this criterion seems to be taken with remarkable seriousness in the post-1970 obstetrics and gynecology literature.

The transactional aspects of surgical decisions also demand investigation. Little is known, for example, about any trade-offs that may be made during negotiations between surgeons and their prospective clients. Current American estimates of nonessential surgery and the well-known phenomenon of persons who inexplicably have had multiple operations suggest that more than just obvious health needs enter into surgeons' decisions.

Since the choice of contraceptive surgery is a decision usually made by couples, one can also wonder why women have so often had to bear the brunt. Could this have to do with surgeons' possible latent hostility toward women or with sexism? Could it be that gynecologists are simply more aggressive than urologists about such surgery? Do the two disciplines avail themselves of consultation with one another when presented with a request for contraceptive surgery? If not, what factors enter into the failure to communicate?

The high female:male ratio apparently reflects the limited recognition by surgeons of the inherently complex nature of the decision to operate. From the perspective of medical/surgical outcome this is unfortunate, as we shall see in the next section.

*Determinants, Consequences, and their Feedback*

A complex social-medical system of the type posited in this section is not unidirectional in its effects. A factor at one level in this construct, in addition to influencing subsequent steps, also provides feedback effects. A change in outcome rates (such as complications), for example, once known by clients and surgeons, would make for better informed decisions. At another level, were data available about some late complications of women's contraceptive surgery (obesity, psychoneurotic symptomatology, or increased ectopic pregnancy rates), more couples might choose vasectomy.

**Analysis of Relevant Research**

Problems associated with outcomes of contraceptive sterilization have been rather clearly identified. Five major problem categories exist:

1. Mortality.
2. Morbidity.
3. Surgical complications, without morbidity.
4. Surgical failure, without full-term pregnancy.
5. Full-term pregnancy.

*Mortality*

Estimates of surgical contraceptive mortality vary somewhat, but most reports place the death rate between twenty-five and thirty-five deaths per 100,000 tubal ligations. Presser (1970), analyzing the combined mortality rate from ten large studies since 1960, reported five deaths in 20,058 operations (24.4 per 100,000). Barnes (1970) reviewed the Johns Hopkins experience over an unspecified period of time. The combined death rate was thirty-five per 100,000, higher for women over age thirty-five. A recent report estimates mortality rate in the United States to be thirty per 100,000 (Hulka, Soderstrom, Larson, and Brooks, 1972); this figure agrees closely with that of Bruhl (1967) in his review of almost 69,000 European total laparoscopies.

When the expected number of deaths is so low, clinical experience must be aggregated across studies. In the largest sample cited by Presser (1970), Lu and

Chun (1967) reported only one death in a series of 5,968 women; the expected number of deaths (based on thirty per 100,000) would have been approximately 1.8. With such low rates of expected mortality prevailing even in so large a study, the need becomes manifest for collaborative research among a number of cooperating institutions and investigators over periods of time. (The research approaches will be further discussed in the last two sections of this chapter.)

Tubal ligation may still be more hazardous than other fertility control procedures. Table 2-1 presents figures on a variety of contraceptive methods.

In comparison with the other methods, the risk of death is sufficiently greater with tubal ligation to warrant consideration of strategies of contraception other than surgery. As Presser (1970) has noted, however, the mortality rates for tubal ligation have seemed to decrease in recent years. In the fifties, for example, some studies had reported rates as high as 400 per 100,000 (McElin, Buckingham, and Johnson, 1967); with greater experience, as the previous discussion showed, the rates have dropped markedly. Whether the present rates will continue to drop remains to be seen. Presser has also noted, in defense of surgery, that the risks need be assumed only once, whereas in other methods the exposure to risk is multiple.

*Morbidity*

The factors associated with contraceptive surgical morbidity are many. As a

**Table 2-1**
**Estimated Annual Mortality Rates by Method of**
**Female Contraception, United States**

| Method | Estimated Annual Mortality Rates (per 100,000 users) |
|---|---|
| Oral Contraception | 3 – 5 |
| Induced abortion, first trimester | 2.5 – 3 |
| Induced abortion, second trimester | 27 |
| Vaginal delivery, full term pregnancy | 20 |
| Tubal ligation | 25 – 35 |

Source: Data estimated from A. C. Barnes, "Discussion." *American Journal of Obstetrics and Gynecology* 106 (1970): 1050-52; and C. Tietze, "Mortality with Contraception and Induced Abortion." *Studies in Family Planning* 45 (September, 1969): 6-8.

reference point in reviewing the literature, one can use the combined morbidity for the three United States studies reported since 1960 and tabulated by Presser (1970, p. 6) as 11.6 percent.[c]  A partial list of the practically significant factors includes:

**Age.**  According to Barnes (1970), older women (over 35 years) have higher rates of postoperative morbidity and mortality than do younger women, particularly the morbidity associated with anesthesia and with bed rest (Barnes, 1970).  The influence of age has not been sufficiently taken into account in the literature reporting and analyzing morbidity rates.

**Parity.**  The frequent stretching of the pelvic tissues in higher parity women increases their postoperative risk of bladder infections and pelvic thromboses.

**Postabortion Status.**  Tietze's (1972) JPSA (Joint Program for the Study of Abortion) data indicated that tubal ligation done in conjunction with induced abortion carries a higher risk of complication than does abortion alone.  Sogolow (1971), however, found a 14 percent morbidity rate for postabortion tubal ligations among 124 women, a rate that compares favorably to the overall postoperative tubal ligations morbidity rate of 10 percent.

**Postpartum Status.**  Turner and Hooper (1971) reported a statistically significant difference in postoperative tubal ligation morbidity that favors other than immediately postpartum women.  Mabray, Malinak, and Flowers (1970), however, found no such difference.  The literature, which has few controlled studies, suggests that unless surgery is possible in the first seventy-two hours postpartum, a reduction in morbidity is best achieved by waiting until the sixth week postpartum (Rubin, 1970).

Factors other than morbidity, however, may recommend tubal ligation soon after childbirth, particularly when nonmedical issues are considered; for example, motivation for surgery is noted to be high at parturition and surgical care costs may be reduced.

**Post-Cesarean Section.**  Cesarean sections occur at a rate of approximately four per 1000 live births (Barnes, 1970).  According to prevailing gynecological opinion, a woman having once had a Cesarean should deliver subsequent children by that route, but more than three such operations are discouraged.  After the third birth, many women undergo tubal ligation; some have hysterectomies,

---

[c]Presser (1970) has noted the marked difference between the reportedly low morbidity rates in the United States and those in other countries.  Medical customs in reporting, she believed, are probably the principal source of the disparity.  Little is directly known about this, however.

however. Bopp and Hall (1970) found in their experience that combining tubal ligation with Cesarean section increased the overall postoperative morbidity from 4 percent to 27 percent. Brenner, Sall, and Sourieblick (1970) found a 20 percent morbidity rate in nearly 200 cases.

**Postpartum Hysterectomy.** In the gynecological literature, there are advocates for the use of hysterectomy solely for sterilization purposes (Haynes, 1970; Hibbard, 1972; Laufe, 1971; Muldoon, 1972; Van Nagell, 1971). Such arguments are often accompanied by faintly concealed derogation of the lower socioeconomic class, minority group women who are frequently lost to follow-up postpartum counseling on contraception. Fairly typical of this sentiment are Roach, Krolak, Powell, Lorens, and Duebler (1972) and McElin, Malinak, and Flowers, (1967) who urged hysterectomy especially for those who usually fail to comply with medical and contraceptive management. Hysterectomy, whether by a vaginal or an abdominal route, carries a much higher morbidity rate than does tubal ligation. Between 30 percent and 50 percent of such patients have complications, with infections and bleeding being most significant. Perhaps Speidel, Perry, and Duncan (1973) have best summarized the role of hysterectomy in surgical contraception: "It is debatable whether hysterectomy for the single indication of sterilization is a justifiable procedure." (p. 9)

**Laparoscopic Sterilization.** This is the newest technique in surgical contraception, virtually "key-hole" or "band-aid" surgery (Jordan, 1971; Larson, 1972; Wadhwa, 1972). The latter name comes from the size of the postoperative dressing that can be used for the small surgical wound. The procedure involves one or two abdominal incisions and the introduction of a laparoscope (Wheeless, 1972) into the insufflated peritoneal cavity. The scope is a long, slender, tubular device through which a surgeon can visualize the oviducts (because of a self-contained light source) and perform the surgery either through crushing the oviduct, by placing a metal clip, or by cauterizing. Morbidity associated with laparoscopy has recently been found by Hulka, Soderstrom, Larson, and Brooks (1972) to be 1.6 percent, the major morbidity resulting from anesthesia, insufflation, or electrocoagulation. In terms of postoperative morbidity, laparoscopy would seem (based on these data) to be the safest procedure currently in use for female sterilization.

*Complications*

As the term is used surgically, *complications* are postoperative problems not necessarily associated with morbidity, but which must be treated by the surgeon nevertheless. A good example is postlaparoscopic subcutaneous emphysema which occurs when air leaks into the tissue between the abdominal muscles and

skin, thereby inadvertently inflating the skin. The condition subsides spontaneously as the tissues absorb the air, usually with no residual effect. Subcutaneous emphysema is cosmetically problematical, consumes health care
resources, and is considered a complication. Its exact incidence is currently
unknown.

Accidental surgical perforation of the bowel, discovered postoperatively,
is another example of a complication. While the patient usually suffers only
minimal discomfort, it is a potentially serious event requiring medical observation until the perforation heals and all residual signs have disappeared. As
already mentioned, the public health significance of such complications is
their potential link to subsequent conditions and their social and organizational
implications for the process of contraceptive sterilization.

A new complication of vasectomy has recently been reported: the presence of sperm antibodies in the serum. In approximately 50 percent of men
examined in special clinical studies, antibodies have been noted to appear by
six weeks postoperatively (Ansbacher, Keung-Yeung, and Wurster, 1972). Their
serological persistence or long-term health implications are not yet understood.
This complication bears further study because of its potential significance for
future clinical and laboratory research.

*Failures*

Failures is a term usually reserved for persons that have undergone surgical
contraception and yet remain fecund postoperatively. The failure rates for tubal
ligation are low (Gaal, 1971). On the basis of aggregating over 26,000 cases in
eighteen studies, Presser (1970) estimated failures at 0.1 per 100 operations. In
these studies, failures ranged from 0 to approximately 2 percent (Presser, 1970,
pp 7-8.)[d]

Among men, the postvasectomy failure rate is considerably higher. From
six studies with a total of 2,300 men, Presser (1970) derived a failure rate of
0.9 per 100 cases. The usual definition of vasectomy failure is the presence of
motile sperm in the ejaculate one week or more postoperatively (Temple, 1970).

The reason for the male-female difference in failure rates is not well understood. The literature is usually unclear as to the length of time the cases have
been followed (Thompson, 1968). Comparability is therefore difficult to
achieve, because failure rates are at least in part a function of time and coital
exposure, neither of which have been controlled in published studies.

There may be an anatomical basis for the male-female differences, as well.

---

[d]One source of failure in females is mistaken ligature of the round ligament rather than the
tube (they are anatomically contiguous and have the same embryological origin).

The small surgical incision used for vasectomy does not permit direct exploration. Some men have more than two vas deferens; unless searched for, the auxiliary vas may easily be overlooked. If not found, of course, the vas retains its function in conveying sperm. The frequency of this anatomic variant in human populations is not currently known, but may account for some of the vasectomy failures.

*Fertility*

Full-term pregnancies after tubal ligation have been reported by Presser (1970, p. 9) to be in the range of 0.04 to 0.08 per 100 person-years. The difference between the failure rate and the slightly lower fertility rate is primarily attributable to induced abortions and ectopic pregnancies (Thelin, 1972). Some post-surgery pregnancies will be terminated voluntarily, others spontaneously. That distinction, as a component of failure, is not fully clarified in the literature, however.

Among men, the postoperative fertility rate is higher, 0.15 per 100 person-years' use (Presser, 1970). The higher rate for men is related to the postoperative presence of viable sperm in the proximal vas deferens. Craft and McQueen (1972) have found positive sperm counts fifteen weeks postoperatively in 25 percent of men who underwent simple vasectomy, and in 6 percent of the men even after vasectomy and irrigation of the vas with sterile water. Despite these pregnancy rates, contraceptive sterilization has much lower postmethod failure rates than other methods of contraception (Presser 1970, Table 6, p. 9).

**Future Research**

Before launching into descriptive research on the public health aspects of surgical contraception, five fundamental methodological issues need exploration:

1. Definition, in research terms, of the major independent variables associated with morbidity, mortality, complication, failure, and fertility rates. Some of these variables have been suggested in the pardigm (see Figure 2-1).
2. Use of longitudinal study designs for investigating failure and pregnancy rates. These could be either retrospective or prospective, and follow specific population groups postsurgery, or could examine consecutive cases of complications frequently attributed to sterilization. Ectopic pregnancies and their determinants could be a subject for one such study. (One estimate is that 25 percent of all ectopics occur in posttubectomized women [Thelin, 1972] ).
3. Development of controlled studies, using either population groups as controls or using individuals (case-control design).

4.  Implementation of analytical models appropriate to extant theory.  Examples include age-adjustment of morbidity, mortality, and complication rates as well as the application of correlation techniques, multiple regression, or cluster analyses in handling the often complex data.
5.  Specification in public health research reports of the study design used in evaluating surgery results, as well as the categories of variables investigated, making possible large scale aggregations of data from several studies.

These five suggestions constitute the field's rather basic research needs before it can begin to function effectively at a scientific level.  The general impression from the surgical literature is that these larger research and public health issues have not been fully recognized as important.  Exceptions exist, of course.  The conferences convened on voluntary sterilization over the last several years have, in fact, given more attention to these public health problems.

Yet another research problem is cross-disciplinary.  The surgical literature is generally bereft of input from epidemiologists or biostatisticians when the public health issues are considered.  The addition of one or two members from these disciplines would not be a panacea; the problems are too complex.  A commitment must, however, be made by those organizing conferences or annual meeting sections on obstetrics and gynecology to include in their programs, on the program committees or as program consultants, individuals well-versed in public health research.  Unless steps are undertaken, we shall continue to read comparative studies in which rates are not age-standardized, and follow-up criteria and independent variables have not been specified.  Moreover, the absence of controlled studies will continue.  Without the influence and collaboration of epidemiologists and biostatisticians, an understanding of the public health factors in contraceptive sterilization will fail to progress at the rate required to meet the projected needs.

Gynecologists, of course, are not alone in their separatist research urges.  The social science literature does not yet contain sufficient cross-disciplinary research on these problems to set a good example to others.  The convergence of investigational objectives on the part of public health, surgery, gynecology, and the social sciences would be desirable.  Emerging from these shared interests would be collaborative studies directed toward resolving the methodological and theoretical issues associated with the health consequences of surgical contraception.

**Summary**

The public health (medical) determinants and consequences of surgical contraception are complex; though reasonably well documented, they are not particularly well understood.  An examination of the literature finds the present level of scientific study to be low both in theory and in methodology.

Five principal dependent or outcome issues are recognized as associated with postoperative contraceptive sterilization: mortality, morbidity, complications, surgical failures, and fertility.

In two categories—mortality and fertility—contraceptive surgery can be compared to other forms of contraception, including abortion. For women, crude mortality rates for surgery appear to be from two to seven times higher than other contraception. Undesired fertility or pregnancy rates after surgery, however, are only a small fraction of those for other forms of contraception, ranging from 0.04 to 0.08 per 100 person-years for women and around 0.15 for men. Fertility rates with other procedures are in the order of 1 to 2 percent (pill) to perhaps 40 percent (foams and jellies).

Mortality, morbidity, and failure rates for surgical contraception are reasonably well-documented as crude rates. Controlled comparative studies, however, are needed to develop risk profiles for surgery in epidemiological terms or to define risk status for various sub-groups of women seeking voluntary surgical contraception. On the latter, the need for such work is greater for women than for men.

A paradigm has been presented to clarify some readily apparent factors that affect outcome. One variable—surgical judgment—is central, but seems rather inaccessible to study. The surgeon's judgment influences whether, when, by whom, and by what procedure the operation will be performed. As the literature adequately demonstrates, the elements included in the paradigm have considerable impact on the crude rates of mortality, morbidity, complications, failure, and pregnancy.

Surgeons must become professionally concerned about the public health issues associated with sterilization and joint biosocial studies of these problems must be undertaken. Until such developments occur, the many public health research questions about surgical contraception will persist.

## References

Anonymous. *Sterilization* (an annotated bibliography) Washington, D.C. Department of Medical and Public Affairs, George Washington University Population Report C-D Number 1 (February 1973).

Ansbacher, R., Keung-Yeung, K. and Wurster, J. C. "Sperm Antibodies in Vasectomized Men." *Fertility and Sterility* 23 (1972): 640-43.

Barnes, A.C. "Discussion." *American Journal of Obstetrics and Gynecology.* 106 (1970): 1050-52.

Bopp, J.R. and Hall, D.G. "Indications for Surgical Sterilization." *Journal of Obstetrics and Gynecology* 35 (May 1970): 760-64.

Brenner, P. Sall, S. and Sourieblick, B. "Evaluation of Cesarean Section Hysterectomy as a Sterilization Procedure." *American Journal of Obstetrics and Gynecology* 108 (1970): 335-39.

Bruhl, W. "Complications of Laparoscopy and Liver Biopsy under Vision: The Results of a Survey." *German Medical Monthly* 12 (1967): 31-32.

Claman, A.D., Wakeford, J.R., Turner, J.M., and Blayden, B. "Impact on Hospital Practice of Liberalizing Abortions and Female Sterilizations." *Canadian Medical Association Journal* 105 (July 10, 1971): 35-41.

Craft, I. and McQueen, J. "Effect of Irrigation of the Vas on Postvasectomy Semen Counts." *Lancet* 1 (March 4, 1972): 515.

Droegemueller, W., Makowski, E. and Macsalka, R. "Destruction of the Endometrium by Cryosurgery." *American Journal of Obstetrics and Gynecology* 110 (1971): 467.

Gaal, R.J. "The Position of Tubal Ligation in Family Planning." *Medical Journal of Australia* 2 (1971): 772-74.

Haskins, A.L. "Oviductal Sterilization with Tantalum Clips." *American Journal of Obstetrics and Gynecology* 114 (1972): 370-77.

Haynes, D.M. and Wolfe, W.M. "Tubal Sterilization in an Indigent Population. Report of 14 Years Experience." *American Journal of Obstetrics and Gynecology* 106 (1970): 1044-53.

Hibbard, L.T. "Sexual Sterilization by Elective Hysterectomy." *American Journal of Obstetrics and Gynecology* 112 (1972): 1076-1083.

Hulka, J.F. and Davis, J.E. "Vasectomy and Reversible Vas Occlusion." *Fertility and Sterility* 23 (1972): 683.

Hulka, J.F. and Omran, K.F. "Cauterization for Tubal Sterilization." In Richart, R. M. and Prager, D.J. (Eds.) *Human Sterilization.* Springfield, Illinois: Charles C. Thomas (1972): 313-333.

Hulka, J.F., Soderstrom, P.M., Larson, S.L., and Brooks, P.G. Complications Committee of the American Association of Gynecological Laparoscopists, First Annual Report. Report from Las Vegas Meeting of the American Association of Gynecological Laparoscopists, November 13-14, 1972.

John, A.H., and Dunster, G.D. "Sterilization by Posterior Culpotomy." *Journal of Obstetrics and Gynecology of the British Commonwealth* 79 (1972): 381-382.

Johnson, Diana S. "Report on the Conference, Female Sterilization: Prognosis for Simplified Outpatient Procedures." *Contraception* 5 (1972): 155-163.

Jordan, J.A.; Edwards, R.L.; Pearson, J; and Maskery, D.J.K. "Laparoscopic Sterilization and Follow-up Hysterosalpingogram." *Journal of Obstetrics and Gynecology of the British Commonwealth* 78 (1971): 460-466.

Larson, S.L. "Laparoscopic Sterilization." *Minnesota Medicine* 55 (April 1972): 369-371.

Laufe, L.E., and Kreutner, A.K. "Vaginal Hysterectomy: A Modality for Therapeutic Abortion and Sterilization." *American Journal of Obstetrics and Gynecology* 110 (1971): 1096-1099.

Laufe, L.E. and Summerson, S. "Internal Vaginal Tubal Ligation in Duncan," G.W.; Falb, R.D., and Speidel, J.J. (Eds.) *Female Sterilization Prognosis for Simplified Procedures.* New York: Academic Press (1972): 73-76.

Lu, T., and Chun, D. "Long Term Follow-up Study of 1055 Cases of Postpartum Tubal Ligation." *Journal of Obstetrics and Gynecology of the British Commonwealth* 74 (1967): 875-880.

Mabray, C.R.; Malinak, L.R.; and Flowers, L.E. "Tubal Sterilization: Morbidity on a Charity Hospital Service." *Obstetrics and Gynecology* 36 (August, 1970): 204-207.

McElin, T.W.; Buckingham, J.C.; and Johnson, R.E. "Tubal Sterilization." *American Journal of Obstetrics and Gynecology* 97 (1967): 479.

Muldoon, M.J. "Gynecological Illness After Sterilization." *British Medical Journal* 1 (1972): 84-85.

Payne, B.C. *Hospital Utilization Review Manual.* Ann Arbor: University of Michigan Medical School; Department of Post-graduate Medicine (1968).

Presser, H.B. "Voluntary Sterilization: A World View." *Reports on Population/ Family Planning,* No. 5, 1970.

Roach, C.J.; Krolak, J.D.; Powell, J.L.; Lorens, A.S.; and Duebler, K.F. "Vaginal Hysterectomy for Sterilization." *American Journal of Obstetrics and Gynecology,* 114 (1972): 670-673.

Roe, R.E.; Laros, R.K.; and Work, B.A. "Female Sterilization: The Vaginal Approach." *American Journal of Obstetrics and Gynecology,* 112 (1972): 1031-1036.

Rubin, A, and Czernobilsky, B. "Tubal Ligation: A Bacteriological, Histological, and Clinical Study." *Obstetrics and Gynecology* 36(2) (August 1970): 199-203.

Sogolow, S.R. "Vaginal Tubal Ligation at Time of Vacuum Curettage for Abortion." *Obstetrics and Gynecology* 38 (1971): 888-892.

Speidel, J.J.; Perry, M.I.; and Duncan, G.W. "Research Approaches to New Sterilization Technology." Paper presented at the 2nd International Conference on Voluntary Sterilization. February 25-March 1, 1973, Geneva, Switzerland.

Temple, J.G., and Jameson, R.M. "Semen Examination after Vasectomy." *Lancet* 2 (December, 1970): 1258.

Thelin, T.J. and Van Nagell, J.R. "Ruptured Ectopic Pregnancy After Bilateral Tubal Ligation." *Obstetrics and Gynecology* 39 (1972): 589-590.

Thompson, B., and Baird, D. "Follow-up of 186 Sterilized Women." *Lancet* 1: (May 1968) 1023-1027.

Tietze, C. "Mortality With Contraception and Induced Abortion." *Studies in Family Planning,* 45 (September 1969): 6-8.

Tietze, C. and Lewit, S. "Joint Program for the Study of Abortion (JPSA): Early Medical Complications of Legal Abortion." *Studies in Family Planning,* 3 (June 1972): 97-122.

Turner, G. and Hooper, N. "Sterilization and Thromboembolism." *Journal of Obstetrics and Gynecology of the British Commonwealth.* 78 (1971): 737-740.

Van Nagell, J.R. Jr., and Roddick, J.W. "Vaginal Hysterectomy as a Sterilization Procedure." *American Journal of Obstetrics and Gynecology.* 111 (November 1971): 703-707.

Wadhwa, R.K. and McKenzie, R. "Complications of Band Aid Surgery for Sterilization." *Journal of the American Medical Association.* 222 (December 1972): 1558.

Wheeless, C.R. Jr. "OPD Laparoscope Sterilization Under Local Anesthesia." *Obstetrics and Gynecology* 39 (May 1972): 767-770.

Yuzpe, A.A.; Allen, H.; and Collins J.A. "Tubal Sterilization: Methodology, Postoperative Management and Follow-up of 2934 Cases." *Canadian Medical Association Journal.* 107 (July 1972): 115-117.

Zipper, J.A.; Stachetti, E.; and Medel, M. "Human Fertility Control by Transvaginal Application of Quinacrine on the Fallopian Tube." *Fertility and Sterility* 21 (1970): 581-589.

**Part II
Social–Demographic and Family Planning
Aspects of Contraceptive Sterilization**

**3**

# Contraceptive Sterilization as a Grassroots Response: A Comparative View of the Puerto Rican and United States Experience
*Harriet B. Presser*

The practice of contraceptive sterilization to limit family size has become increasingly popular throughout the world. In some countries, this has been the result of organized efforts on the part of governmental family planning programs to encourage individuals to choose the option of sterilization. In other countries, interest in the method has gained momentum at the grassroots level without much institutional encouragement. Puerto Rico and the United States fall into the latter category. As the two countries in which contraceptive sterilization is most widely practiced relative to their total population, Puerto Rico and the United States are worthy of detailed analysis.

This chapter describes the trend in the practice of sterilization in each country, explains why—from a demographic and social perspective—individuals have been so receptive to its practice, and determines the structural supports for and constraints against sterilization within the two societies. The demographic effectiveness of sterilization in each country is also considered. Finally, in comparing and contrasting the experience of Puerto Rico with that of the United States, suggestions are made about the relevance of various demographic and social factors and about areas for further research. The discussion throughout this chapter relies heavily on the existing literature.

**Puerto Rico[a]**

*Trend in Practice*

The practice of female sterilization in Puerto Rico began in the early 1930s at a highly reputable hospital in San Juan; in the decades to follow the operation was performed in many government and private hospitals. Little hard data on incidence are available on an annual basis. In government district hospitals from 1944 to 1950, the annual number of sterilizations doubled (Stycos, 1954). By 1950, in these institutions alone, close to 7,000 women had been sterilized (Cordero, 1966). Statistics on contraceptive sterilization in government hospitals

---

[a]The following discussion of Puerto Rico is drawn largely from the author's *Sterilization and Fertility Decline in Puerto Rico* (Berkeley, Calif.: University of California Press, 1973).

were no longer published after 1950, probably in part because of the unfavorable publicity they caused (Back, Hill, and Stycos, 1960).

Private hospitals undoubtedly experienced a similar, if not more pronounced, increase in the number of sterilizations performed in the late 1940s. Indeed, many private clinics and small hospitals were established during this period, primarily, or solely, for the purpose of performing sterilizations (Satterthwaite, personal communication, 1968). A conservative estimate is that in 1949, 17.8 percent of all hospital deliveries (both government and private) were followed by sterilization, representing about 7 percent of all deliveries (hospital or elsewhere) during that year in Puerto Rico (Stycos, 1954).

Island-wide fertility surveys conducted in 1947-1948 and 1953-1954 verify the rising popularity of sterilization over these years. A study conducted in 1947-1948, based on a sample of 6,000 households, found that 6.6 percent of women who had ever married were sterilized (Hatt, 1952, p. 444, Table 318). This estimate is also considered to be conservative (Back, Hill, and Stycos, 1960). Six years later (1953-1954), another study revealed that 16.5 percent of the married women were sterilized among a "stratification sample" of 999 household heads (Hill, Stycos, and Back, 1959, p. 167, Table 80). Although the samples in the two surveys are not strictly comparable, the sizeable differences in prevalence suggest that the incidence of sterilization had risen considerably over the six-year period. In the 1940s, women of relatively high socioeconomic status—as indexed by a dichotomous classification of monthly home rental value—seemed especially likely to have been sterilized (Hatt, 1952). By the mid-1950s, however, adoption of the procedure had reached all socioeconomic groups, as suggested by the high rates of sterilization at all educational levels (Hill, Stycos, and Back, 1959, p. 168, Table 81).

Between the mid-1950s and the mid-1960s, there were no estimates of the incidence or prevalence of female sterilization in Puerto Rico. It would have been difficult, if not impossible, to obtain such data on an island-wide basis from hospital records. It was commonly believed, moreover, that other contraceptive methods were replacing sterilization and that only under very special circumstances was the operation performed. (Vazquez, personal communication, 1966). The facts, however, were otherwise. A secondary analysis of the Master Sample Survey of Puerto Rico in 1965 (when additional questions on sterilization were added) revealed that contrary to expectations the practice of sterilization had reached an extremely high level. In a sub-sample of over 1,000 ever-married Puerto Rican women aged twenty to forty-nine, 31.9 percent—or 34.0 percent of the mothers in this age range—had been sterilized (Presser, 1969). The prevalence of sterilization had apparently doubled since the mid-1950s, exceeding by far the experience of any other country. It was being practiced widely by women of all educational levels, but most notably among women with moderate levels of schooling (four to eleven years). These findings, which many initially treated with disbelief, were verified by the 1968 Master Sample Survey; again, about one-third of the women were found to have been sterilized (Gutiérrez, 1972, p. 391, Table 3).

It is important to note the above estimates of female sterilization include those performed for therapeutic, as well as contraceptive, reasons. Although the precise proportion of all sterilizations that were at least partly contraceptive in intent cannot be ascertained, it seems reasonable to assume that the great majority of the procedures were prompted by the desire to limit births. A breakdown by types of sterilizing operations performed (oopherectomy, hysterectomy, or tubal ligation) in Puerto Rico is not possible; however, hospital records studied in depth by the writer reveal the predominant method to have been postpartum tubal ligation.

The practice of male sterilization in Puerto Rico is not nearly so widespread as female sterilization. On an island-wide basis, it is estimated that, as of 1968, less than 2 percent of Puerto Rican men had been sterilized (Gutiérrez, 1972). From 1956 to 1966, the Family Planning Association of Puerto Rico subsidized vasectomy for about 3,000 men—a special attempt on the part of the Association's Medical Director, Dr. M.E. Paniagua, to encourage couples who requested female sterilization to choose male sterilization instead. He succeeded in over one-fourth of the cases. Vasectomy in recent years has been offered by goverment-supported family planning clinics.

*Receptivity to Sterilization*

Why did so many Puerto Rican women want to become sterilized? An explanation of this phenomenon requires answering at least three other questions. First, why were Puerto Rican women so highly motivated to limit their family size? Second, why did they choose sterilization as the principal means of achieving this end? Third, why female rather than male sterilization?

**Demographic Conditions and the Desire to Limit Family Size.** According to demographic theory, a widespread desire for smaller families is initiated by a sharp decline in mortality at a time of high fertility, accompanied by rapid industrialization (Davis, 1963). Puerto Rico was at this early phase of demographic transition in the 1940s and 1950s. Infant mortality had been declining rapidly; unless fertility control practices increased, family size would have become larger. Small family size ideals prevailed. Despite a strong preference for only two children (Hill, Stycos, and Back, 1959), however, many women were exceeding their preferences by at least two or more children. Economic development was rapid, offering the prospect of a higher standard of living and possibly reducing the number of children desired by the family.

The increased rate of employment of Puerto Rican women outside the home was an aspect of industrialization that may have been particularly relevant to the desire for smaller families. For an employed woman an additional child is more costly; it generally involves the loss of a job and salary—at least temporarily. And unlike women who work at home, return to the labor force after having a child usually adds to the cost of a job in terms of child care.

In Puerto Rico, there has been a notable shift in female employment from home needlework to work outside the home. Labor force participation rates for women, as such, have remained fairly constant in recent decades—they declined between 1940 and 1960 from 25 percent to 20 percent, and rose again to 23 percent in 1970 (U.S. Bureau of the Census, 1963; 1972b). In 1940, however, 35 percent of the female labor force had been employed in home needlework; this decreased to 23 percent in 1950 and to 4 percent in 1960 (Weller, 1968; data for 1970 are as yet unavailable).

Insofar as work outside the home exposes women to nonfamilial sources of satisfaction, interest in having an additional child may be reduced. This is particularly likely for women who hold "good" positions, that is, white collar as compared to manual jobs. In Puerto Rico, the percentage of women employed in white collar jobs has notably increased over past decades—from 12 percent of all employed women in 1940, to 29 percent in 1950, 38 percent in 1960, and 51 percent in 1970 (U.S. Bureau of the Census, 1943; 1953; 1963; 1972b). So rapid a shift in the nature of female employment is remarkable for a developing country.

In summary, several reasons seem to have motivated Puerto Rican women to limit their family size: the reduction in infant mortality, the rising standard of living, the increased employment of women outside the home, and the shift in female employment from manual to white collar jobs.

**Choice of Sterilization.** The widespread practice of sterilization depends not only on the desire to limit family size but on the awareness that sterilization is a safe, effective, and available means of achieving that end. Physicians in Puerto Rico seem to have played a key role in making surgery a viable option for women interested in family planning.

A few physicians in Puerto Rico initially promoted the practice of female sterilization. The process by which the technical knowledge and acceptability was diffused to other physicians has been described by Stycos (1954):

A good many physicians on the island were already aware of the problems of population, the prestige of the private hospital was great, and a number of physicians came informally to learn more about operative techinques. At the same time, the efforts of Dr. José Belaval, head of the Pre-Maternal Health program (a division encompassing the birth control clinics) made many physicians interested in the pressing need for sterilization and birth control. Many physicians thought, and still think, that contraceptive methods are too difficult for lower class Puerto Ricans and regarded postpartum sterilization as the most feasible solution to the problems (p. 3).

Although the physicians may have been principally interested in the welfare of lower class women, women of all social classes responded to the availability of sterilization.

The rapidity with which Puerto Rican physicians endorsed sterilization for other than strictly therapeutic reasons is revealed in the results of a questionnaire sent to physicians in 1952. Although only half of the 900 questionnaires were returned, 80 percent of those responding favored sterilization for reasons of health, 66 percent for reasons of poverty, and 63 percent when women had had more children than they desired (Belaval, Cofresi, and Janer, 1953).

Clearly, the practice of sterilization was dependent upon the approval of physicians; without such approval, the growing demand for the operation could not have been met. However, the diffusion process may also be viewed in the reverse direction; that is, the growing demand for the operation may have expedited approval by physicians. (This was the impression gained by Kingsley Davis [personal communication] during his visit to Puerto Rico in the late 1940s). Women had found sterilization acceptable and were frequently asking physicians to perform it. To what can one attribute this growing demand?

A major consideration is that women, as pointed out earlier, were highly motivated to restrict their family size and were not being offered effective contraceptive options. Prior to the mid-1960s, the island's birth control clinics were not actively promoted. Those women who did attend the clinics were provided with relatively ineffective family planning methods, mostly foam and condoms. Had the physicians not introduced sterilization, perhaps Puerto Ricans would have relied essentially on the traditional methods of withdrawal and (illegal) induced abortion, as did other countries during the early phase of demographic transition. Since physicians did, however, offer an alternative that was safe and highly effective (sterilization), Puerto Rican women were very receptive. By the early 1950s, the demand for sterilization had far exceeded the facilities (Stycos, 1954).

Although most Puerto Ricans are Catholic (over 80 percent), the stance of the church against sterilizations performed for contraceptive reasons does not seem to have discouraged the adoption of the procedure. For one thing, Puerto Rican Catholicism, if measured by church attendance, may be only nominal insofar as strict adherence to ritual and doctrine are concerned. It could also be argued that if religious beliefs play any discernible role concerning the acceptability of sterilization it is that of enhancing the popularity of contraceptive surgery over other birth control methods. Sterilization could be relatively less provoking of religious guilt since it involves the patient only passively—the operation is performed by the physician. As Back, Hill, and Stycos (1960) have pointed out, moreover, sterilization is resorted to only once; if there is sin, the sin is never repeated, unlike the transgression that accompanies other methods of family planning. Physicians may also help their patients avoid the religious issue by providing health reasons for the surgery (the only legal basis for sterilization in Puerto Rico), thus making it easier for the women to view the operation as a therapeutic (religiously permissible) rather than a contraceptive endeavor.

Other reasons have also been adduced to explain the apparent lack of impact of Catholic sanctions against sterilization. The procedure can, of course, easily be kept secret (Alvarado and Tietze, 1947), thereby avoiding a public confrontation with the church or with one's neighbors. Finally, religious beliefs are, after all, only one of a number of cultural influences upon the individual; given the significant tradition in Puerto Rican society of modesty, sterilization—a contraceptive procedure dissociated from the immediate sex act—may be considered suitable to the family planning needs of the society (Hill, Stycos, and Back, 1959).

There have been no recent studies of medical opinion in Puerto Rico regarding sterilization in Puerto Rico. The Catholic church may have influenced medical opinion in recent years into becoming less favorable toward the method. Whether this is the case, and, if so, whether it will be sufficient to stifle future demand for the operation remain to be seen.

**Female Versus Male Sterilization.** Why is it that Puerto Rican women, rather than men, chose to become sterilized? It may be significant that obstetricians and gynecologists—not urologists—initially introduced and promoted the practice of sterilization. Moreover, it was pospartum sterilization that was promoted. Female patients did not have to be recruited; they were already patients because of their pregnancy. With continued child-bearing considered a health risk, birth control may have been viewed by both the woman and the physician as the woman's responsibility.

Another impediment to the practice of male sterilization in Puerto Rico may be the prevailing "machismo" complex. The need of Puerto Rican men to assert their masculinity, and the insecurity this may reflect, may minimize the appeal of an operation that would produce sterility. The acceptability of vasectomy in Puerto Rico may, however, be underrated. As previously noted, the Medical Director of the Family Planning Association, who advocated vasectomy over female sterilization, succeeded in convincing one-fourth of the couples wishing to become sterilized to choose vasectomy. The success of vasectomy clinics in some Latin American countries (Goldsmith, Goldberg, and Echeverria, 1973) also suggests that "machismo" need not be a significant deterrent.

### Structural Supports and Constraints

It would seem that for sterilization to become so popular in Puerto Rico, structural conditions within the society would have had to have been highly supportive of the practice. This was not always the case. A historical analysis of the medical, legal, religious, and political developments from the early 1930s to the mid-1960s indicates that structural support for the practice of sterilization was, in fact, generally lacking (Presser, 1973). Medical facilities were limited relative to the demand; sterilization was legal for health reasons only; and there was considerable religious opposition and political indifference.

Structural conditions are not immutable; although they may fix limits on the practice of sterilization, they may also change in response to demand—as, indeed, happened in Puerto Rico. Medical facilities expanded as many private clinics and small hospitals were established to perform postpartum sterilizations. Physicians responded to the opportunity for increased fees when the operation was performed in private facilities (fifty dollars or more, plus the fee for delivery). The broad interpretation of "health reasons" given by physicians was never challenged in the courts, thereby circumventing legal obstacles. Religious opposition, which was highly publicized, actually boomeranged; the church's exhortations served to educate the population about the nature and availability of the operation. Government indifference to sterilization, finally, was merely an extension of its lack of support for birth control practice in general. Had birth control clinics (which did not offer sterilization) been more actively promoted by the government, the grassroots demand for sterilization might never have achieved such high levels.

Although many of the physicians in Puerto Rico may have been trained on the mainland, it is difficult to argue that policies then current in the United States were instrumental in promoting the practice of sterilization on the island. Indeed, there is evidence to the contrary. When Puerto Rican hospitals in the 1950s and 1960s sought to become accredited, the Joint Commission for Hospital Accreditation (constituted by the American College of Physicians, the American College of Surgeons, the American Hospital Association, and the American Medical Association) seems to have imposed a 10 percent limit on sterilization in proportion to all deliveries as one criterion for accreditation. This stipulation was frequently reported to the writer by Puerto Rican hospital administrators, but there is no official documentation of this policy. (The restriction seems to have led to considerable underreporting of the operation in hospitals, which may partly explain the general unawareness of its remarkably widespread prevalence in the mid-1960s.) Negative attitudes toward sterilization prevailed in American government circles, as well. In 1966, the Family Planning Association of Puerto Rico, having accepted federal funds from the Office of Economic Opportunity (OEO), found it necessary to end its subsidies for contraceptive surgery because of OEO policy against such support. (OEO changed its rules regarding contraceptive sterilization in 1971; the debate since then has centered on determining appropriate guidelines for implementing federally sponsored sterilization programs).

*Demographic Effectiveness*

The extent to which the practice of sterilization has averted births in Puerto Rico depends upon the age and parity at which women were sterilized and an estimate of their subsequent fertility behavior had they not undergone the procedure. The latter is highly speculative and can only be indirectly evaluated.

The demographic impact of sterilization on Puerto Rican fertility in the late 1940s and early 1950s seems to have been minimal. In 1948-1949, sterilization was not practiced extensively, although, among those who had the surgery, many seemed to have chosen the procedure early in their fertility history. In 1953-1954, the operation was practiced extensively, but those sterilized were sterilized later. By 1965, however, sterilization was practiced extensively *and* women were sterilized early; the majority had three or fewer children (Presser, 1969).

It does not seem that sterilized women would have practiced contraception widely or effectively had they not become sterilized, for they were not doing so prior to the operation. There is some evidence that lower-class women sterilized in 1966 were more likely to have been using contraception in the year preceding pregnancy than were nonsterilized women of similar age and parity, but the great majority of women in both groups were non-users (Presser, 1973). The relationship between abortion experience (induced and spontaneous combined) and the practice of sterilization is unclear—which may simply reflect the poor quality of data on induced abortion in Puerto Rico.

It has been conservatively estimated that, among women sampled in 1965, about two to three births per mother were averted by sterilization (Presser, 1969). The demographic impact of female sterilization on Puerto Rican fertility in the 1960s would thus appear to have been substantial.

## United States

### Trend in Practice

Surgical sterilization was performed for eugenic reasons in the United States as early as 1897—probably on women, although the type of operation was not specified by Hordern (1971). The historical origins of sterilization solely for contraceptive reasons (male or female) in the United States have not been documented. Its practice seems to have been popular in North Carolina in the late 1940s, but no precise information is available (Woodside, 1950). The national fertility surveys, conducted every five years from 1955 to 1970, have provided data upon which estimates have been made about the incidence and prevalence of contraceptive sterilization for the total United States.

The 1955 national fertility survey (Growth of American Families, or GAF) asked only if wives or their husbands had had an operation which made pregnancy impossible. Operations that were contraceptive in intent were not distinguished from other operations, nor was the type of operation specified (that is, women were not asked whether they had had an oopherectomy, hysterectomy, or tubal ligation). A total of 9 percent of the couples were sterilized. Sterilization was about twice as common among couples in which the wife was not a high school graduate as among high school and college graduates (Freedman, Whelpton, and Campbell, 1959).

Using the 1955 GAF data, Tietze (1960) produced what he considered a conservative estimate of the prevalence of contraceptive sterilization (male and female combined) among white couples for that year: 1 percent when the wife was aged 18-29 and 7 percent when the wife was 30-39. As for the annual incidence of the procedure during the decade preceding 1955, Tietze made the following observation:

Extrapolating the results of our computation to the total population of the United States, we may conclude that there were in 1955 at least 1,200,000 persons of reproductive age, mainly women, who had chosen permanent surgical protection against unwanted pregnancy. The corresponding minimum estimate of the annual number of sterilizations during the decade preceding 1955 is on the order of 75,000 including operations other than salpingectomy and vasectomy, but performed for the purpose of family limitation (Tietze, 1960, p. 441).

The 1960 GAF Study and the two National Fertility Studies (NFS) since then have asked specifically whether operations to prevent further pregnancies were at least partly contraceptive in intent. From the 1960 GAF study, Campbell (1964) estimated the annual incidence of contraceptive sterilization between 1955 and 1960 in the total United States among both whites and nonwhites at about 110,000. This estimate suggests a substantial increase in incidence over the previous decade.

Estimates of the prevalence of contraceptive sterilization in the United States have not been as speculative as those of annual incidence, which are difficult to determine from cross-sectional data. Estimates of prevalence relate specifically to the population represented by the sample. In 1955 and 1960, the GAF samples comprised white married couples, husband present, with wife aged 18 to 39; in 1965 and 1970, nonwhites were included in the sample. (In 1970, previously married women were part of the sample for the first time; data on this group have not been analyzed in relation to sterilization.)

Table 3-1 presents the trend from 1955 to 1965 in the prevalence of contraceptive sterilization among white married couples by sex of the sterilized spouse. The prevalence of contraceptive sterilization appears to have doubled during the ten-year period, from 4 percent to 8 percent. Moreover, male sterilization was increasing at a more rapid rate than was female sterilization. Whereas one-fourth of all contraceptive sterilizations were male in 1955, three-eighths were male in 1965.

Between 1965 and 1970, the trend in the prevalence of contraceptive

**Table 3-1**
**Prevalence of Contraceptive Sterilization by Sex of Sterilized Spouse for White Married Couples, Currently Married, Husband Present, with Wife Aged 18 to 39: United States, 1955, 1960, and 1965**

| Year | Total Couples Surveyed | Contraceptively Sterilized Couples | | |
|------|------|------|------|------|
| | | % Total | % Male | % Female |
| 1955[a] | Not available | 4 | 1 | 3 |
| 1960 | 2,414 | 6 | 2 | 4 |
| 1965 | 2,919 | 8 | 3 | 5 |

Source: P.K., Whelpton, A.A. Campbell, and J.E. Patterson *Fertility and Family Planning in the United States* (Princeton: Princeton University Press, 1966), Tables 84 and 86, pp. 145, 150; C. Westoff and N.B. Ryder, "Family Limitation in the United States," Proceedings of the International Population Conference, London, Vol. II, Session 4:3, 1969, pp. 1307.

[a]Estimate derived from 1960 survey of women who were married and 18-34 years old as of 1955.

sterilization can be assessed for the total population of currently married couples, including blacks. Table 3-2 indicates that over that five-year period the prevalence of contraceptive sterilization rose from 8 percent to 11 percent. Once again, the rate of increase was greater for male sterilization (vasectomy) than for female sterilization (tubal ligation, hysterectomy, and other surgical procedures). By 1970, 45 percent of all contraceptive sterilizations were male. Although the overall prevalence of sterilization is similar across races, there is a marked difference by race in the sex of the sterilized spouse: in 1965 and in 1970, almost all sterilizations among blacks were female, whereas male and female sterilization are about equal among whites.

The increase in the prevalence of contraceptive sterilization between 1965 and 1970 is more marked when one considers only the risk population—that is, couples who intend no more children and are not sterile except for contraceptive reasons. As indicated in Table 3-2, for this population the prevalence of contraceptive sterilization grew by almost one-half over five years—from 13 percent in 1965 to 18 percent in 1970. The sharp rise is apparent for both blacks and whites.

It has been estimated that, overall, in 1970 the United States had about 2.75 million couples (with the husband present and the wife under forty-five years of age) who had chosen sterilization as a contraceptive method. Including separated couples, the estimated number is just under three million. In 1970 alone, about

**Table 3-2**

**Prevalence of Contraceptive Sterilization, by Race and Type of Operation, for Couples Currently Married, Husband Present, With Wife under 45 Years of Age: United States, 1965 and 1970**

| Year and Race | Total N | Couples with Contraceptive Sterilization | | | | Couples at Risk with Contraceptive Sterilization | | | | |
|---|---|---|---|---|---|---|---|---|---|---|
| | | % Vasectomy | % Tubal Ligation | % Other[b] | Total Percentage[c] | Total N at Risk[a] | % Vasectomy | % Tubal Ligation | % Other[b] | Total Percentage[c] |
| 1965 | | | | | | | | | | |
| Total | 4,666 | 3 | 4 | 1 | 8 | 2,892 | 6 | 6 | 1 | 13 |
| White | 3,659 | 4 | 3 | 1 | 8 | 2,269 | 6 | 6 | 1 | 13 |
| Black | 937 | 0 | 8 | 1 | 9 | 609 | 0 | 12 | 2 | 14 |
| 1970 | | | | | | | | | | |
| Total | 5,793 | 5 | 4 | 2 | 11 | 3,361 | 8 | 7 | 3 | 18 |
| White | 4,906 | 5 | 4 | 1 | 11 | 2,901 | 9 | 6 | 2 | 18 |
| Black | 761 | 1 | 9 | 3 | 12 | 460 | 1 | 15 | 4 | 21 |

Source: Presser and Bumpass "Demographic and Social Aspects of Contraceptive Sterilization in the United States: 1965-1970." In Commission on Population Growth and the American Future, Research Reports, Vol. I, 1972, Table 19, p. 533. Corrections made in 1970 figures for risk population. For total population, previously unpublished data added on type of operation.

Note: Numbers reported are the actual sample cases upon which the statistics are based. All statistics for the total population have been appropriately weighed to adjust for the over-sampling of blacks. Other nonwhites are included in the total.

[a]Couples who intend no more children and are not sterile except for contraceptive reasons.

[b]Includes hysterectomies and other contraceptive operations.

[c]Due to rounding, totals may not correspond to the sum of the categories.

700,000 contraceptive operations (male and female) were performed. Based on the 1970 NFS, Bumpass and Presser (1972) put the total of vasectomies performed in 1970 in the United States at 320,000—a figure much lower than the highly publicized claim of 750,000 advanced by Lea, Inc. in a survey prepared for the Association for Voluntary Sterilization (AVS) (1971). Like the estimate of Davis and Hulka (1970) of only 37,000 male sterilizations performed in 1967, the AVS projection for 1970 was based on the practice of a sample of physicians.

While the practice of contraceptive sterilization has clearly gained relative popularity throughout the United States, it is particularly prevalent in some geographical regions. A small area study revealed an especially high prevalence, for example, among subscribers to the Kaiser Foundation Plan in the Walnut Creek area of California (Phillips, 1971). A mail survey in 1968 (with a 92 percent response rate!) showed that 23 percent of all white couples, with wife aged twenty through fifty-four, had had contraceptive operations. Two-thirds of these procedures were vasectomies and one-third, tubal ligations. Education was inversely related to contraceptive practice among both husbands and wives.

The 1960 NFS also showed a clear inverse relationship between education and contraceptive sterilization (Whelpton, Campbell, and Patterson, 1966). This negative correlation persisted in 1965, but became less apparent in 1970 (Presser and Bumpass, 1972a) because of the increasing popularity of vasectomy among the better educated.

*Receptivity to Sterilization*

Findings about the practice of sterilization in the United States came as a surprise to those who first investigated the matter. As Freedman and his associates, commenting on their 1955 survey findings, acknowledged:

That almost 1 out of every 10 couples in the child-bearing years had such an operation, was considered so startling a finding that all the interviews involving them were carefully reread to make certain that the question was not misunderstood. On the contrary, in most cases the wives volunteered comments about the nature or circumstances of the operation, which strengthened confidence in validity of the information (Freedman, Whelpton, and Campbell, 1959, p. 27).

The "1 out of every 10" finding referred to all operations, contraceptive and therapeutic combined. Nevertheless, it is apparent that at least as early as the mid-1950s—and possibly earlier—substantial numbers of couples were opting for sterilization as a contraceptive method on a very private and individualized basis. The notable increase in the practice of sterilization was given minimal attention, however, by family planners and demographers alike. The fact that by 1970

sterilization had become the most popular method of contraception currently
used by older couples (wife aged thirty to forty-four) therefore became "one of
the most dramatic findings in the NFS (National Fertility Study)" (Westoff,
1972, p. 10).

In considering why couples in the United States became increasingly receptive to sterilization as a method of birth control, we shall first explore, as we
did for Puerto Rico, some of the demographic factors that may have affected
motivation to limit family size. We shall then speculate about the reasons for
choosing sterilization, in particular, and why both male and female sterilization
became popular.

**Demographic Conditions and the Desire to Limit Family Size.** In the mid-1950s,
the United States was in the final phase of demographic transition. Mortality was
low, the country was highly industrialized, and fertility was at a moderately low
level. The baby boom, which had begun at the end of World War II, was nearing
an end. Between 1955 and 1965, expected family size did not change very
much, averaging slightly over three children per woman. Between 1965 and
1972, there was a steady decline in expected family size for women aged eighteen
to thirty-four, averaging about half-a-child less per woman; for women aged
thirty-five to thirty-nine, there was little change (United States Bureau of the
Census, 1973, p. 1, Table A).

Labor force participation rates for women rose steadily after World War II.
Whereas 26 percent of women aged fourteen and over were in the labor force in
1940, the figure was 40 percent in 1970 (United States Bureau of the Census,
1972a. Table 78, p. 1-37). The percentage of women employed in white collar
jobs shifted notably between 1940 and 1950, from 45 percent to 54 percent,
but did not change markedly in subsequent decades; by 1970, 58 percent of employed women were in white collar occupations (Knudsen, 1969, Table 1,
p. 185; United States Bureau of the Census, 1972a, Table 81, p. 1-375). This lack
of change in the occupational composition of the female labor force may be related to the stability in expected family size. In 1970 the labor force participation of women in the United States was at a rate almost twice that of Puerto
Rico, yet there was little difference between the countries in the occupational
status of employed women, as measured by the percent in white collar occupations (58 percent in the United States and 50 percent in Puerto Rico).

Although the increased practice of sterilization in the United States was
not concomitant with a decrease in expected family size, motivation not to exceed expectations may have become stronger between 1955 and 1965. The
choice of sterilization during this period may reflect an increasing demand among
couples who had achieved their desired family size for a contraceptive method
more effective than that previously used, and perhaps a decreasing willingness to
rely on abortion, which was then illegal. More recently, the trend toward smaller
family size expectations, along with the desire for highly effective—and safe—

contraception, may have added impetus to the practice of sterilization. Interestingly, even after the pill and the IUD were introduced in the early 1960s, many couples still preferred sterilization.

**Choice of Sterilization.** Very little is known about the process by which men and women in the United States have come to learn about contraceptive sterilization. Little publicity was given in the mass media to its practice prior to the late 1960s; family planning clinics, as well, were not actively promoting the method for either men or women. Except for the promotional efforts of the Association for Voluntary Sterilization (formerly the Human Betterment Association), which maintained a speaker's bureau and a registry of physicians willing to perform the operation, historically no organized support has existed for its practice. Not until the media became interested in the population and environment issue in the late 1960s did contraceptive sterilization become highly publicized and vasectomy clinics open. Before then, the increasing popularity of contraceptive surgery seems to have resulted from word-of-mouth diffusion among individuals, their physicians, and friends.

For the practice of contraceptive sterilization to have become so widespread, medical opinion must have become increasingly favorable. Unfortunately, because of the paucity of data on physicians' attitudes toward contraceptive sterilization in the United States, the trend in attitude over time cannot be determined. Two studies in the 1960s indicate substantial support for vasectomy among physicians.

In 1964, Landis (1966) surveyed physicians in two counties in the East Bay Area region of San Francisco about their attitudes toward vasectomy and their experience in performing the operation. The response rate—58 percent—compares well with other mailed questionnaires, but is sufficiently low to question the representativeness of the sample. Among those responding, at any rate, 60 percent approved of vasectomy for contraceptive reasons. There was considerable uncertainty about the legality of the operation; only one-third of the physicians considered it clearly legal. Thirty percent of the physicians from all specialities had performed the operation; for urologists, the percent was 84. Many of these urologists were performing vasectomies, but were unsure of its legal status.

In 1968, Davis and Hulka (1970) sent a questionnaire to all urologists in the United States listed in the Directory of Medical Specialists, asking about the number of vasectomies they had performed in 1967 and the requests for vasectomies they had rejected. The response rate of the urologists was low (40 percent) and, again, prompts some caution about the findings. Although many urologists appeared to have been performing vasectomies in 1967 (64 percent of those responding), the rejection rate was high (42 percent of all requests). The major reasons reported for not performing vasectomy were "legal" and "ethical and religious."

If the number of studies on physicians' attitudes toward vasectomy are scant, there are no empirical studies at all of physicians' attitudes toward female sterilization. Medical practice suggests that gynecologists and obstetricians have been more favorable in their attitudes toward female sterilization than urologists are toward male sterilization, but the urologists' attitudes have changed markedly in recent years.

From the perspective of the couple, why choose sterilization? Couples in the United States have had considerable experience with other contraceptive methods, with induced abortion often serving as a back-up for not using birth control or for contraceptive failures. Not until couples have achieved (or exceeded) their desired family size does sterilization become a viable option. At this stage, many couples may prefer sterilization to alternative methods. They may not be so willing then as during the childspacing stage of marriage to tolerate an unplanned pregnancy, an abortion, or the possible risks and side effects of the pill and the IUD. For those who strongly feel they want no more children, the advantages of sterilization—that it is a one-time, safe, and effective method—may outweigh the disadvantages—that it is a surgical procedure and its reversibility cannot be assured. The general acceptability of sterilization is high even among fecund (nonsterilized) couples who intend no more children. Among such couples in 1970, 39 percent of the wives said they would seriously consider female sterilization and 28 percent thought their husbands would feel similarly about undergoing vasectomy (Presser and Bumpass, 1972a).

The increasing acceptability of contraceptive sterilization in recent years may reflect, in part, better public understanding of the nature of the operation. In the minds of many, sterilization has long been confused with castration. A small study of college students in the late 1940s revealed that 38 percent of the respondents felt that vasectomy resulted in the loss of male sexual potency and 52 percent thought that tubal ligation ended menstruation (Woodside, 1950). In a more recent study of college students and faculty, 49 percent confessed ignorance or uncertainty about the effects of vasectomy on sexual performance and 37 percent were sure or thought it probable that tubal ligation interfered with the menstrual cycle (Eisner, van Tienhoven, and Rosenblatt, 1970). There is some evidence, on a national basis, that knowledge about the nature of vasectomy has improved between 1965 and 1970—at least among women. Whereas 25 percent of the women in the 1965 NFS thought vasectomy would interfere with a man's physical ability to have sexual intercourse, the percentage dropped to 15 in 1970 (Presser and Bumpass, 1972a). It may well be that as sterilization became widespread there was considerable communication between the sterilized and the nonsterilized—the former educating the latter about the nature of the operation.

**Female Versus Male Sterilization.** As noted earlier, female sterilization in the United States has historically been more prevalent than has been the male procedure. The practice of vasectomy has been increasing at a rapid rate, however, and is approaching a one-to-one ratio with female sterilization. Changes in male and female attitudes toward responsibility for birth control may be relevant to the shift toward vasectomy. In the 1970 NFS, all women were asked: "If a couple decides on sterilization in order to prevent unwanted children, should it be the husband or the wife who gets sterilized?" Considerably more women felt it should be the husband rather than the wife—62 percent versus 38 percent, respectively (Presser and Bumpass, 1972a, p. 534).

From a strictly medical perspective, vasectomy is safer than female sterilization. It is also less expensive and does not require hospitalization. If there is increasing rationality about birth control practice, this may get expressed by a continuing shift from female sterilization toward vasectomy—unless, of course, female methods themselves become safer, cheaper, and are performed without risk on an outpatient basis. Whether the trend toward vasectomy will continue also depends on the role that physicians and the media play in reducing unwarranted fears about the physiological consequences of the operation, as well as the extent to which the option of vasectomy is presented to couples by obstetricians and gynecologists who perform only female sterilization.

*Structural Conditions: Support and Resistance*

Although some physicians may have been favorably disposed toward the practice of contraceptive sterilization when it was first becoming popular, they were undoubtedly deterred by institutional constraints imposed by the medical profession that determined who could and could not be sterilized for contraceptive reasons. Female sterilizations, in particular, have until recently been subject to hospital specifications about eligibility, and to committee review. Hospital policy has often involved minimum age-parity standards, usually derived from those "suggested" by the official manual of the American College of Obstetricians and Gynecologists (1965):

1. At least twenty-five years of age and five living children.
2. At least thirty years of age and four living children.
3. At least thirty-five years of age and three living children.

Hospitals could also impose stricter age-parity standards or refuse to perform any sterilizations at all for contraceptive reasons.

In addition to the American College of Obstetricians and Gynecologists, other medical organizations also seem to have concerned themselves with the extent to which hospitals were performing the operation for contraceptive purposes. Woodside, in her study of a sample of hospitals in North Carolina in the late 1940s, gave the following report of her observations:

The number of sterilizations performed is apparently a matter of some concern to the executive of professional bodies such as the American College of Surgeons. One gynecologist stated that pressure was being brought by this authority to stop "sterilizations of convenience" in hospitals accredited to the College, and that admonitory letters would be written if too many operations of this type appeared in the records. Two other gynecologists also mentioned a veto from the College and a third referred to "restrictions" on sterilizations, saying that word had gone forth unofficially from the American Medical Association warning doctors "not to be too free with tubal ligations." It was not possible to obtain concrete evidence about this alleged attitude of the professional authorities, since no doctor produced any written statements and a letter of inquiry to the College of Surgeons was not acknowledged. Nevertheless, it seems improbable that spontaneous mention of restrictions would be made by doctors in different areas without some factual foundation (Woodside, 1950, p. 55–56).

As has already been mentioned, the writer's experience in Puerto Rico was similar when investigating the "informal" rule that no more than 10 percent of all hospital deliveries were to be followed by sterilization.

The practice of vasectomy is usually not subject to hospital policy. Nevertheless age-parity and other nonmedical standards are often arbitrarily imposed by physicians who perform vasectomies in their private offices.

In recent years, professional bodies have shifted their positions toward sterilization. After the 1969 manual of the American College of Obstetricians and Gynecologists removed their age-parity guidelines, many hospitals seemed to relax their standards. In 1970, the College dropped its recommendation that consultation with another physician be made for patients requesting contraceptive sterilization.

Medical organizations have recently not only removed past obstacles but have given their support to the practice of contraceptive sterilization. An editorial in the *Journal of the American Medical Association* (1968) endorsed its practice, focusing on the merits of vasectomy. In 1972, the American Public Health Association issued a program guide for voluntary sterilization (male and female) that stressed the removal of administrative constraints (*The Nation's Health,* 1972). In response to criticism from groups outside the Association, an editorial of the *American Journal of Public Health* (1973) reaffirmed its position and discussed at length the issue of irreversibility, which was the focus of criticism. The Commission on Population Growth and the American Future (1972) also recommended that administrative restrictions be eliminated and asked for the support of the national hospital and medical associations and their state chapters to implement this policy.

The change in hospital policy toward sterilization is probably partly because of recent court decisions—such as *McCabe* v. *Nassau Medical Center* (Eastern District, New York, 1971)—holding the hospital liable for proven damages resulting from the refusal to provide contraceptive surgery upon request. For the individual physician, the legal ramifications of the operation were all too often unclear in the past. Uncertainty among physicians about the legality of contraceptive sterilization seems to have served as a major deterrent to its practice. The previously cited studies by Landis (1966) and Davis and Hulka (1970) support this view with regard to vasectomy. Until recently, professional associations have made no special effort to educate physicians about the legality of either vasectomy or tubal ligation. At present, contraceptive sterilization is, in fact, legal in all states.

Having adequate facilities to perform contraceptive sterilization has never been a major issue in the United States. For many decades, most women have been giving birth to their children in hospitals; postpartum sterilization requires only one or two additional days of hospitalization. Family planning clinics have generally not offered their clients the option of contraceptive sterilization, although vasectomy—and some techniques of female surgery—can be performed on an out-patient basis. Vasectomy clinics have recently become popular, however. Since 1969, when the first clinic opened in New York, about 150 additional bona fide vasectomy clinics and at least another 150 hospitals have begun to provide out-patient vasectomy services. Again, demand will apparently serve to expand facilities.

Only recently has there been political support for any type of family planning service. Contraceptive sterilization was specifically endorsed in 1967 by the Department of Health, Education, and Welfare, the Department of Defense, and Medicaid (as reported by the Association for Voluntary Sterilization [1967]). Although the federal government is willing to match state funds for contraceptive sterilizations performed under Medicaid, states apparently have some leeway in deciding whether the method is to be covered under the program (Richter, 1973).

In reviewing the actions and attitudes of the various medical, legal, and governmental bodies, one may conclude that in the United States, as in Puerto Rico, there have been numerous structural constraints on the practice of contraceptive sterilization, despite the growing popularity of the method. In recent years, however, public demand seems to have brought about increasing institutional support for the practice.


*Demographic Effectiveness*

The increasing prevalence of contraceptive sterilization in the United States suggests that the method may be playing a significant role in controlling fertility. In addition to its widespread use, in recent years the surgery has been chosen relatively early in the reproductive history of adopters. Data from the 1970 NFS indicate that among couples sterilized between 1965 and 1970 the median age of the wife at the time of sterilization was 31.8 and of her husband, 35.1; the wife had a median of 2.8 children.

An analysis of the previous contraceptive experience of these couples, how-ever, suggests that many had been using effective contraceptive methods prior to sterilization and perhaps would have continued such use had they not undergone the surgery. Only 22 percent had used no contraception in the interval preceding or following the last birth. More than half (51 percent) used the pill or the IUD as their most recent method; 15 percent employed the diaphragm or condom; and 11 percent resorted to other methods. Of those sterilized who used any contra-ceptive method, in other words, only 14 percent had practiced methods generally considered relatively ineffective in preventing pregnancy, such as foam, jellies, rhythm, and withdrawal (Presser and Bumpass, 1972b).

We are clearly in a transitional state in the United States with respect to con-traceptive practice. Increasingly, couples are using more effective contraceptive methods and may be relying more upon induced abortion as a back-up. What-ever the demographic impact of contraceptive sterilization has been in the past, it seems as though its impact in the future may be minimal.

## Implications for Further Research

Contraceptive sterilization gained widespread popularity at a much earlier stage in the demographic transition in Puerto Rico than it did in the United States. In Puerto Rico, women were having moderately large families but desired smaller ones. We have speculated about the factors motivating women to have smaller families: the reduction in mortality, rising standards of living, the increased em-ployment of women outside the home, and the shift from manual to white collar employment for women. Further research is needed on the variables affecting motivation to restrict family size at the early phase of demographic transition.

In the United States, unlike Puerto Rico, contraceptive sterilization became popular at a time when family size desires were moderately small and unchang-ing. In recent years, when family size desires began to change and women wanted fewer children, the practice of sterilization increased markedly. It thus appears that the grassroots acceptance of sterilization is not contingent upon a *change* in family size desires, but that the appeal of sterilization (or the appeal of any birth control method, for that matter) may be enhanced when family size desires are on the decline.

Lack of previous contraceptive experience does not seem to deter the accep-tance of contraceptive sterilization, nor does experience with effective alternative methods. An individual may wish to become sterilized because she (or he): (1) does not know about other contraceptive methods, (2) does not want to use ineffective contraceptive methods, (3) does not want to rely on induced abortion (legal or illegal) as back-up, or (4) is not satisfied with other highly effective con-traceptive measures. Many combinations of previous birth control experience can lead to the practice of contraceptive sterilization. This chapter has specu-lated about the particular appeal of contraceptive sterilization in Puerto Rico

and the United States relative to other contraceptive methods; the matter requires further investigation.

The relative appeal of male versus female sterilization is also worthy of further study. At a grassroots level, female sterilization seems to have greater appeal—
at least initially. Acceptance of male sterilization in the absence of large-scale
promotional efforts may be highly dependent on the individual's level of education, as is suggested by the recent increase in vasectomy among the better educated in the United States. A question worthy of pursuit is how attitudes about
male and female responsibility for birth control, as well as sex-role attitudes in
general, relate to couples' choices between vasectomy and tubal ligation.

It is apparent from the experience of both the United States and Puerto Rico
that people of all educational levels may find contraceptive sterilization appealing—at least female sterilization—given the desire to have no more children.
More information is required, however, about factors associated with resistance
to the practice, as well as to its acceptance, and the extent to which negative
attitudes are related to a misunderstanding of the nature of the operation (male
or female).

There is clearly a need to keep questions on contraceptive sterilization in
our national fertility studies. These studies provide a continuing source of data
on the prevalence of contraceptive sterilization, attitudes of the general population toward its practice, and some of the demographic and social characteristics
of sterilized and nonsterilized persons. Items in the Master Sample Survey of
Puerto Rico—although essentially a health survey—serve a similar purpose for
sterilization data concerning the Commonwealth.

Besides relating the choice of sterilization to various individual demographic
and social characteristics, structural factors that provide the social context for
the practice should be explored. Favorable medical opinion seems the most
important of these factors, given strong couple motivation to limit family size.
What motivates physicians to support sterilization? Do they regard lower class
couples differently from those of higher social class? A study of physicians'
knowledge, attitudes, and practice (both personal and professional) regarding
birth control methods in general, and including contraceptive sterilization, would
seem to be a research area of high priority. Practitioners in the specialties of ob-
stetrics/gynecology and urology are of particular interest.

Among the areas involving the physician that are worthy of research interest
are the following:

1.  The physician's perception of his or her role in providing birth control
    services.
2.  Practitioners' reasons for approving or disapproving of contraceptive steril-
    ization, male and female, relative to other contraceptive methods and induced
    abortion.
3.  Among physicians who approve of contraceptive surgery, an examination of

the doctor-patient relationship, differentiating between the more "coercive" promotion of the practice and the more "responsive" stance which caters to the expressed needs of the men and women coming for consultation.

4. Why some physicians prefer hysterectomy over tubal ligation as a method of contraception, although the former is at least four times more risky.

Comparative studies on the practice of contraceptive sterilization are also lacking. It would be of both theoretical and practical interest to compare countries in which the method has been widely accepted at the grassroots level, with countries in which its popularity can be attributed to highly organized family planning programs. The comparative approach would highlight the relative contributions of individual motivation to terminate fertility and the structural conditions that affect the availability of contraceptive surgery.

*Recent Developments: 1975*

The practice of contraceptive sterilization in the United States has risen dramatically in the early 1970s. Since the writing of this chapter, preliminary findings on sterilization were reported from the 1973 National Survey of Family Growth (Pratt, 1975). The population of currently married couples with contraceptive sterilization rose from 11 percent in 1970 to 16 percent in 1973; considering only the "risk population" (those who intend no more children and are not sterilized for therapeutic reasons), the increase was from 18 percent in 1970 to 29 percent in 1973. Motivation to limit family size may have increased during this period, but there may also have been growing dissatisfaction with alternative methods of fertility control and greater awareness of sterilization as a viable option.

## References

Alvarado, C.R. de and Tietze, C. "Birth Control in Puerto Rico." *Human Fertility* 12, 1 (1947): 15-17, 24-25.

Association for Voluntary Sterilization. *News* (Spring 1967).

Association for Voluntary Sterilization. *Progress Report* (March 25, 1971-May 19, 1971). Mimeo.

Back, K.W., Hill, R., and Stycos, J.M. "Population Control in Puerto Rico: The Formal and Informal Framework." *Law and Contemporary Problems* 25 (1960): 562-65.

Belaval, J., Cofresi, E., and Janer, J. "Opinion de la Clase Medica de Puerto Rico sobre el Uso de Esterilizacion y los Contraceptivos." Mimeographed private release (1953). (As cited in Stycos, 1954, p. 3).

Bumpass, L.L. and Presser, H.B. "Contraceptive Sterilization in the U.S.: 1965 and 1970." *Demography* 9,4 (1972): 531-48.

Campbell, A.A. "The Incidence of Operations that Prevent Conception." *American Journal of Obstetrics and Gynecology* 89 (1964): 694-700.

Commission on Population Growth and the American Future. "Population and the American Future." Washington, D.C.: U.S. Government Printing Office, 1972.

Cordero, Rafael de J. "The Future of an Island." Paper presented at the symposium Time for Decision: The Biological Crossroads held at the University of California Medical Center, San Francisco, January 14-16, 1966.

Davis, J.E. and Hulka, J.F. "Elective Vasectomy by American Urologists in 1967." *Fertility and Sterility* 21 (1970): 615-21.

Davis, K. "The Theory of Change and Response in Modern Demographic History." *Population Index* 29, 4 (1963): 345-66.

Eastern District New York, 1975. *McCabe* v. *Nassau County Medical Center*, 453 F 2nd 698.

Editorial. "Voluntary Male Sterilization." *Journal of the American Medical Association* 204, 9 (1968).

Editorial. "Voluntary Sterilization." *American Journal of Public Health* 63, 7 (1973): 573-75.

Eisner, T., van Tienhoven, A., and Rosenblatt, F. "Population Control, Sterilization, and Ignorance." *Science* 167, 391, 7 (1970): 337.

Freedman, R., Whelpton, P.K., and Campbell, A.A. *Family Planning, Sterility and Population Growth.* New York: McGraw-Hill Book Company, Inc., 1959.

Goldsmith, A., Goldberg, R.J., and Echeverria, G. "Vasectomy in Latin America." *IPPF Medical Bulletin* 7, 2 (1973): 1 and 2.

Gutiérrez, O. "Algunos factores asociados con la fecundidad en Puerto Rico." In Lerner, S. and R. de la Peña, eds. *Conferencia Regional Latinamericana de poblacion.* Actos 1, pp. 387-92.

Hatt, P.K. *Backgrounds of Human Fertility in Puerto Rico.* Princeton: Princeton University Press, 1952.

Hill, R., Stycos, J.M., and Back, K.W. *The Family and Population Control.* Chapel Hill: University of North Carolina Press, 1959.

Hordern, A. *Legal Abortion: The English Experience.* Elmsford, New York: Pergamon Press, 1971.

Knudsen, D.D. "The Declining Status of Women: Popular Myths and the Failure of Functionalist Thought." *Social Forces,* 48, 2 (1969): 183-92.

Landis, J.T. "Attitudes of Individual Californian Physicians and Policies of State Medical Societies on Vasectomy for Birth Control." *Journal of Marriage and the Family* 28 (1966): 277-83.

Phillips, N. "The Prevalence of Surgical Sterilization in a Suburban Population." *Demography* 8 (1971): 261-70.

Pratt, William. "The Practice of Sterilization in the United States: Preliminary
    Findings from the 1973 National Survey of Family Growth." Paper
    presented at the annual meeting of the Population Association of America,
    Seattle, Washington, 1975.
Presser, H.B. "The Role of Sterilization in Controlling Puerto Rican Fertility."
    *Population Studies* 23, 3 (1969): 343-61.
Presser, H.B. *Sterilization and Fertility Decline in Puerto Rico.* Berkeley:
    University of California, Institute of International Studies, 1973.
Presser, H.B. and Bumpass, L.L. "Demographic and Social Aspects of Contra-
    ceptive Sterilization in the United States: 1965-1970." In *Commission
    on Population Growth and the American Future,* Research Reports, Vol-
    ume I, Demographic and Social Aspects of Population Growth, edited by
    C.F. Westoff and R. Parke, Jr., 1972a, pp. 506-568.
Presser, H.B. and Bumpass, L.L. "The Acceptability of Contraceptive Steriliza-
    tion among U.S. Couples: 1970." *Family Planning Perspectives* 4, 4
    (1972b): 18-26.
Richter, A.J. Personal communication to Association for Voluntary Steriliza-
    tion, May 23, 1973.
Satterthwaite, A.P. As reported in a personal interview, 1968.
Stycos, J.M. "Female Sterilization in Puerto Rico." *Eugenics Quarterly*
    1 (1954): 3-9.
*The Nation's Health.* The official newspaper of the American Public Health
    Association (August 1972).
Tietze, C. "The Current Status of Fertility Control." *Law and Contemporary
    Problems* 25 (1960): 426-44.
U.S. Bureau of the Census. Census of Population: 1940. Puerto Rico: Occupa-
    tions and Other Characteristics by Age, 1940. Washington, D.C.: U.S.
    Government Printing Office, 1943.
U.S. Bureau of the Census. Census of Population: 1950. Puerto Rico: Detailed
    Characteristics. Vol. 2, Part 53. Washington, D.C.: U.S. Government
    Printing Office, 1953.
U.S. Bureau of the Census. Census of Population: 1960. Characteristics of the
    Population. Puerto Rico. Vol 1, Part 53. Washington, D.C.: U.S. Govern-
    ment Printing Office, 1963.
U.S. Bureau of the Census. Census of Population: 1970. General Social and
    Economic Characteristics. Final Report PC (1) —C1, United States Sum-
    mary. Washington, D.C.: U.S. Government Printing Office, 1972a.
U.S. Bureau of the Census. Census of Population 1970. General Social and
    Economic Characteristics. Final Report PC (1) —C53, Puerto Rico.
    Washington, D.C.: U.S. Government Printing Office, 1972b.
U.S. Bureau of the Census. Current Population Reports, Series P-20, No. 248.
    Birth Expectations and Fertility: June 1972. Washington, D.C.: U.S.
    Government Printing Office, 1973.

Vázquez, J.L. Personal communication, August 31, 1966.

Weller, R.H. "A Historical Analysis of Female Labour Force Participation in Puerto Rico." *Social and Economic Studies* 17 (1968): 60-69.

Westoff, C.F. "The Modernization of U.S. Contraceptive Practice." *Family Planning Perspectives* 4, 3 (1972): 9-12.

Westoff, C. and Ryder, N.B. "Family Limitation in the United States." In Proceedings of the International Population Conference, London, Vol. II, Session 4:3 (1969), pp. 1301-1318.

Whelpton, P.K,, Campbell, A.A. and Patterson, J.E. *Fertility and Family Planning in the United States.* Princeton: Princeton University Press, 1966.

Woodside, M. *Sterilization in North Carolina.* Chapel Hill: University of North Carolina Press, 1950.

# 4

## Sterilization in India, 1965–1975: An Overview of Experience and Research Results
### Moni Nag

After slackening during the three years from 1973-1974 to 1975-1976, the sterilization program in India is again being strengthened considerably. By the middle of 1976, a few states in India were in the process of making sterilization compulsory for couples with three or more living children, unless all children are of the same sex. The primacy of sterilization for Indian family planning is reflected in the fact that at the end of March 1976, of 16 percent of couples (of reproductive ages) protected by contraceptive methods, 12 percent were protected by sterilization, while 4 percent were protected by other methods. The annual variation in the number of sterilizations and the percentage of males sterilized is shown in Table 4-1.

The sharply increased acceptance of sterilization in 1971-1972 and 1972-1973 was mostly due to the response to vasectomy camps organized in various states. The sudden reduction in the number of contraceptive sterilizations in 1973-1974 can be attributed to the following factors: (1) discontinuation of mass vasectomy camps and the associated incentive programs of the central government as "counterproductive"; (2) public uproar following eleven post-vasectomy deaths caused by tetanus infection, all occurring within one locality of Uttar Pradesh state during a vasectomy campaign in February-March 1972; (3) realization of the need for more systematic and sustained follow-up of sterilization acceptors; and (4) a drastic cut in the budget of family planning programs (Jain, 1975, p. 13; Franda, 1972, pp. 1, 7). Some of the budget cuts were restored in 1974-1975.

It has generally been the policy of the Indian government to encourage male, rather than female, contraceptive sterilization, because vasectomy has several advantages over its counterpart among women. Table 4-1 shows that the percentage of male sterilization gradually increased after 1957 until it reached a peak of 89.6 percent in 1967-1968. The percentage declined in the subsequent three years (1968-1971), rose once more between 1971-1973 and declined again in 1973-1975, but there is no clear reason for these shifts. The percentages of male sterilization in separate states and union territories for the period January 1956 to March 1975 are presented in Table 4-2. There is a remarkable variation among the states in the percentage of male sterilization, ranging from 16.5 percent for Nagaland to 94.4 percent for Orissa.

---

This chapter represents a shortened version of the paper Dr. Nag presented to the workshop.

**Table 4-1**
**Sterilization Performance in India through Governmental Programs,**
**1956 to 1974-1975[a]**

| Year[b] | Number of Sterilizations | Percent of Male Sterilizations |
|---|---|---|
| 1956 | 7,153 | 33.5 |
| 1957 | 13,736 | 30.2 |
| 1958 | 25,148 | 36.5 |
| 1959 | 42,302 | 41.7 |
| 1960 | 64,338 | 58.4 |
| 1961 | 104,585 | 61.1 |
| 1962 | 157,947 | 71.1 |
| 1963 | 170,246 | 67.3 |
| 1964 | 269,565 | 74.6 |
| 1965 | 476,889 | 84.2 |
| Jan.-March 1966 | 193,934 | 90.2 |
| 1966-1967 | 887,368 | 88.5 |
| 1967-1968 | 1,839,811 | 89.6 |
| 1968-1969 | 1,664,817 | 83.1 |
| 1969-1970 | 1,422,118 | 74.2 |
| 1970-1971 | 1,329,914 | 66.1 |
| 1971-1972 | 2,187,336 | 74.1 |
| 1972-1973 | 3,121,856 | 83.7 |
| 1973-1974 | 942,402 | 42.8 |
| 1974-1975 | 1,349,045[c] | 45.2[c] |
| Total | 16,270,510[c] | 74.6[c] |

Source: Data up to 1971-1972 taken from India, Ministry of Health and Family Planning (no date, p. 42). Data for 1972-1973, 1973-1974, and 1974-1975 provided by P. Singha of the Department of Family Planning, Government of India.

[a]Does not include relatively insignificant number of sterilizations in private facilities.

[b]Based on calendar year (January to December) for 1956-1965; From 1966-1967, based on financial year (April 1 to March 31).

[c]Provisional.

*Variation by States*

The figures for the states of India as of March 31, 1974, are given in Table 4-3. Maharashtra state leads all others in the percentages of couples protected through sterilization (21.6 percent) as well as through all methods (22.9 percent). Rajasthan had the lowest percentage. Because contraceptive sterilization accounts for so large a proportion of family planning strategies, the pattern for this one method essentially is synonymous with the relative popularity of all contraceptive practices in the various states.

Several studies have identified the factors that explain the variation among

**Table 4-2**

**Percentages of Males Among Persons Sterilized in India, by Governmental Sponsor, from January 1956 to March 1975[a]**

| Sponsor | Total Sterilized | Total Males Sterilized | Percentage of Males |
|---|---|---|---|
| *States* | | | |
| 1. Andhra Pradesh | 1,805,388 | 1,120,110 | 62.0 |
| 2. Assam | 242,934 | 195,404 | 80.4 |
| 3. Bihar | 951,017 | 886,908 | 93.3 |
| 4. Gujarat | 1,127,402 | 640,932 | 56.9 |
| 5. Haryana | 292,711 | 210,762 | 72.0 |
| 6. Himachal Pradesh | 66,789 | 40,133 | 60.1 |
| 7. Jammu and Kashmir | 77,197 | 55,746 | 72.2 |
| 8. Kerala | 776,589 | 539,512 | 69.5 |
| 9. Madhya Pradesh | 1,228,551 | 998,322 | 81.3 |
| 10. Maharashtra | 2,842,659 | 1,948,423 | 68.5 |
| 11. Manipur | 3,659 | 2,780 | 76.0 |
| 12. Meghalaya | 2,569 | 796 | 31.0 |
| 13. Karnataka | 740,076 | 444,639 | 60.1 |
| 14. Nagaland | 345 | 57 | 16.5 |
| 15. Orissa | 809,339 | 764,152 | 94.4 |
| 16. Punjab | 370,131 | 167,323 | 45.2 |
| 17. Rajasthan | 371,628 | 288,331 | 77.6 |
| 18. Tamil Nadu | 1,833,527 | 1,549,037 | 84.5 |
| 19. Tripura | 20,685 | 19,327 | 93.4 |
| 20. Uttar Pradesh | 1,287,631 | 1,151,461 | 89.4 |
| 21. West Bengal | 1,020,064 | 861,937 | 84.5 |
| *Union Territories* | | | |
| 22. A. and N. Islands | 1,393 | 734 | 52.7 |
| 23. Arunachal Pradesh | 165 | 74 | 44.9 |
| 24. Chandigarh | 5,940 | 1,713 | 28.8 |
| 25. D. and N. Haveli | 954 | 679 | 71.2 |
| 26. Delhi | 101,871 | 53,450 | 52.5 |
| 27. Goa, Daman and Diu | 16,648 | 3,161 | 19.0 |
| 28. L.M. and A. Islands | 256 | 255 | 99.6 |
| 29. Mizoram | 849 | 39 | 4.6 |
| 30. Pondicherry | 18,659 | 13,516 | 72.4 |
| *Central Government Institutions* | | | |
| 31. Ministry of Defence | 77,153 | 53,626 | 69.5 |
| 32. Ministry of Railways | 175,731 | 123,085 | 70.0 |
| *Total* | 16,270,510 | 12,136,424 | 74.6 |

Source: India, Ministry of Health and Family Planning (personal communication dated February 16, 1976).

[a]Figures exclude relatively insignificant number of sterilizations in private facilities.

Table 4-3
Couples Protected through Sterilization and All Methods in Various States of
India as of March 31, 1974

| State | Relative to the Whole of India, Percent of Couples of Reproductive Age (15-44) Living in the State | Percent of Couples Protected by Sterilization, All Methods | |
|-------|------|------|------|
| Maharashtra | 9.4 | 21.6 | 22.9 |
| Kerala | 3.2 | 16.8 | 19.2 |
| Punjab | 2.2 | 11.4 | 18.8 |
| Tamil Nadu | 7.4 | 16.2 | 17.7 |
| Haryana | 1.6 | 11.0 | 17.3 |
| Andhra Pradesh | 8.2 | 16.1 | 17.2 |
| Gujarat | 4.8 | 15.5 | 17.1 |
| Orissa | 4.2 | 13.2 | 15.9 |
| Madhya Pradesh | 8.2 | 10.8 | 12.2 |
| Karnataka | 5.1 | 10.1 | 11.4 |
| West Bengal | 7.5 | 9.9 | 10.7 |
| Himachal Pradesh | 0.7 | 6.7 | 8.4 |
| Assam | 2.4 | 7.9 | 5.8 |
| Jammu and Kashmir | 0.9 | 5.9 | 7.5 |
| Uttar Pradesh | 16.7 | 5.6 | 7.2 |
| Bihar | 10.9 | 5.8 | 6.6 |
| Rajasthan | 4.9 | 5.2 | 6.3 |

Source: S.P. Jain, "The Indian Family Planning Programme: An Assessment of Past
Performance." *Journal of Family Welfare* 21, 4 (1975): 18-19.

the states in family planning program performance (Agarwala, 1972, pp. 27-50;
Misra, 1973, pp. 1769-79; Srikantan, 1974; Jain and Sarma, 1974). A recent
study by the World Bank using regression analysis shows that on the whole
program input variables explain a higher proportion of the variation (1971-
1972) than do socioeconomic variables (King et al., 1974, pp. 149-57). (It
should be noted that inter-state variation in the birth rate, on the other hand,
is more related to socioeconomic factors.)

*Socio-Demographic Characteristics of Individuals*
*Undergoing Contraceptive Sterilization*

In sixteen studies, each with a sample size of over 200 males (Soni, 1971;
Thakor and Patel, 1972, pp. 186-92; Krishnakumar, 1971; Thiyagarajan and
Narayanaswami, 1971, pp. 46-51; Nair and Ayyappan, 1967; Rajagopal and
Sukumaran, 1968; Nair and Pillai, 1966; Nair and Nair, 1966; Bhatnagar, 1964,
pp. 1-14; Sinha, Jain, and Prasad, 1969, pp. 69-77; Varma and Boparai, 1971,

pp. 655-59; Rao, 1968, pp. 2-5; Chitre, Saxena, and Ranganathan, 1964, pp. 36-49), the mean number of living children of sterilized men ranges from 3.5 to 5.4. With the exception of four of these studies (Thiyagarajan and Narayanaswami, 1971, pp. 46-51; Bhatnagar, 1964, pp. 1-14; Rao, 1968, pp. 2-5; Chitre, Saxena, and Ranganathan, 1964, pp. 36-49), the data show that more than 70 percent of the men had four or more children.

The mean number of living children for sterilized females ranged from 4.4 to 5.4 in seven studies, each of which included a sample size of at least 100 (Saigal, 1963, pp. 58-60; Rajagopal and Sukumaran, 1968; Kumaran and Khan, 1966; Nair and Nair, 1966; Nair and Ayyappan, 1967; Sally and Bhardwaj, 1966; Lippitt, Ranganathan, and Hulka, 1969, pp. 434-39). In all but one study (Rajagopal and Sukumaran, 1968), more than 70 percent of the women had four or more children.

There are studies that show that couples with no living son volunteered less frequently for sterilization than did those with no living daughter. Among a sample of 3,465 vasectomized men reported by Dandekar (1963, p. 151), for example, there were only four men with no son, but 287 with no daughter.

Because the reproductive capacity of the female ends before that of the male, the wife's age at the time of her husband's or her own sterilization is more relevant to birth prevention than is the age of her husband. In general, contraceptive sterilization finds the woman considerably younger than her husband, but still not early in her own reproductive career. In twelve studies using sample sizes of over 200 (Population Council, 1970, pp. 4-18; Krishnakumar, 1971; Thiyagarajan and Narayanaswami, 1971, pp. 46-51; Sundaram, 1969, pp. 48-56; Poffenberger, 1967, pp. 48-51; Sinha, Jain, and Prasad, 1969, pp. 69-77; Halder, 1968; Rao, 1968, pp. 2-5; Chitre, Saxena and Ranganathan, 1964, pp. 36-49), the mean age of wives of sterilized males varied from 28.7 to 33.5 years. The mean age of husbands at the time of their sterilization ranged from 36.5 to 44.0 years.

In 1961, the illiteracy rate among the males and females aged twenty-five and over in India was 57 percent and 86 percent, respectively. Among those undergoing sterilization in the 1960s, however, the rate was much lower. In nine of the ten male studies in India cited by Presser (1970), the percentage of illiterates ranged from 3 to 37 percent. Six studies of female acceptors cited by Presser showed an illteracy rate ranging from 2 to 40 percent.

Data are not available on the religious composition in the localities in which contraceptive sterilizations were performed. From the all-India figures on religious composition, Hindus seem overrepresented among sterilization acceptors in the studies discussed by Presser (1970) but underrepresented in the studies that Kumar (1972, pp. 42-45) has presented.

*Physical Complications of Contraceptive Sterilization*

No other deaths except the eleven mentioned above (which were secondary to tetanus) have been directly related to vasectomy in India. Only two cases of death related to female sterilization have been reported so far (Coyaji, 1964).

Well-designed longitudinal studies that follow sterilized persons for a reasonable period after surgery are rare. Sterilized men are usually asked to return to the clinics if there are complications, but, according to at least one report (Pai, 1969), about 80 percent of the cases did not come even for a postoperative check-up. In only a few studies has follow-up been highly emphasized.

In fifteen of seventeen reports that included samples of over 100 subjects (Dandekar, 1963, pp. 212-24; Sundaram, 1969, pp. 48-56; Saxena, 1973, pp. 188-98; Phadke, 1959, pp. 342-45; Bhatnagar, 1964, pp. 1-14; Venkatacharya, 1971, pp. 491-505; Srinivasan and Kachiravan, 1968, pp. 13-32; Rao, 1968, pp. 2-5; Sinha, Jain, and Prasad, 1969, pp. 134-41; Saxena, Chitre, and Lobo, 1965, pp. 1-12; IRHPF n.d.; Sawhney and Langoo, 1969, pp. 2-5; Wig and Singh, 1970; Apte and Gandhi, 1970, pp. 3-17; Sandhu and Bhardwaj, 1968, pp. 17-20; Katti and Hasalkar, 1970; Sandhu and Bhardawaj, 1969), the percentage of persons who complained of side effects postsurgery ranged from 18.1 to 40.5. In the two remaining studies, the corresponding percentages were 2.7 and 3.6. Pain in the testicle and at the site of operation was the most frequent complaint.

Is there a change in general health following vasectomy? In the seventeen selected studies, it was found that 70.2 to 84.6 percent reported no change, 0.0 to 23.9 percent reported improvement, and 1.6 to 21.6 percent reported worsening of their general health. The wide range of variability may in large part be a function of the timing of the interview, previous feeling toward sterilization, psychological preparedness for sterilization, or the vagueness of the term "general health" as used both by the sterilized persons and by the interviewers.

Sterilized women seem to have more immediate physical complications and discomfort than do sterilized men. In three selected studies of females (Chakravarty, 1966, pp. 418-22; Ghatikar and Bhoopatkar, 1966, pp. 572-78; Rao, Saha, and Sadasivaiah, 1968), immediate complaints were voiced by 50.6 to 80.0 percent of the samples. Menstrual disturbances and dysfunctional uterine bleeding seem to persist among some women even two years after sterilization (Chakravarty, 1966, pp. 418-22).

*Change in Sexual Desire and Activity after*
*Contraceptive Sterilization*

In eight of twelve selected studies in which ninety or more subjects were interviewed (Dandekar, 1963, pp. 212-224; Bhatnagar, 1964, pp. 1-14; Varma and Boparai, 1971, pp. 1-12; Wig and Singh, 1970; Apte and Gandhi, 1970, pp. 3-17;

Katti and Hasalkar, 1970; Sinha, 1965; Kakar, 1970, pp. 37-46; Rathore, 1972, pp. 20-25), the percentages of sterilized men reporting *no* change in their sexual desire after sterilization ranged from 2.5 to 95.5. Sexual desire was reported to have increased among 0.0 to 23.3 percent and weakened among 0.9 to 53.1 percent. Variation across studies is considerable, perhaps because factors other than vasectomy entered into the judgment of the respondents.

Like reports of sexual desire, changes in coital frequency varied widely across studies. In six of seven selected studies (Bhatnagar, 1964, pp. 1-14; Sinha, Jain, and Prasad, 1969, pp. 134-41; Wig and Singh, 1970; Apte and Gandhi, 1970, pp. 3-17; Sinha, 1965; Kakar, 1970, pp. 37-46; Rathore, 1972, pp. 20-25) with a sample size of over ninety, the percentage of sterilized men reporting no change in frequency of coitus ranged from 68.9 to 95.5; 41.6 percent in the other study indicated no change. The percentage reporting increase of coital frequency ranged from 4.0 to 17.7. Decreased frequency characterized from 4.5 to 40.6 percent of the respondents.

One study (Kakar, 1970, pp. 37-46) found sexual desire weakened in 40.9 percent of forty-four male respondents aged thirty-five to forty-four; the figure was 70.0 percent among twenty respondents in the forty-five to fifty-four age group. Another study (Dandekar, 1966, pp. 435-38) found sexual desire weakened in 52.2 percent of 601 respondents in the thirty-eight to forty-seven age group and in 65.8 percent of the 193 respondents aged forty-eight and over. Apparently, advanced age at the time of surgery is directly related to postoperative diminution of sexual desire.

Educational status is significantly related to outcome. At least two studies (Kakar, 1970, pp. 37-46; Dandekar, 1963, pp. 212-24) have shown that weakened sexual desire is more frequent among illiterates.

Expectation seems to play an important role in postsurgical sexual behavior. According to Pai (1969), preoperative discussion with the acceptor of the possibility of sexual after effects "might precipitate the condition." In a comparison of vasectomies performed in hospitals and camps, he found a much higher percentage among the hospital cases who reported postoperative "sexual weakness." It was the hospitals, interestingly enough, which had spent a good deal of time on psychological preparation of prospective acceptors.

Kakar (1970) has empirically compared anticipated changes in sexual desire and activity with changes actually experienced. Of the respondents aged twenty-five to thirty-four, 32 percent experienced weakened sexual desire after sterilization although none had anticipated any change. Among those fifty-five years of age and older, however, anticipation and later experience were more closely linked.

Very few studies have been done in India on changes in sexual desire and behavior among sterilized women. In two studies (Dawn, 1966; Rao, Saha, and Sadasivaiah, 1968), it was found that the percentages of women reporting increased sexual desire and activity were higher than those reporting a negative change. For both studies, it is not possible to distinguish nonresponse from no change, since the investigator did not do so.

*Reversal (Reanastomosis) after Surgery*

Requests for reversal after surgery seem to be rather rare. According to one report (Krishnakumar, 1971), of 62,913 vasectomized in one area in 1971, 117 (0.002 percent) cases were registered for reversal. Another study (Pai, 1969) reported only 135 (0.001 percent) of about 100,000 vasectomy cases requesting reversal. Three selected studies (Kar, 1969; Krishnakumar, 1971; Phadke and Phadke, 1967) show the following reasons to be given most commonly for requesting reversal of vasectomy: (1) death of wife and/or remarriage; (2) death of one or more children; and (3) desire for more children. These reasons are not mutually exclusive, of course. In two studies (Kar, 1969; Krishnakumar, 1971), 9.6 percent and 6.0 percent of men requesting reversal were reported to be unmarried.

The degree of success of vasectomy reversal in India is not well known. Two separate studies (Kar, 1969; Phadke and Phadke, 1967) on a total of 163 men show sperm reappearance in 70.0 and 86.3 percent of the cases, a proportion higher than the 60 percent figure derived by Lee (1966) from a number of earlier studies in different countries. The success rate of reversal is likely to be inflated unless the total number of persons who requested it are taken into account. These numbers are not known for the two studies mentioned above. It is difficult to explain why the percentages of successful impregnations in the Indian studies were so different (20.0 and 57.6). The average was about 30 percent in the studies reviewed by Lee.

*Use-Effectiveness of Contraceptive Sterilization*

Use-effectiveness can be estimated by measuring the occurrence of pregnancy among the wives of sterilized men. In a follow-up study in Maharashtra state (Dandekar, 1963), only four of 1,191 wives of vasectomized men were found to have given birth within twelve to twenty-four months after the operation. The failure rate (0.3 percent) was less than the rates (2.0 and 4.1 percent) found in two American studies (Chaset, 1966; Ferber, Tietze, and Lewit, 1967).

A few studies of the failure rate of female sterilization have been done in India but they are not strictly comparable with one another. The percentages range from 0.1 to 1.9 in four selected studies (Coyaji, 1964; Adatia and Adatia, 1966; Chakravarty, 1966; Ghatikar and Bhoopatkar, 1966).

*Demographic Effectiveness*

The methods used by Haynes et al. (1969) for estimating the number of future births prevented by sterilization represent a definite improvement over those used previously by others (Dandekar, 1959; Gopalaswami, 1968; Sarma, 1963; Agarwala, 1966). The investigators selected two samples for comparison. The first consisted of 1,081 women in two districts of Kerala state who were either sterilized or were the wives of sterilized men. The control sample comprised 1,000 women on whom data were available from the files of a continuing demographic survey conducted for a different purpose in the same districts. Using the number of births occurring at each age-level of women in the control sample, they estimated that 2.48 future births were prevented per sterilization. The conclusions of Simmons (1971) are roughly similar.

Despite different assumptions and methods, Jain's (1969) estimate of 2.489 births prevented per sterilization in India is very close to that of Haynes et al., although Jain appears to have generally underestimated the ages of women at the time of sterilization.

An estimate of the demographic effectiveness of sterilization in India from 1956 to 1969 has been prepared by Venkatacharya (1971) based on matrices of annual birth probabilities specific to the age of women at the time of their own or their husband's sterilization. His matrices provided a refined correction for the susceptibility of women to the risk of pregnancy at various ages.

*Motivation and Incentives*

A study conducted in the early phase of a sterilization program found that the relative unpopularity of vasectomy in West Bengal compared to a few other states of India was due to some misinformation among the people regarding the effects of vasectomy. When an adequate campaign was launched, the number of acceptors increased considerably in West Bengal. Similar results were obtained in a village study in Haryana state (Oswal, 1973).

India has had a very intensive experience with financial and other kinds of incentives (often referred to officially as "compensation for loss of earnings") for involvement in family planning programs. Most of the research on incentives was conducted in Tamil Nadu state. From 1956 to 1966, the Tamil Nadu government changed its policy several times regarding payment to the acceptors and the canvassers. On the basis of two studies (Repetto, 1968; Srinivasan and Kachirayan, 1968) regarding the effects of changes in the incentive programs of Tamil Nadu, as well as other related investigations, Rogers (1971) has made some significant generalizations about the role of incentives in diffusing family planning innovations.

*Needed Research*

Although many studies have been done in India using routine records kept on sterilized persons, well-designed follow-up studies are very few in number. As a result, considerable information is available on the socio-demographic characteristics of the sterilized persons, but our knowledge about the physical and psychological effects of sterilization is not at all satisfactory. The use-effectiveness of sterilization and the role of incentive-disincentives in influencing the motivation for sterilization are topics in urgent need of research in view of the government of India's recent reemphasis of its sterilization program.

## References

Adatia, M.D. and Adatia, S.M. "A Ten Year Survey of Sterilization Operations (in Women)." *Journal of Obstetrics and Gynecology of India* 16 (1966): 423-26.

Agarwala, S.N. "The Arithmetic of Sterilization in India." *Eugenics Quarterly* 13, 3(1966): 209-13.

_____ . *Family Planning Performance in India, 1967-70: A District-wise Study.* Bombay: International Institute for Population Studies, 1972, pp. 27-50, (mimeo).

Apte, J.S. and Gandhi, V.N. "A Follow-up Study of Vasectomy Cases." *Journal of Family Welfare* 7, 1 (1970): 3-17.

Bhatnagar, N.K. "Vasectomy — A Study of Effects and Reactions." *The Journal of Family Welfare* 11, 2 (1964): 1-14.

Chakravarty, S. "Follow-up Studies of Surgical Sterilisation in Women with Special Reference to Ovarian Changes." *Journal of Obstetrics and Gynaecology of India* 16 (1966): 418-22.

Chaset, N. "Male Sterilization." *Journal of Urology* 87 (1962): 512-17.

Chitre, K.T., Saxena, R.N., and Ranganathan, H.N. "Motivation for Vasectomy." *Journal of Family Welfare* 11 (1964): 36-49.

Coyaji, B.J. "Report on 2847 Sterilizations." *Journal of Obstetrics and Gynaecology of India* 14 (1964): 485-93.

Dandekar, K. "Sterilization Programme: Its Size and Effects on Birth Rate." *Artha Vijnana* 1 (1959): 220-32.

_____ . "Vasectomy Camps in Maharashtra." *Population Studies* 17, 2 (1963): 147-54.

_____ . "After-effects of Vasectomy." *Artha Vijnana* 5, 3 (1963): 212-24.

Dawn, C.S., "Late Effects of Sterilization." *Journal of Obstetrics and Gynecology* 16 (1966): 435-38.

Dubey, D.C. and Bardhan, A. "Mass Acceptance of Vasectomy: The Role of Social Interaction and Incentives in Social Change," In *Population and*

*Social Organization*, ed. Moni Nag. The Hague: Mouton Publishers, 1975, pp. 295-305.

Ferber, A.S., Tietze, C., and Lewit, S. "Men with Vasectomies: A Study of Medical, Sexual, and Psychosocial Changes." *Psychosomatic Medicine* 29 (1967): 354-66.

Franda, M.F. "Mass Vasectomy Camps and Incentives in Indian Family Planning." *Fieldstaff Reports of the American Universities, South Asia Series 16, 7,* India, Hanover, American Universities Field Staff (1972).

Ghatikar, N.V. and Bhoopatkar, I. "Aftermaths of Puerperal Sterilisation." *Journal of Obstetrics and Gynaecology of India* 56 (1966): 572-78.

Gopalaswami, R.A. "Advantages of Vasectomy." Directorate General of Health Services, Ministry of Health, New Delhi. *Family Planning News* 3, 2 (1962): 34-35.

Halder, B.N. "Follow-up Study of 250 Vasectomy Cases in Madhya Pradesh." *Family Planning News* (October 1968).

Haynes, M.A. , Immerwahr, G.E., George, A., and Nayar, P.S.J. "A Study on the Effectiveness of Sterilizations in Reducing the Birth Rate." *Demography* 6 (1969): 1-11.

India, Ministry of Health and Family Planning. *Family Welfare Planning in India: Year Book 1972-73.* New Delhi, Government of India, n.d.

IRHPF (Institute of Rural Health and Family Planning). *A Brief Report on the Study of Persons Who Have Undergone Vasectomy in the Institute Area.* Gandhigram: (Mimeographed), n.d.

Iyer, H.P. and Selvaraj, S.R. *Demographic Particulars of Sterilised Persons in Cannanore District, 1965-1966.* District Report Series (F.P.). Papers. No. 4 Kerala: Demographic Research Centre, Trivandrum, 1968.

Jain, Anrudh K. and Sarma, D.V.H. *Some Explanatory Factors for Statewise Differential Use of Family Planning Methods in India.* New York: The Population Council, 1974 (mimeo).

Jain, S.C. *The Canvassar System: A Study of A Policy Pertaining to Delivery of Family Planning Services,* Draft: Research Proposal, 1969 (manuscript).

Jain, S.P. "The Indian Family Planning Programme: An Assessment of Past Performance." *Journal of Family Welfare* 21, 4 (1975): 10-27.

Kakar, D.N. "After-effects of Vasectomy on Sex Behaviour: An Exploratory Investigation." *Journal of Family Welfare* 17, 2 (1970): 37-46.

_____. "Sexual Problems Related to Vasectomy: Suggested Guidelines for Future Research." *Journal of Family Welfare* 21, 3 (1975): 16-20.

Kar, J.K. "Surgical Correction of Post-vasectomy Sterility." *Journal of Family Welfare* 15, 3 (1969): 50-53.

Katti, A.P. and Hasalkar, J.B. *A Follow Up Study of Sterilised Males.* Dharwar, Demographic Research Centre, Institute of Economic Research (mimeographed), 1970.

King, Timothy et al. *Population Policies and Economic Development.* Baltimore:

Johns Hopkins University Press, 1974, pp. 149-57.

Krishnakumar, S. *Ernakulam District Janapperuppa Pratirodha Yajna (Crusade for Control of Population Growth): A Report on the Massive Vasectomy Camp at Ernakulam.* Cochin (Ernakulam District) (mimeographed), 1971.

_____. *The Story of the Ernakulam Experiment in Family Planning.* Cochin, Government of Kerala, 1971.

Kumar, A. *An Over-view of Sterilization Studies in India.* Bombay: International Institute for Population Studies (mimeographed), 1972.

Kumaran, N.O. and Khan, M.S.S. *Report on the Demographic Particulars of Sterilised Persons in Cannanore District for 1964-1965.* Paper No. 40. Trivandrum (Kerala): Demographic Research Centre (mimeographed), 1966.

Lee, H.Y. "Studies on Vasectomy, III: Clinical Studies on the Influences of Vasectomy," *Korean Journal of Urology* 7 (1966): 15-29.

Lippitt, T. Ranganathan, K.V., and Hulka, J.F. "Tubal Ligation as Part of Family Planning in India." *American Journal of Obstetrics and Gynecology* 105 (1969): 434-39.

Misra, Bhaskar D. "Family Planning: Differential Performance of States." *Economical and Political Weekly* 8 (1973): 1769-79.

Murty, D.V.R. *Estimated Reductions in Birth Rate Resulting from Different Combinations of Sterilisation and Contraception Programmes in India.* Paper presented at the United Nations World Population Conference, Belgrade, 1965.

Nag, M. "Attitudes Towards Vasectomy in West Bengal." *Population Review,* 10, 1 (1966): 61-64.

Nair, G.S. and Nair, K.N.R. *Report on the Demographic Particulars of Sterilized Persons in Kozhi Kode District 1964-65.* Paper No. 37. Trivandrum: Demographic Research Centre, 1966.

Nair, K.R. and Pillai, N.K. *A Report on the Demographic Particulars of Sterilised Persons in Kottayam District, 1964-65.* Paper No. 35. Trivandrum: Demographic Research Centre, 1966.

Nair, P.S.G. and Ayyappan, K.S. *Demographic Particulars of Sterilised Persons in Trichur District, 1965-66.* District Report Series (Family Planning), Paper No. 1. Trivandrum: Demographic Research Centre (mimeographed), 1967.

Oswal, M.G. "Factors Influencing Acceptance of Vasectomy in an Indian Village." *International Journal of Health Education* 16, 1 (1973): 43-50.

Pai, D.N. "Discussion." In Richart, R.M. and Prager, D.J., eds., *Human Sterilization.* Springfield, Ill.: Charles C. Thomas, 1969.

Phadke, G.M. "Vasectomy." In *Report of the Sixth International Conference On Planned Parenthood,* held at Delhi, 1959. Bombay: Family Planning Association of India, 1959, pp. 342-45.

Phadke, G.M. and Phadke, A.G. "Experiences in the Reanastomosis of the Vas Deferens." *Journal of Urology* 97 (1967): 888-90.

Poffenberger, T. "Age of Wives and Number of Living Children of a Sample of Men Who Had the Vasectomy in Meerut District, U.P." *Journal of Family Welfare* 13, 4 (1967): 48-51.

Poffenberger, T. and Poffenberger, S.B. "A Comparison of Factors Influencing Choice of Vasectomy in India and the U.S." *The Indian Journal of Social Work* 25, 4 (January 1965).

Pohlman, E. *Incentives and Compensations in Birth Planning.* Carolina Population Center Monograph 11. Chapel Hill: University of North Carolina, 1971.

Population Council. "India: UN Mission Evaluation of the Family Planning Program." Studies in Family Planning 56 (1970): 4-18.

Presser, H. "Voluntary Sterilization: A World View." (Population Council) *Reports on Population/Family Planning* 5 (July 1970).

Rajagopal, T.P. and Sukumaran, K.K. *Demographic Particulars of Sterilized Persons in Ernakulam District (1964-65 and 1965-66).* (Two Issues). Trivandrum: Demographic Research Centre, Government of Kerala, 1968.

Rao, H.K. "A Study of Vasectomy Cases Around Ramanagaram." *Family Planning News* 9, 8 (1968): 2-5.

Rao, H.K., Saha, S.K. and Sadasivaiah, K. "A Follow-up of Tubectomy Operations: Pilot Study at Vanivilas Hospital," Bangalore, Regional Health Office (Southern Region), *Family Planning News,* November 1968.

Rathore, H.S. "After-effects of Vasectomy and Its Social Acceptance." *The Journal of Family Welfare* 19, 2 (1972): 20-25.

Repetto, R. "India: A Case Study of the Madras Vasectomy Program." *Studies in Family Planning* 31 (1968): 8-16.

_____. *Temporal Aspects of Indian Development.* Ph.D. Thesis. Cambridge, Massachusetts: Harvard University, 1969.

Research and Marketing Services. *A Study on the Evaluation of the Effectiveness of the Tata Incentive Programme for Sterilization.* Bombay, Unpublished Report, 1970.

Rogers, E.M. "Incentives in the Diffusion of Family Planning Innovations." *Studies in Family Planning* 2, 12 (1971): 241-48.

Saigal, M.D. "Tubectomy Operations in Kaira District." *Family Planning News* 4, 3 (1963): 58-60.

Sally, K.P. and Bhardwaj, K.S. *A Report on Demographic Particulars of Sterilized Persons in Alleppey District, 1964-65.* Paper No. 41. Trivandrum: Demographic Research Centre, 1966.

Sandhu, S.K. and Bhardwaj, K.S. "Follow-up Study of Vasectomised Cases in Meharauli Block." *Family Planning News* 9, 12 (1968): 17-20.

_____. *Report on Follow-up Study of Vasectomized Cases in Paharganj Area.* New Delhi: Central Family Planning Institute, 1969.

Sarma, R.S.S. "Demographic Effects of a Large-scale Sterilization Policy." *Artha Vijnana* 5, 1 (March 1963): 17-23.

Sawhney, J.L. and Langoo, P.N. "A Study of Male Sterilisation in Jammu and Kashmir." *Family Planning News* 10, 1 (1969): 2-5.

Saxena, D.N. "Vasectomy: What Are the Qualitative Gains?" *International Journal of Health Association* 16 (1973): 188-98

Saxena, R.N., Chitre, K. and Lobo, J.A. "Follow-up of Vasectomy." *Journal of Family Welfare* 11 (1965): 1-12.

Simmons, G.B. *The Indian Investment in Family Planning.* An Occasional paper of the Population Council. New York: Population Council, 1971.

Sinha, S.N. *An Exploratory Study of One Hundred Urban Sterilized Males in Lucknow.* Paper presented in the Seminar on Sterilization, Gokhale Institute of Politics and Economics, Poona (mimeographed), 1965.

Sinha, S.N., Jain, P.C., and Prasad, B.G. "A Sociomedical Study of Urban Sterilized Males in Luchnow." Part I. Socio-demographic Data and Pre-Operative Phase Reactions. *Journal of the Indian Medical Association* 53, 2 (1969): 69-77.

———. "A Sociomedical Study of Urban Sterilized Males in Lucknow." Part II. Postoperative Effects and Reactions. *Journal of the Indian Medical Association* 53, 3 (1969): 134-41.

Soni, V. *The Ernakulam Camps: An Analysis.* New Delhi: The Ford Foundation, 1971.

Srikantan, K.S. *Comparative Analysis of Family Planning Programs in the Context of Socio-Economic Infrastructure: States of India.* New York: The Population Council, 1974 (mimeo).

Srinivasan, K. and Kachirayan, M. "Vasectomy Follow-up Study: Findings and Implications." *Bulletin of the Institute of Rural Health and Family Planning* 3, 1 (1968): 13-32

Sundaram, C. "A Follow-up Study of Sterilised Male Industrial Workers in Bombay." *Journal of Family Welfare* 16, 1 (1969): 48-56.

Thakor, V. H. and Patel, V.M. "The Gujarat State Massive Vasectomy Campaign," *Studies in Family Planning* 3, 8 (1972): 186-92.

Thiyagarajan, B. and Narayanaswami, S.S. "A Statistical Study of the Vasectomised Persons at Government General Hospital, Madras, 1967-68." *Journal of Family Welfare* 17, 3 (1971): 46-51

Varma, R.N. and Boparai, M.S. "Vasectomy in the Army." *Indian Journal of Medical Research* 59 (1971): 655-59.

Venkatacharya, K. "A Model to Estimate Births Averted Due to IUCDs and Sterilizations." *Demography* 8, 4 (1971): 491-505.

Wig, N.N. and Singh, S. *A Psychological Study of Symptoms Following Vasectomy* (mineographed), 1970.

# 5

## Demographic-Social and Family Planning Aspects of Contraceptive Sterilization in Countries Other Than the United States, Puerto Rico, and India
*Dorothy Nortman*

### Changed Attitudes Toward Contraception

For this chapter — essentially a worldwide view of sterilization — it is necessary to consider the procedure within the context and from the perspective of practices, policies, and attitudes relating to *all* means of fertility control.

In the past decade, there has been a radical change in governmental and other institutional attitudes toward the practice of contraception, a shift from historical positions of overt or covert hostility to the present general advocacy, support, and sponsorship of family planning programs (Symonds and Carder, 1973). The revision in official attitude has produced a revolution in contraceptive practice. Not only is contraception now more widespread, but it has also been transformed in nature and quality. Traditional, back-fence, and often ineffective methods are being replaced by sophisticated, modern, and reliable techniques, including sterilization, requiring delivery through the medical profession, to a large degree.

In the recent development of institutional support for contraceptive practice and research in improved technology, the health benefits of family planning, now almost universally acknowledged, played a legitimating, not a predisposing, role. That is, the stimuli for the change in public policy have been mainly demographic, economic, and political. The major forces that have led to the worldwide reversal in public attitude toward contraception in general and sterilization in particular can be briefly summarized as follows:

1.  Concern over high rates of population growth that are regarded as serious obstacles to economic modernization and improvement in levels of living in the developing world (United Nations, Department of Economic and Human Affairs, 1971);
2.  Increasing realization that a world population growth rate of 2 percent per year, at which numbers double in thirty-five years, cannot long endure; that unless birth rates fall, it will not be long before death rates rise;
3.  Growing awareness that many couples want fewer children and that present day contraceptive technology, while far from ideal, is nevertheless sufficiently

63

advanced to enable even the poor and illiterate effectively to space and limit births;

4.  Concern over the environmental deterioration, pollution, congestion, tension, and resource depletion engendered by the production, distribution, and consumption patterns of advanced societies; and, finally,

5.  The emergence as dominant themes in the conduct of human affairs of the rights of the individual to respect, dignity, freedom of choice, and equality of opportunity regardless of sex, age, or ethnic origin (Callahan, 1972).

The new attitudes that have legitimated various means of fertility control, including induced abortion, have also made acceptable sterilization upon request for contraceptive purposes. In the past, when sterilization had been performed, it was as a by-product of a medical procedure considered necessary to protect the life or health of the patient (Potts, 1973). Today, in both developed and developing countries, not only are the incidence and prevalence of sterilization increasing, but the operation is available free of charge in many parts of the world. Because vasectomy is technically much simpler than tubal ligation or other female procedures, males as well as females are requesting and receiving contraceptive surgery.

**Why Focus on Sterilization?**

Contraceptive methods vary greatly in their cost, effectiveness, potential demographic impact, need for medical delivery, ease of application, appeal, and relation to the sex act. For several reasons, however, sterilization is in a class by itself.

Sterilization's most obvious distinction lies in its virtual permanence and therefore almost 100 percent effectiveness in preventing conception. With a near perfect continuation rate, sterilization is superior to the two modern contraceptive methods, the IUD and the pill, which, experience has shown, have discontinuation rates of 25 to 50 percent per year, respectively (Mauldin, Nortman, and Stephan, 1967). Yet, the very permanence of sterilization limits the potential demand for it, because it is appropriate only for those ready to make an irrevocable decision to have no more children.

The second feature peculiar to sterilization is its surgical nature. As such, it has a high initial cost relative to other methods and requires medical facilities and personnel which in many countries are unavailable for any large-scale demand. In the developing world, this may be the greatest obstacle to providing sterilization for those ready to request it (Potts, 1973).

Sterilization also suffers uniquely from the stigma still attached to the method because of its historical use for eugenic and punitive reasons. In Eastern Europe, in particular, the memory of sterilizations performed under pre-World

War II totalitarian regimes remains fresh. A further deterrent to the adoption of sterilization is the widespread ignorance and misconceptions about the procedure. Among the educated as well as the uneducated, in developed as well as in developing societies, the nature and consequences of sterilization are misunderstood. The very term is often erroneously identified with castration and the method is often assumed to produce loss of libido.

Because of its permanence, technique, and somewhat unfortunate associations, therefore, sterilization is subject to strong forces both for its adoption and for its rejection. The uniqueness of the method is a factor in the deliberations not only of individual couples but also of administrators concerned with the demographic impact of their family planning programs and the health of their clients.

Although the characteristics of sterilization acceptors have been studied (see Chapters 3 and 4), little is known as to why some couples and some programs accept the method, while others—in seemingly similar circumstances—do not. Even quite fundamental questions remain to be answered. In the case of individuals, how is the acceptance of sterilization linked with factors such as motivation, socioeconomic status, access to other methods, and the local medical delivery system? For publicly supported family planning programs, how do demographic pressures, ethnic considerations, religious and cultural factors, legal constraints, and the distribution of the public health network affect the promotion of sterilization? The remainder of this chapter discusses some of these issues, with the awareness that such issues constitute major areas for future research.

### The Potential Market for Voluntary Sterilization

Except perhaps in Africa, survey findings have yielded surprisingly high proportions of people knowledgeable about sterilization as a contraceptive procedure. The extent of public knowledge is particularly impressive when one considers the limited grounds upon which sterilization was traditionally practiced: to protect the patient's life or health or for eugenic or punitive reasons.

According to a 1963 survey in Dacca, Bangladesh (then East Pakistan), for example, female sterilization was known by over 90 percent of both husbands and wives and vasectomy by 82 percent of the husbands and by 63 percent of the wives (Green, Gustafson, Griffiths, and Yaukey, 1972). In a rural area of Thailand (Pho-tharam), a 1964 survey found that "among those who claimed some knowledge of contraception. . . , 80 percent of the knowledge was limited to vasectomy and ligation" (Hawley and Prachuabmoh, 1966, p. 329). In another Thai survey, this one in a Bangkok suburb in 1967-1968 involving 960 women of reproductive age, not only were respondents knowledgeable, but 15 percent of the probability sample had been sterilized and another 8 percent had sterilized husbands (Cowgill, Keovichit, Burnight, Udry, and Yamarat, 1971). There is substantial public awareness of sterilization in Latin America, as well. Surveys conducted during 1964-1966 of nine metropolitan areas disclosed that an average of two-thirds of the women respondents had heard of contraceptive sterilization; the percentages ranged from 37 percent in Bogota to 92 percent in Panama City (where 20 percent of the respondents also said they had been sterilized) (CELADE, 1972).

Although even local data on China are unavailable, family planning is unanimously reported to be strongly promoted there. All contraceptive methods are emphasized, including vasectomy, which is performed by "barefoot" doctors. According to recent information provided by Potts (1973), in a Chinese factory commune with 7,600 workers, 1,384 females and 789 males were sterilized, yielding a rate of 29 percent.

Unlike Asia and Latin America, the evidence from Africa indicates that there is very limited knowledge of sterilization there—although the situation may be changing. A 1963 survey among the urban elite in Ghana found that only 3 percent of the males, and no females, knew of surgical sterilization; it should be noted, however, that 44 percent of the respondents knew of no method at all (Caldwell, 1968). A finding in Turkey in 1963 that 10 percent had heard of sterilization, with 2 percent then using the method, was perhaps predictable (Berelson, 1964).

In the developed countries, contraceptive sterilization is not only well known, but is gaining widespread acceptance. The indications of this popularity are many.

In the United States, more than half the respondents expressed approval of the operation in 1970 compared with one-third in 1965 (Presser and Bumpass, 1972). In the United Kingdom, under the National Health Services Amendment Act of 1972, local health authorities may give advice on vasectomy and arrange for the procedure. In Canada, an as yet unpublished estimate is that three times as many vasectomies were performed in 1972 as in 1969.

In Japan, sterilization has been readily available since passage of the Eugenic Protection Law in 1948. The official figures show an increase in the number of sterilizations performed from 5,695 in 1949 to a maximum of 44,485 in 1956. Since then, performance has declined (14,104 in 1971, for example). The decline is suspect, however, since Japan, as is well known, is highly successful at controlling its fertility. If official statistics are to be believed, Japan is maintaining a low birth rate mainly with the Ota ring and traditional contraceptives—not the more modern orals and IUDs—and with declining sterilization and abortion. The likelihood is rather that both abortion and sterilization are grossly underreported in the official statistics.

Despite their limitations (Population Council, 1970), knowledge, attitude, and practice (KAP) surveys of fertile couples who want no more children suggest an enormous potential demand for an acceptable permanent contraceptive method.  Even in the developing world, where rational birth control is little practiced and high fertility is still the norm, substantial proportions of couples in all age brackets want to stop having children.

A 1967 KAP survey in rural Morocco, for example—a region of very high fertility where women still wear the veil—26 percent of women in their twenties and 48 percent of those in their thirties said they wanted no more children (Lapham, 1970).  In the more urban areas of developing countries, interest in terminating childbearing approaches levels evinced in developed countries of low fertility.  The 1967 Bangkok suburb KAP survey, for instance, reported that two-thirds of all the women interviewed, and more than 80 percent of those over age thirty, said they had all the children they wanted (Cowgill, Keovichit, Burnight, Udry, and Yamarat, 1971).  Unequivocal evidence of the potential demand for an acceptable permanent contraceptive lies in the extensive use of induced abortion by women who want no more children—a practice that has been documented in Latin America, the countries of Eastern Europe, Japan, and the United States.

With excess fertility estimated at 20 to 30 percent of the world's births, it is clear that not only contraceptive sterilization but the whole array of present contraceptive technology is failing to meet people's requirements for birth control.

## Prevalence and Incidence of Contraceptive Sterilization in Developing Countries with Government Family Planning Programs

As a medical procedure, the performance of sterilization usually entails reports and records, but these are not generally aggregated to provide regional or national data on prevalence and incidence.  In the absence of a registry, surveys are the major source of information, but they do not often include questions on sterilization.  For most countries in which contraception is widespread and practiced largely with services and supplies obtained through the private sector of the economy, data on sterilization are only conjectural or inferential.  Ironically, information is more readily available in developing countries in which government supported family planning programs try to keep a count of acceptors, by method, and through follow-up surveys, of continuing users.  For sterilization acceptors, an attrition rate of about 5 percent per year is generally allowed to take account of mortality, other marriage dissolution, and passing beyond the reproductive ages.  An estimate of the worldwide prevalence of sterilized couples of fertile ages is thus a wild guess, but some figure approaching 10 percent is within the realm of possibility.

By the end of 1977, sixty-three countries in the developing world supported the principle of family planning, all of them on the grounds of

health and family welfare, and thirty-four for the explicit purpose of reducing
the population growth rate. Most subsidize a family planning action program,
often integrated within the country's health network, that offers a variety of
methods; it is not uncommon, however, for one method to predominate. Only
about a dozen of the programs (all in Asia, except for Tunisia) report contraceptive sterilization. The remainder of the programs, mostly in Africa and
Latin America, do not offer sterilization at all or consider the number performed
to be too small for separate reporting. Tables 5-1 and 5-2 present data on
sterilization users and acceptors, respectively, in countries providing usable
information.

Two programs, those of Bangladesh and India, rely heavily on sterilization—
mostly vasectomy—largely because of disappointment with IUDs. The Singapore and Fiji programs are also strongly oriented toward sterilization, which
accounts for a substantial proportion of acceptors and about one-third of the
current users enrolled in the family planning program. The South Korean and
Tunisian programs are IUD-oriented and Thailand seems to be emphasizing
use of the pill; sterilization is nonetheless prominent in all three countries and
is considered important in South Korea and Thailand. Although the Taiwan
program does not offer sterilization, the method is apparently popular among
those who procure services and supplies through private channels, with 29
percent of current users in the private sector thought to be sterilized (see
Table 5-1).

Because of high drop-out rates among acceptors of IUDs and orals, for the
three methods combined, the percent of sterilization users exceeds that of
sterilization acceptors. According to Table 5-1, a sterilized spouse accounts in
Fiji for 31 percent of users of the three modern contraceptive methods, 10 percent in Hong Kong, 15 percent in Taiwan, 11 percent in South Korea, 10 percent in Thailand, and not readily quantifiable but probably sizeable proportions
in Bangladesh, India, Nepal, and Singapore. Relative to other methods, then,
in countries with programs offering contraceptive sterilization, its prevalence
and incidence are not unimpressive.

Table 5-2 presents the trend in sterilization acceptors in national family
planning programs and their proportions relative to the total number of clients
using modern contraceptive methods (contraceptive sterilization, IUD, and the
pill). The upward trend is clearly visible, with India having achieved three
million sterilization acceptors in fiscal 1972 and Singapore, Sri Lanka (formerly Ceylon), and Thailand showing substantial increases in 1972 over figures
from the previous year. The decline in Bangladesh can be attributed to a large
extent to the wartime disruption of its program; the proportion of program
acceptors represented by sterilized persons makes it clear that sterilization is
the dominant method offered. In Thailand, the number of acceptors is increasing but the proportion is going down because of the great popularity of orals
which, since mid-1969, can be dispensed by midwives.

**Table 5-1**

**Users, by Method and Source of Supplies and Services, for Ten Countries[a] with National Family Planning Programs: January of Specified Year**

| Country, Year and Contraceptive Method | Users as Percent of Married Women of Reproductive Age | | | Percent Distribution of Users | | |
|---|---|---|---|---|---|---|
| | All Users | Public Sector | Private Sector | All Users | Public Sector | Private Sector |
| *Fiji: 1973* | 36.4 | 32.0 | 4.4 | | | |
| Sterilization | 11.3 | 11.3 | 0.0 | 31 | 36 | 0 |
| IUDs | 9.7 | 9.7 | 0 | 27 | 30 | 0 |
| Orals | 10.6 | 7.9 | 2.6 | 29 | 25 | 60 |
| Other | 4.8 | 3.0 | 1.8 | 13 | 9 | 40 |
| *Hong Kong: 1973* | 52 | 25.6 | 27.1 | | | |
| Sterilization | 6 | 0.4 | 5.3 | 10 | 2 | 20 |
| IUDs | 6 | 5.6 | 0.7 | 12 | 22 | 2 |
| Orals | 23 | 11.8 | 11.1 | 44 | 46 | 41 |
| Other | 18 | 7.8 | 10.0 | 34 | 30 | 37 |
| *India: 1973* | u | 13.6 | u | | | |
| Sterilization | u | 10.2 | u | u | 75 | u |
| IUDs | u | 1.4 | u | u | 10 | u |
| Other | u | 2.0 | u | u | 15 | u |
| *Nepal: 1971* | u | 2.5 | u | | | |
| Sterilization | u | 0.4 | u | u | 16 | u |
| IUDs | u | 0.1 | u | u | 6 | u |
| Orals | u | 0.6 | u | u | 25 | u |
| Other | u | 1.3 | u | u | 53 | u |
| *Pakistan: 1971[b]* | u | u | u | | | |
| Sterilization | 5 | 5 | 0.0 | u | u | u |
| IUDs | 7 | 7 | 0.0 | u | u | u |
| Orals | u | 0 | u | u | u | u |
| Other | u | u | u | u | u | u |
| *Singapore: 1973* | u | u | u | | | |
| Sterilization | 6 | 5.9 | 0.0 | u | u | u |
| IUDs | u | u | u | u | u | u |
| Orals | 12 | 12.1 | 0.0 | u | u | u |
| Other | u | u | u | u | u | u |
| *South Korea: 1972* | 25-30 | 20-24 | 5-6 | | | |
| Sterilization | 2-3 | 2-3 | 0 | 11 | 14 | 0 |
| IUDs | 11-12 | 11-12 | 0 | 42 | 52 | 0 |
| Orals | 7-9 | 4-5 | 3-4 | 30 | 19 | 74 |
| Other | 5-6 | 3-4 | 2 | 17 | 15 | 26 |
| *Taiwan: 1973* | 58 | 27 | 30 | | | |
| Sterilization | 9 | 0 | 9 | 15 | 0 | 29 |
| IUDs | 34 | 23 | 10 | 58 | 85 | 34 |
| Orals | 4 | 3 | 1 | 7 | 11 | 3 |
| Other | 11 | 1 | 10 | 20 | 4 | 34 |

**Table 5-1** — *(Continued)*

| Country, Year and Contraceptive Method | Users as Percent of Married Women of Reproductive Age | | | Percent Distribution of Users | | |
|---|---|---|---|---|---|---|
| | All Users | Public Sector | Private Sector | All Users | Public Sector | Private Sector |
| *Thailand: 1973* | 26 | 17.7 | 8.0 | | | |
| Sterilization | 3 | 2.6 | u[c] | 10 | 15 | u[c] |
| IUDs | 5 | 4.8 | u[c] | 19 | 27 | u[c] |
| Orals | 15 | 10.3 | 4.9 | 59 | 58 | 62 |
| Other | 3 | u[c] | 3.1 | 12 | u[c] | 38 |
| *Tunisia: 1973* | u | 6.4 | u | | | |
| Sterilization | u | 1.3 | u | u | 20 | u |
| IUDs | u | 3.4 | u | u | 53 | u |
| Orals | u | 1.3 | u | u | 20 | u |
| Other | u | 0.4 | u | u | 7 | u |

Source: D. Nortman, "Population and Family Planning Programs: A Factbook." Reports on Population/Family Planning, The Population Council, New York. September 1973. Table 16.

Note:  "u" data unavailable.  Subcategories may not add up to totals because of rounding.

[a]Selected on the basis of available data on sterilization in public or private sector of economy. National family planning programs that do not report sterilization include those of Egypt, Indonesia, Iran, Kenya, Morocco, Philippines, and Turkey, plus Latin American countries that support family planning services.

[b]Includes Bangladesh, formerly East Pakistan.

[c]Figures too small to affect totals significantly.

It is striking that all countries with sizeable proportions of sterilized couples are in Asia.  Is there something about Asian culture that predisposes individuals or programs toward the choice of sterilization?  Or is the readiness to undergo sterilization a reaction to disappointment with the IUD and with orals?

It may well be that the overrepresentation of Asian countries is simply an artifact of time and/or political considerations.  Among the sixty-three nations that support family planning, many that are committed to the principle of family planning have only recently begun to translate their goals into action. The African countries, particularly, tend to fall into this category.  Latin American countries, while more advanced in their programs, do not feature sterilization because of the influence of the Roman Catholic church.  Nevertheless, survey data in Latin America indicate that sterilization is widely known and often performed by private doctors.  In San José, Costa Rica, for example, as early as 1964, 6 percent of females aged fifteen to forty-four (in a sample of over 1,300) were found to be sterilized, representing 12 percent of those using

Table 5-2
**Annual Acceptance of Contraceptive Sterilization in Family Planning Programs of Twelve Developing Countries, 1967-1972**

| | Number of Sterilization Acceptors (Thousands) | | | | | |
| | Year | | | | | |
| Country | 1967 | 1968 | 1969 | 1970 | 1971 | 1972 |
|---|---|---|---|---|---|---|
| Bangladesh | 150.0 | 365.0 | 370.0 | 186.0 | 42.0 | u |
| Fiji | 0.5 | 0.7 | 0.9 | 1.2 | 1.5 | 1.7 |
| Hong Kong | 1.0 | 1.0 | 1.0 | 0.9 | 0.5 | 0.4 |
| India[a] | 1,840.0 | 1,665.0 | 1,422.0 | 1,329.0 | 2,185.0 | 3,019.0 |
| Malaysia (West) | 0.6 | 2.6 | 2.7 | 3.5 | 4.0 | 3.9 |
| Nepal | 0.3 | 1.7 | 3.6 | 4.2 | u | u |
| Pakistan (West) | 1.8 | 50.1 | 28.0 | 8.0 | u | u |
| Singapore | 0.7 | 1.0 | 1.4 | 2.3 | 3.9 | 6.2 |
| Sri Lanka | 3.6 | 3.9 | 2.9 | 5.0 | 4.3 | 9.5 |
| South Korea | 20.0 | 16.0 | 15.0 | 17.0 | 19.0 | u |
| Thailand | 12.0 | 12.1 | 15.3 | 18.6 | 23.5 | 31.5 |
| Tunisia | 0.7 | 1.6 | 2.5 | 2.3 | 2.3 | 2.5 |

*Sterilization Acceptors as Percent of Total Program Acceptors[b]*

| | | | | | | |
|---|---|---|---|---|---|---|
| Bangladesh | 33 | 48 | 50 | 54 | 61 | u |
| Fiji | 11 | 27 | 39 | 41 | 47 | 52 |
| Hong Kong | 10 | 5 | 4 | 4 | 2 | 2 |
| India[a] | 73 | 77 | 75 | 73 | 82 | 90 |
| Malaysia (West) | 3 | 4 | 4 | 6 | 8 | 7 |
| Nepal | 8 | 32 | 24 | 24 | u | u |
| Pakistan (West) | 0.5 | 10 | 7 | 3 | u | u |
| Singapore | 4 | 4 | 7 | 15 | 28 | 39 |
| Sri Lanka | 12 | 10 | 6 | 10 | 9 | 16 |
| South Korea | 6 | 6 | 4 | 4 | 4 | u |
| Thailand | 25 | 21 | 12 | 8 | 6 | 7 |
| Tunisia | 5 | 10 | 13 | 10 | 10 | 9 |

Source: Nortman, "Population and Family Planning: A Factbook," Table 13.

Note: "u" data unavailable.

[a]Data based on fiscal year, April 1 to March 31.

[b]Total comprises acceptors of IUDs, orals, and sterilizations only.

any contraception. A national rural sample in Costa Rica in 1969 gave 4.2 percent sterilized, or 17 percent of the total of 25 percent using any method (Thein and Reynolds, 1972). Another indication of the acceptability of surgical contraception in Latin America was the recent opening of International Planned Parenthood Federation (IPPF) vasectomy clinics, in San José, Costa Rica and in Bogotá, Colombia.

## Cultural, Legal, and Ethical Considerations

Cultural factors, particularly religion, do influence the disposition to accept contraceptive sterilization. Only one major religion, the Roman Catholic, is unambiguously opposed to surgery as a contraceptive technique, which explains the absence of sterilization in the national programs of Latin America—although, as we have seen, the practice through the private sector is not insignificant. Given sufficient motivation, people apparently manage to overcome or explain away the theological objections.

Lacking a pyramidal hierarchy akin to that of Roman Catholicism, the Moslem religion permits a divergence of views on family planning. Among followers of Islam, therefore, socioeconomic and psychological factors are likely to be more decisive than doctrine in shaping the actions of couples or country-wide programs. Evidence for the diversity of acceptable policy among predominantly Moslem countries lies in the vigor with which Pakistan has pursued a vasectomy program, the availability but muted role of sterilization in the Tunisian program, and the emphasis in Egypt, Iran, and Morocco on pills, to the total exclusion of sterilization.

In Asian cultures, the pragmatism of their Buddhist and Confucian heritage has led to the ready acceptance of both the principle and the practice of contra-ceptive sterilization in China, Korea, Sri Lanka, Taiwan, Thailand, and, of course, Japan. The countries of Asia, including those with strong Moslem influence, like Bangladesh, Indonesia, Malaysia, and Pakistan, are not constrained by religious doctrine in the choice of birth control techniques; induced abortion, as well as sterilization, is therefore available in government-sponsored family planning programs throughout the continent.

Protestant and Jewish orthodoxy is sometimes interpreted as imposing con-straints on contraceptive sterilization. Whatever the official policies, however, the adherents of these religions tend to choose contraceptive methods on the basis of convenience, effectiveness, and other articulated, nontheological grounds.

Legal and administrative barriers operate more directly than do religious factors to limit the practice of contraceptive sterilization. Even for expressedly medical or eugenic reasons, sterilization is not universally legal—Italy and Spain forbid the procedure outright, no matter what the justification. Table 5-3 summarizes replies to a questionnaire circulated by the European Region of the International Planned Parenthood Federation on the legal status of contra-ception and abortion. It will be noted that in ten of the twenty-seven countries listed, sterilization is available upon request. In the remaining thirteen in which the practice is legal, restrictive conditions are imposed. Some of the stipula-tions are meaningful—for example, that the operation be performed by a physician in an appropriate place. Others, like Denmark's 1967 law, empower

**Table 5-3**
**Sterilization Laws in Twenty-Seven European Countries**

| Country | Legal? | Legal Grounds | | |
|---|---|---|---|---|
| | | On Request | Medical-eugenic | Other |
| Austria | Yes | No | Yes | No |
| Belgium | Yes | Yes | Yes | Yes |
| Bulgaria | Yes | No | Yes | Yes |
| Britain | Yes | Yes | Yes | Yes |
| Czechoslovakia | Yes | No | Yes | No |
| Denmark | Yes | No | Yes | No |
| Finland | Yes | No | Yes | Yes |
| France | Yes | Yes | Yes | Yes |
| German Democratic Republic | Yes | Yes | Yes | Yes |
| German Federal Republic | Yes | No | Yes | No |
| Greece | Yes | No | Yes | No |
| Hungary | Yes | Yes | Yes | Yes |
| Iceland | Yes | No | Yes | No |
| Ireland | Yes | Yes | Yes | Yes |
| Italy | No | — | — | — |
| Luxembourg | Yes | Yes | Yes | Yes |
| Malta | Yes | No | Yes | No |
| Netherlands | Yes | Yes | Yes | Yes |
| Norway | Yes | No | Yes | No |
| Poland | Yes | Yes | Yes | Yes |
| Portugal | Yes | No | Yes | No |
| Romania | Yes | No | Yes | Yes |
| Spain | No | — | — | — |
| Sweden | Yes | No | Yes | No |
| Switzerland | Yes | Yes | Yes | Yes |
| Turkey | Yes | No | Yes | No |
| Yugoslavia | Yes | No | Yes | No |

Source: Adapted from IPPF (1973, Appendix 2).

a committee to make the arbitrary determination of whether "the living conditions of the applicant and family render it necessary to avoid the birth of more children."

Committees, usually comprising doctors, tend to be conservative in approving permanent contraception. In Australia, for example, some surgeons apply the "120 rule"—that a woman's age times her parity exceed 120—to qualify a patient for surgical contraception (Potts, 1973). The legal constraints upon the practice sometimes lead surgeons to perform a hysterectomy instead of tubal ligation in an attempt to legitimate the operation medically.

The legal status of sterilization and abortion in Southeast Asia was summarized by delegates from that region to the January 1973 meeting of the

Expert Group on Sterilization and Abortion of the Inter-Governmental Coordinating Committee on Family and Population Planning. For the most part, they reported, there are no legal restrictions on sterilization procedures, except where French and other Catholic influence still prevails; unless official policy has incorporated the method into family planning programs, however, physicians tend to be conservative about performing sterilization for contraceptive purposes. Laos, for example, has no law, but official policy discourages sterilization for fertility control. The laws of the Khmer Republic, as well, do not mention sterilization, but female surgery runs fourth in acceptability—after pills, IUDs, and condoms. In other parts of Southeast Asia, the future for sterilization seems more promising. Although the original French statutes of 1930 banning contraceptives are still on the Vietnamese books, attitudes toward all family planning methods are becoming more liberal in that country. In the Philippines, a Presidential Decree in December 1972 greatly broadened the grounds for sterilization. In Malaysia, Nepal, Singapore, and Thailand, finally, sterilization is already part of national family planning programs.

Across the world, as the foregoing suggests, there is a distressing lack of uniformity in the codes governing the performance of contraceptive sterilization. In an attempt to bring some international coherence to the legal status of the procedure, a model law was drafted in February 1973 by a workshop at the Geneva meeting of the Association for Voluntary Sterilization. The government's obligation, according to the proposed statute, is to permit and to provide adequate services for sterilization. The medical profession is obliged to explain the nature and consequences of the operation and to make a carefully balanced decision in the case of men and women legally incompetent to decide for themselves about sterilization. The model also ensures the right of a surgeon with conscientious objections to refuse to perform the operation.

Besides cultural and legal issues, the practice of sterilization also involves ethical considerations. A major question in this regard concerns the use of incentives to attract clients. In the Indian, Korean, and Pakistan sterilization programs, both the recruiters and the clients receive a cash payment (Nortman, 1973). In Korea, when the budget was increased in 1966 and the vasectomy target was raised to 20,000 for the year (it is now 30,000), payment to acceptors for work lost was budgeted at $3.20 (U.S.) and a $.40 referral fee was provided for recruiters. Whether payments to acceptors are incentives or merely compensation for travel and time lost from work is a moot point.

The primary ethical issue is whether the payments are coercive. If they are too small to be meaningful, why pay clients at all? If the inducement is large enough to be attractive, are the poor being "forced" into accepting an offer they cannot refuse? It has also been charged that by paying anyone who brings in a client, one encourages the recruitment of men for whom vasectomy is in fact inappropriate, such as the simple-minded or those who do not meet the age requirements. Field staff, under pressure to fulfill high and sometimes unreasonable quotas, have similarly been accused of permitting vasectomies among those who should be disqualified.

## Other Barriers to the Adoption of Contraceptive Sterilization

In the developing world, it may well be that the public demand for contraceptive sterilization greatly exceeds the supply of trained personnel and appropriate facilities. In South Korea, the program itself trained 500 physicians to do vasectomies. This was relatively simple for Korea, with its well-distributed health network and adequate supply of medical personnel. In many countries of Asia, Africa, and Latin America, however, the acute shortage of trained personnel and facilities is enough to explain the limited prevalence of contraceptive sterilization.

The psychological barriers to the acceptance of contraceptive sterilization need not be explored here since they are discussed in Chapters 6 through 11 in this volume. Obviously, the finality of the act and the necessity for surgery have important psychological meanings for the potential adopter. In all societies, moreover, regardless of the level of education, there is also widespread ignorance of the nature and consequences of the procedure—for example, its identification with castration and the concern over loss of libido—constituting another important obstacle to the adoption of sterilization.

## Potential Demographic Impact of Contraceptive Sterilization

The potential demographic impact of contraceptive sterilization is a function of two major variables: (1) the age-parity characteristics of the wife and (2) her estimated fertility from the time of surgery to the end of her reproductive age. (For other methods, a third factor is the duration of use of the technique adopted; in the case of contraceptive sterilization, it is assumed that the effects will endure to the end of the fertile period.)

The first factor, age-parity, is a measure of natural fecundity, usually defined as the biological capacity to reproduce, modified by cultural practices like the proscription of sexual intercourse during certain religious holidays among Moslems or the Indian practice of returning to one's native village for the birth of a child. The second factor attempts to gauge the efficacy of the alternative birth control methods—if any— that might have been used had the surgery not been performed.

Thus, although contraceptive sterilization can be regarded as an almost 100 percent effective method, the number and timing of births averted by sterilization depend on the effectiveness of alternative practices. In societies in which women successfully control their fertility by many methods, including induced abortion if necessary, contraceptive sterilization may be preferred for its convenience and on grounds of health, since it may preclude repeated induced abortions; but the sheer demographic impact of a switch to contraceptive sterilization is small. Where fertility is high, on the other hand, implying rather ineffective contraceptive practice, the adoption of contraceptive sterilization can have a major demographic impact, provided that substantial numbers of potentially high-fertility women or their husbands become sterilized. For a meaningful decline in fertility to occur, both high prevalence and acceptance at young ages are required. As it now stands, sterilization apparently is chosen relatively late in the fertility careers of most adopters.

The data in Table 5-4 indicate that acceptors of sterilization in family planning programs are older and have more children than those choosing either IUDs or orals. The postpartum approach seems to reach younger, lower-parity women, at least among acceptors of IUDs and orals. There is reason to speculate that acceptors have higher-than-average fertility expectations than do non-acceptors of comparable age-parity, but for a strong demographic impact, effective contraception in the developing countries has to be practiced earlier and more widely than it is at present. As long as fertility norms remain high, sterilization is not likely to be attractive for the high proportions of younger, lower-parity couples required to practice contraception if the reduced fertility targets in developing countries are to be met.

**Future Research**

It has already been suggested that little is known about why couples or countries adopt sterilization. Medical facilities and personnel would seem to be a necessary condition, yet India and Bangladesh—countries in which health services are not abundantly available—have actively and successfully promoted this particular method of contraception. Also little studied is the relationship between sterilization and other methods. Do they substitute for each other or do they show trends in the same direction? How does the relationship vary with age, with an individual's status in life, and with the different stages of a country's socioeconomic development?

If more were known about the determinants of sterilization acceptance and its relation to other methods, human welfare as well as potential demographic impact could conceivably be increased. Research is necessary on how to simplify the procedure, make it reversible, clarify its nature and consequences to the potential user, and motivate men as well as women to accept the method.

The moral and ethical questions are also important areas for future

**Table 5-4**

**Average (Median) Age of Wife and Average Number of Living Children Among Family Planning Program Acceptors, by Method Adopted: Countries Reporting on Sterilization Acceptors**

| Country and Method | Dates | Acceptor Sample (Thousands) | Wife's Median Age | Median Number of Living Children |
|---|---|---|---|---|
| *Bangladesh* | | | | |
| Sterilization | 1967-1968 | 9.4 | 31.6 | 4.8 |
| IUDs | 7/65-12/66 | 1.2 | 30.4 | 4.7 |
| *Pakistan* | | | | |
| Sterilization | 1967-1968 | 6.8 | 33.8 | 4.4 |
| IUDs | 7/65-12/66 | 1.6 | 34.6 | 5.0 |
| *Tunisia* | | | | |
| Sterilization | 1969 | 1.9 | 35.6 | 5.8 |
| IUDs | 1966 | 2.1 | 34.4 | 5.0 |
| IUDs | 1969 | 8.6 | 31.4 | 4.6 |
| *International Postpartum Program* | | | | |
| *Hong Kong* | | | | |
| Sterilization | 7-12/71 | 2.0 | 32.8 | unavailable |
| Orals | 7-12/71 | 5.9 | 24.6 | 1.4 |
| All methods | 7-12/71 | 9.4 | 27.0 | 1.9 |
| *Indonesia* | | | | |
| Sterilization | 1-6/71 | 0.5 | 36.2 | 7.1 |
| IUDs | 1-6/71 | 7.9 | 30.2 | 4.5 |
| Orals | 1-6/71 | 2.3 | 29.3 | 4.0 |
| All methods | 1-6/71 | 11.8 | 30.3 | 4.4 |
| *Thailand* | | | | |
| Sterilization | 7-12/71 | 6.6 | 30.9 | 4.3 |
| IUDs | 1/68-6/69 | 2.3 | 27.3 | 3.0 |
| IUDs | 7-12/71 | 20.0 | 28.2 | 3.2 |
| Orals | 7-12/71 | 7.6 | 26.9 | 2.4 |
| All methods | 7-12/71 | 34.7 | 28.6 | 3.4 |
| *Venezuela* | | | | |
| Sterilization | 7-12/71 | 0.5 | 34.4 | 7.3 |
| IUDs | 7-12/71 | 7.2 | 26.6 | 3.8 |
| Orals | 7-12/71 | 5.0 | 24.7 | 3.4 |
| All methods | 7-12/71 | 13.2 | 26.2 | 3.7 |

Source: Nortman, "Population and Family Planning Programs: A Factbook," Tables 15A and 15B.

research and exploration. Are governments justified in promoting sterilization through incentives? Is the ethical justification contingent upon the nature and amount of the incentive? Conversely, should laws and/or the medical profession impose restraints upon the right of an individual to the operation upon request?

The issues are obviously complex and demand an interdisciplinary approach involving contributions from the fields of biomedicine, psychology, economics, demography, sociology, and computer science.

## References

Berelson, B. "Turkey: National Survey on Population." *Studies in Family Planning* 1, 5 (December 1964): 2.

Caldwell, J.C. *Population Growth and Family Change in Africa: The New Urban Elite in Ghana.* Canberra: Australian National University Press, 1968, pp. 162-68.

Callahan, D. "Ethics and Population Limitation." *Science*, 175, 4021 (February 4, 1972): 487-94.

CELADE, "Fertility and Family Planning in Metropolitan Latin America," Community and Family Study Center, University of Chicago, 1972. Table 8.1, p. 155.

Cowgill, D.O. Keovichit, S., Burnight, R.G., Udry, J.R., and Yamarat, C., "Sterilization a Case of Extensive Practice in a Developing Nation." Milbank Memorial Fund Quarterly XLIX 3, Part 1, July 1971.

Green, L.W. Gustafson, H.C., Griffiths, W., and Yaukey, D. "The Dacca Family Planning Experiment." School of Public Health, University of California, Berkeley. Pacific Health Education Reports No. 3, 1972, p. 79.

Hawley, A.H. and Prachuabmoh, V. "Family Growth and Family Planning: Responses to a Family-Planning Action Program in a Rural District of Thailand." *Demography* 3, 2 (1966): 329.

Lapham, R.J. "Family Planning Attitudes, Knowledge, and Practice in the Sais Plain," The Population Council, Studies in Family Planning 1 (58) (1970): 12.

Lapham, R.J. and Mauldin, W.P. "National Family Planning Programs: Review and Evaluation" The Population Council, Studies in Family Planning 3, 3 (March 1972), Table 2.

Maudlin, W.P., Nortman, D., Stephan, F.F. "Retention of IUDs: An International Comparison" The Population Council, Studies in Family Planning, 1 (18 and Supplement) (1967): 1-12.

Nortman, D. "Population and Family Planning Programs: A Factbook." Reports on Population/Family Planning, The Population Council, New York. September 1973.

Presser, H. and Bumpass, L. "Acceptability of Contraceptive Sterilization among U.S. Couples, 1970." *Family Planning Perspectives* 4, 4 (October 1972): 19.

Population Council. "A Manual for Surveys of Fertility and Family Planning: Knowledge, Attitudes, and Practice." New York, 1970.

Potts, M. "Current Status of Sterilization in the World—Prevalence, Incidence, Who and Where." In *Advances in Voluntary Sterilization,* Proceedings of the Second International Conference, Geneva, 1973, edited by M.E. Schima, I. Lubell, J.E. Davis, and E. Connell, pp. 97-103. Princeton, N.J.: Excerpta Medica, American Elsevier Publishing Co., Inc., 1974.

Symonds, R. and Carder, M. *The United Nations and the Population Question, 1945-1970.* A Population Council Book. New York: McGraw-Hill Book Co., 1973.

Thein, T.M. and Reynolds, J. "Contraception in Costa Rica: The Role of the Private Sector." Columbia University, International Institute for the Study of Human Reproduction. February 1972.

United Nations, Department of Economic and Human Affairs. "Human Fertility and National Development: A Challenge to Science and Technology." New York, 1971.

**Part III
Psychosocial Aspects of
Contraceptive Sterilization**

# 6

## Psychological Aspects of Contraceptive Sterilization: Theoretical Framework, Methodological Considerations, and Needed Research

*David A. Rodgers*

What are the psychological and sociological antecedents, correlates, and consequences of the voluntary use of vasectomy, tubal ligation, and hysterectomy for contraceptive purposes? Answers to these rather broad questions demand a theoretical framework, permitting an assessment of what is known about the relevant issues so that effective research can be pursued to fill the gaps. This chapter attempts to map the field, at least from one theoretical perspective.

If a vasectomy or tubal ligation were an orderly occurrence in a systematic sequence of events, the description of the entire sequence would, of course, constitute the appropriate theoretical framework for understanding contraceptive sterilization. There are, however, numerous such theoretical frameworks that could be posited. Some, for example, might consider a vasectomy to be the manifestation of self-mutilative tendencies by a man with pathological psychosexual concerns in which he is symbolically castrating himself before he can be castrated by a feared and oppressive father-figure. It is doubtful whether anyone familiar with research in the field would take such a theoretical formulation very seriously, although it may indeed accurately describe a small percentage of vasectomized men. The formulation does highlight, however, a not uncommon tendency: the assumption that there is some unique and fairly precise explanation of the phenomenon of contraceptive sterilization. Other participants in this conference, for example, have proposed standardizing the research methodology and investigational tools that will be used worldwide for vasectomy studies. Such an undertaking would have most meaning if, and only if, there were universal explanations that could be identified and illuminated by the research instruments or strategies chosen. It is somewhat more plausible that explanations may be uniquely related to individual situations, such that different research tools and methodologies would be appropriate in different cultures and countries. A variety of research approaches used at this stage of our ignorance might at least result in a broader net cast into the theoretical waters; the more uniform studies could be left to follow-up the regularities identified by variegated initial exploratory research. The variety of research approaches is of less serious concern than the *absence* of research approaches, which has largely characterized the field to date.

The argument for variety and multiplicity of theoretical frameworks is not necessarily an endorsement of complete randomness and nondirection in research on contraceptive sterilization. Certain types of theories are, in fact, better than others at explaining the research data so far collected. Specifically, utilitarian theories are to be preferred over formulations grounded in psychopathology. The utilitarian approach posits that contraceptive sterilization is chosen as the most satisfactory available solution among a variety of alternatives for a particular functional problem. The choice of surgical procedures is best explained by a functional analysis of the decision, which also makes for a highly individualized conceptualization of considerable explanatory and even predictive power.

**Utilitarian Theory**

An example of utilitarian theory can be found in formulations stemming from the series of studies which began at the Scripps Clinic and Research Foundation on vasectomy and the use of ovulation suppressors (Rodgers and Ziegler, 1968; Ziegler, Rodgers, and Prentiss, 1969). Those who turned to vasectomy, it was hypothesized, were relatively young couples who had had two or three children in quick succession despite their use of contraceptive measures. With a long period of fecundity ahead of them and wishing no more children (for economic or other reasons), the couples saw in vasectomy a permanent, reliable, and highly functional solution to their concern about what was for them "excessive" fecundity. The choice or discontinuance of oral contraceptives by certain women, similarly, also has a functional basis: those who chose and remained on the pill were women who enjoyed sex, who tended to assume primary responsibility for family decisions, and had previously borne the burden of contraception within the family, and whose husbands tended to be somewhat irresponsible and undependable. Wives with the contrary characteristics tended to discontinue oral contraceptive use. These functional hypotheses stem from identifying the problems better solved by a particular contraceptive than by alternative approaches and thereby predicting that persons with those particular problems choose the optimal solution, other factors being equal.

*"Pushes"*

With its emphasis on functionality, the utilitarian theory could lead to a rather systematic research strategy even without further precise specification of the content of the functional relationship. The approach would suggest, for example, studies aimed at identifying certain problems that might be labeled "pushes" which would predispose a person toward use of contraception in general or a particular form of contraception. Numbered among the "pushes" might be: higher fecundity than is desired, various problems (medical, economic, emotional, or sexual) that would be aggravated by a further pregnancy, or goals that might be better served by certainty of contraception (such as desire for sexual activity without liability of pregnancy either extramaritally or within a marriage to a spouse who makes certainty of contraception a condition for sexual access). This list is, of course, not exhaustive, but suggests a domain of exploration that would have a high payoff value in identifying factors predisposing the individual toward contraceptive sterilization.

## "Hurdles"

An additional group of antecedent variables in a functional hypothesis might be called the "hurdles" to use of a particular procedure. With surgical techniques, for example, the anticipation of such unpleasant consequences as pain, cost, injury to processes other than fertility, threat to life, disapproval by related others, and even self-disapproval might constitute an inhibition to the choice of these procedures. The inhibitions in one community or culture might be quite different from those in another. The commitment never to have more children, thereby running the risk that a disaster could leave one childless, for instance, no doubt constitutes more of a "hurdle" in India than in the United States. Identifying the precise dimensions of such hurdles could constitute research studies all in themselves. The conditions that would counteract the inhibiting effect of the "hurdles" are also worthy of study. The cost of a vasectomy operation, for example, might be seen as quite high and therefore an inhibition. Conversely, the costs could be perceived as being quite low when contrasted to those entailed by a possible unwanted pregnancy or the need for oral contraceptives extrapolated over a period of many years.

## "Pulls"

A third class of antecedent variables that could also be considered in functional hypotheses might be labeled the "pulls" to having a particular form of contraception. In contrast to "pushes," which involve the correction of preexisting problems, "pulls" are the anticipated positive gains. Examples include incentive programs, social approval (for instance, in "Population Zero" cultures), and the anticipation of privileges not otherwise obtainable (like "safe" nonmarital sexual experiences, an apparent motivating factor for many U.S. Navy men who obtained vasectomies in Mexico).

## Variables Related to Surgery

The circumstances of the surgery itself may also be analyzed from the functional point of view. The resources upon which the individual must depend for getting the surgery can either interpose additional hurdles or facilitate the adoption of the contraceptive method. Is the community one in which the "120 rule" applies, in which case a twenty-five year old woman with four children could not obtain a tubal ligation even if she were otherwise highly motivated and met all other criteria? Does local usage require, for example, psychiatric evaluation and approval by a eugenics or hospital committee before the operation can proceed? Do the available gynecologists, urologists, and other relevant personnel tend to discourage potential candidates from undergoing the procedures? Or, do governmental bodies provide monetary or other incentives, operating tables in the middle of railroad stations, and the like? Again, a large domain of variables in this regard remains to be mapped and evaluated that may well be unique to the setting in which a study is conducted. Perhaps related to local circumstances is the information network through which individuals learn about the various dimensions of contraceptive sterilization—possibly situationally idiosyncratic and practically important in determining who elects the procedure. In the early sixties, for example, we found vasectomy to be much more common among engineers of a certain group of aerospace companies in the San Diego area than it was among other groups simply because word of mouth was the primary mode by which information about the procedure was transmitted in that particular area. The communication network among this engineering group lent itself to considering such a "structural" solution to birth control problems.

*Outcome*

The functional approach can also be used in the study of outcome. Consideration could be given to three somewhat distinct dimensions.

The utilitarian definition of "satisfaction," first of all, focuses on the adequacy of problem solving. Did the procedure have the anticipated effects in terms of solving the problem that led to the decision, providing the expected incentive, and effectively overcoming the hurdles? Did subsequent experience with the results of the operation show the decision to have been, indeed, functional? To the extent it did, subjects would probably be satisfied with the procedure. To the extent it did not, subjects would probably be dissatisfied. In our research, for example (Ziegler, Rodgers, and Prentiss, 1969), we found that vasectomy resulted in increased frequency of sexual intercourse, a typical goal for many of the men who obtained the operation. The vasectomy seldom led to an improvement of the general marital relationships, however, another factor that was important for some men who saw the procedure as a way of salvaging an otherwise distressed marriage. Systematic follow-up of contraceptive sterilization outcome should appropriately assess the accuracy of the predisposing functional "hypothesis" on the part of the adopters.

A second class of outcome variables that follows logically from a functional theoretical framework is that of the side effects of the surgical procedure, defined, in this context, as any consequence of the operation other than that directly intended (for instance, limiting fecundity).

For example, tubal ligation or hysterectomy by laparotomy involves a somewhat prolonged recovery period which may test many previously unexplored interpersonal dimensions in a marriage. How supportive is the husband when his wife is seriously incapacitated? If he is too supportive, she may "learn" to use sick role-behavior excessively. If he is supportive enough, the wife may become dissatisfied, begin testing for the first time his helpfulness in other areas, and may open fundamental doubts about the marriage that might otherwise not have come to light. If there is the optimal degree of support, on the other hand, the marriage bond may be strengthened by the couple's response to the crisis of recovery, quite apart from the contraceptive effect of the surgical procedure itself. The recovery period also necessitates an alteration in sexual patterns, with various possible consequences. Too early and too vigorous sexual assault by an insensitive husband may result in the development of a fear of intercourse on the part of the woman which could then be stabilized as a disruptive influence. Alternatively, a husband might for the first time in a couple's sexual history become unusually solicitous and gentle in his sexual approach, with a resultant marked improvement in the sexual relationship. Again, subsequent sexual behavior would be an indirect side effect of contraceptive sterilization, rather than a direct consequence of effective fertility control.

Pathological outcomes of contraceptive sterilization generally fall into the side-effect category. A sense of loss of masculinity or of femininity would be a side effect rather than the direct consequence of the surgery, as would feelings of guilt or shifts in bargaining power within the marriage. The "pathological," as opposed to "functional," explanations around contraceptive surgery, as has already been mentioned, seem to contribute little to understanding the decision-making process leading up to the choice of a particular procedure. "Pathology" is better applied as a description of outcome. Dissonance reduction hypotheses, concerns about loss of masculinity or femininity on the part of the adopter or as sensed by the other spouse, conflicts over bargaining rights in the marriage, and related explanatory concepts seem to order important segments of data that can all be termed somewhat "pathological" or at least not inevitable consequences of surgical contraception.

The less immediate and more indirect outcomes of the procedure might also be studied functionally. What are the effects on standard of living, for example, of having two versus four or five children? How is the acceptance of children influenced by having more than a couple had initially wanted? Very little has been done to map systematically the contrasting consequences of relatively large versus relatively small families, although no consequences of effective contraception could be more fundamental. Birth order may even have implications for the kinds of occupations to which third and fourth children aspire and for which they are best fit, as contrasted to the occupational choices of first- or second-borns. Little is known about whether children who are unwanted at the time of conception turn out to be unwanted at a later date and whether there is a deleterious effect on them, their siblings, or their parents.

Other researchable questions come readily to mind. Are there detailed long-term studies in India, for example, of whether persons whose families have been artificially limited by vasectomy suffer more, on the average, than those not similarly limited, granted that the cultural norm suggests such an outcome? There is remarkably little hard data on whether the long-term consequences of vasectomy are, in fact, those assumed and predicted by the population planners and the culture in general. The relationship of effective contraception, especially contraceptive sterilization, to later promiscuity and extramarital activity is yet another long-term consequence that bears study, although it is admittedly a tricky area for research. A major revolution in the cultural institutions surrounding the family is probably one of the ramifications of generally effective contraception. If such is the case, then identifying the parameters of this long-range consequence is fully as important as specifying the individual emotional response to the procedures.

The phenomenon of contraceptive sterilization, from the functional analytic point of view, is, then, probably somewhat individualized—its explanations varying with the individual or group—rather than being a completely homogeneous, universal occurrence with the same dimensions for all subjects. Rational, not irrational, considerations predominate in determining the choice of the procedure, according to the utilitarian approach; the concept of "pathology" is better used in ordering significant amounts of the data regarding subsequent outcomes of the surgery. Research is conspicuously lacking in the long-term and indirect consequences of contraceptive sterilization on the family, its members, and broader societal institutions and practices.

Besides the need to establish a useful theoretical framework, other fundamental questions are evoked by the study of contraceptive sterilization. Of considerable importance are the nature of sexuality and sexual response and research on the cultural attitudes that reflect the *Zeitgeist* and provide the background for individual responses to the procedures.

*Human Sexuality*

Control of fecundity would of course be pointless were it not in the context of a desire for sexual activity independent of procreation. Sexual behavior, when even the possibility of conception has been eliminated with certainty, calls for a re-examination of the phenomenon of sexuality about whose dimensions our knowledge is remarkably primitive.

It is clear that male sexuality is quite different from female sexuality. It is, therefore, altogether likely that the consequences of contraceptive sterilization of the male are different from those of the female, though the details have yet to be elucidated. Novelty, for example, is probably an important dimension in male sexual responsiveness, but may well be a trivial dimension in evoking female sexual arousal. If such is the case, there would be a differential response to surgery on the part of the other spouse. The novelty introduced by tubal ligation or hysterectomy could stimulate the sexual interest of a male partner who has not previously had experience with a surgically contracepted female. The converse may not hold, however; indeed, a woman may be less rather than more sexually aroused by the novelty of a male partner who has had a vasectomy, even if she has not previously had experience with such a partner.

The essential source of sexual satisfaction may also be different for men and women. For most women, a secure and meaningful emotional relationship with a respected and concerned partner is a primary dimension in sexual satisfaction; the relationship factors for most men may not bear upon their achievement of purely sexual satisfaction. The wife's sexual response following tubal ligation or hysterectomy may therefore depend very heavily on her husband's attitude, supportiveness, concern, and respect for her, whereas a man's postvasectomy adjustment may be a great deal more grounded in his own experience of and capacity for sexual performance. The critical variables in a pathological adaptation to contraceptive sterilization may thus vary with the partner undergoing the procedure. Purely sexual experiences could be hypothesized as more important for satisfactory adaptation in the male, whereas the relationship dimensions are relatively more crucial in the female. The place of novelty and the elements providing satisfaction are, at any rate, but two examples of how a comprehensive understanding of sexuality as a phenomenon in itself might modify and clarify the theoretical context in which contraceptive sterilization could be evaluated.

*The Social Field*

Contraception is a distinctly interpersonal phenomenon, obviously, since it presupposes a fertile partner. It is, however, also one of a whole variety of events and relationships (procreation and marriage contracts, for instance) related to and designed for regulating sexuality which are central to many of our social institutions. Social attitudes, therefore, are highly likely to have significant impact on response to contraceptive sterilization. Guilt-inducing, shame-inducing, and approval controls are common vehicles for cultural influence, as are the processes of information transmission. The importance of the social field should prompt our study of cultural attitudes about contraception in general, different contraceptive procedures, family size, and almost all the many other variables influenced by or related to contraceptive sterilization.

Attitudes about surgery, for example, differ markedly from one culture to another. In the United States, surgery is probably seen as a procedure involving high professional expertise and technical competence, such that submitting to the procedures can almost be faddish and fashionable. Throughout Central Africa, in contrast, surgery is apparently viewed as a last resort before death and is something to be greatly feared. Surgical contraception will clearly provoke different, culturally determined reactions, therefore, if only as a specific instance of the societal response to surgery in general. Indeed, if there were some desire to stimulate use of the technique in Africa, the very term *surgical contraception* should probably be replaced by an expression less likely to evoke anxiety and negative feelings. A similar argument has been made (Rodgers and Ziegler, 1973) for dropping the term *voluntary sterilization* in this country in favor of the less negatively connotative *surgical contraception*. The cultural dimensions of contraceptive surgery are, at any rate, numerous. The limits for research in this area are set only by the perceptiveness and sensitivity of the investigators, combined with previously derived evidence of possibly fruitful leads.


*Some Comments on Methodology*


As was noted earlier, the present state of knowledge leads one to favor a multiplicity of approaches over any particular research methodology.

Prospective and large-scale studies using standardized measuring instruments have much to recommend them. However, even these investigative designs involve certain hazards. A study of 10,000 vasectomized subjects might well statistically confirm the "castration" hypotheses at the .05 level of significance. Were the results used to show the universal truth of such formulations, the research community will have been ill-served by such large-scale studies. Indeed, one of the advantages of small sample size is that only powerful hypotheses stand much chance of surviving our standard significance tests. More modest $N$s may thus tend to clarify the more important variables more quickly than do the larger studies in which weak hypotheses of relatively minor importance may reach acceptable significance levels.

The use of standardized instruments, as has been mentioned, risks the inevitable limitation of the range of results that can be obtained. A strong case could be made, for instance, for using the California Psychological Inventory in studies on contraceptive sterilization. Since the CPI is a rather lengthy paper-and-pencil test, however, its use would normally preclude administering other instruments like the Minnesota Multiphasic Personality Inventory, a test of inner-directed versus outer-directed control, or some other inventory that might identify as-yet-unsuspected critical relationships.

The search for ideal designs should not discourage attempts at more practicable efforts. Although it is of course useful to have directly comparable results from more than one research study, it is to be hoped that comparability in so minimally explored a field will not be gained at the expense of unreasonably narrowing the scope of study. Although longitudinal prospective studies are also highly essential, they tend to be quite expensive. Much important data can be generated by good cross-sectional or retrospective studies. Significant research could be done by identifying a target population, going back to school or army records or similar data banks, and retrospectively generating good pseudo-longitudinal studies of variables like the consequences of family size for later socioeconomic status, emotional health, or sexual practice.

Objective tests are in general more dependable research instruments than those whose divination is largely at the mercy of interpreter bias and skill. This is especially true at the end of an era when exaggerated emphasis was placed on the "tea leaf technology" of Rorschach, Szondi, Blacky, and other projective devices. One suspects, nevertheless, that much highly meaningful information could be obtained from carefully done clinical testing in the TAT tradition, using specially prepared pictures (for example, a crying baby, a large family, a pregnant woman, or a person on an operating table).

Other research methods, would probably also be productive. The Haire Market Basket technique (Haire, 1950) has proved useful for rather precise identification of cultural response to variables that are not easily assessed by more direct approaches (see, for example, Rodgers, Ziegler, and Levy [1967]). Interviews involving role playing are another valuable source of research leads. A subject could be asked, for example, to play the role of a citizen being exposed to a particular pitch for or against a certain contraceptive procedure; the findings might suggest dimensions for more direct exploration with specific target populations. The study of personal documents, finally, such as carefully done sexual diaries maintained before and after surgical contraceptive procedures, is long overdue in this and other areas related to population control.

A severe weakness in much of my own methodology—a failing I would strongly urge others not to replicate—is the failure to replicate. Since much of the work in this area is perforce exploratory, significant findings should be immediately subjected to essential replication on comparable groups to determine whether the results are fortuitous or reproducible. For significant contribution to science, there is no excuse for my own failure to follow-up with repeat testing the several hypotheses that Ziegler, other colleagues, and I derived from our rather limited and exploratory studies. Even if others do appropriate critical studies, the responsibility for follow-up should reside with those who initially generated the hypothesis.

Additional detail on methodology is perhaps superfluous. The standard rules for good research are well known and require little review for a sophisticated audience. With particular reference to studies on contraceptive sterilization, it need only be said that the creative use of multiple approaches is far more desirable than is the premature encouragement of conformance to restricted models of investigation.

Throughout the course of this chapter, allusions have been made to needed research. It should be apparent by now that we have barely scratched the surface. As the other chapters in this volume indicate, much remains to be done in defining the problems, the appropriate methodology, and the theoretical framework which will lead to an eventual understanding of the complex phenomenon that is contraceptive sterilization.

## References

Haire, M. "Projective Techniques in Marketing Research." *Journal of Marketing* 14, (1950): 649-56.

Rodgers, D.A. and Ziegler, F.J. "Social Role Theory, the Marital Relationship, and Use of Ovulation Suppressors." *Journal of Marriage and the Family* 30 (1968): 584-91.

Rodgers, D.A. and Ziegler, F.J. "Psychological Reactions to Surgical Contraception." In J.T. Fawcett, (ed.), *Psychological Perspectives on Population.* New York: Basic Books, 1973, pp. 306-326.

Rodgers, D.A., Ziegler, F.J., and Levy, N. "Prevailing Cultural Attitudes about Vasectomy." *Psychosomatic Medicine* 29 (1967): 367-75.

Ziegler, F.J., Rodgers, D.A., and Prentiss, R.J. "Psychosocial Response to Vasectomy." *Archives of General Psychiatry* 21 (1969): 46-54.

# 7

## Psychosocial Effects of Vasectomy: Report of a Study in Progress and a Critical Review of the Literature
### Edward W. Pohlman

To ask whether the psychosocial effects produced by vasectomy are "good" or "bad" is perhaps unavoidable but, nonetheless, primitive. The question is far more complex: for a given subculture at a given time, which kinds of individuals or couples experience what kinds of psychosocial effects and under what circumstances? Ideally we need tests that can predict with validity which candidates, if any, will have sharply negative reactions to vasectomy (or, for that matter, female contraceptive surgery).

This chapter advocates a program of research which would permit comparisons across samples and over time. It voices a strong appeal for using the same basic research instruments and procedures, where possible, in studies of men and women, for comparable studies in different cultures, and for systematic re-testing of hypotheses every five or ten years in view of the rapid changes in the acceptability and incidence of vasectomy among various subgroups.

### The Groundwork of Theory

The breadth of currently available psychological and sociological theory is not visible in most of the studies devoted to the psychosocial effects of contraceptive sterilization. Because concern on this question was raised early and most vigorously by psychotherapists—whose orientation is often Freudian—the research literature deals frequently with the notion that vasectomy may be symbolically associated with castration.

According to psychoanalytic theory, the male is prone to anxiety about the loss of the penis or, more symbolically, the loss of manhood, vigor, sexual appeal, strength, and competence; the preoccupation is known as "castration anxiety." Consciously or unconsciously, according to this formulation, the man and his partner may equate vasectomy with castration, despite a rational understanding that the two are very different. These considerations may suggest that contraceptive surgery is more upsetting to the male than the equivalent procedure is to the female, although she conceivably may also view it as making her less of a woman (Parker, 1967). These extrapolations from depth psychology may apply in individual cases; their generalizability needs to be tested by research.

Freudian theory is not the only framework within which investigators have worked; at least two somewhat more social psychological concepts have been applied to understanding the response to contraceptive surgery. Several investigators (Rosario, 1971; Poffenberger and Poffenberger, 1965), using different terminology, have emphasized the influence of other people on the self-perception of the vasectomized man and especially on his perceptions of what the surgery has done to him. A third body of theory used somewhat in construing data from vasectomy research is that of cognitive dissonance or cognitive consistency (Festinger, 1957). In overly simple terms, this theory can be said to hold that the individual strives for consistency and harmony in his or her cognitions and attempts to avoid discordancies. Having undergone the painful and/or expensive process of surgery, for example, makes one the more likely to value, defend, or try to convince others to adopt the practice.

To explain research findings, these theories in their various combinations can sometimes be integrated and blended. One view of the Freudian castration anxiety hypothesis, for example, is that castration anxiety is inescapably rooted in the biological reality that girls have no penises. No matter what culture he lives in, according to this school of thought, the boy observes this lack, decides for himself that all children started life with penises but some lost theirs, and fears such a loss himself. It is possible, however, to place much more emphasis on the culture and on social learning and to stress that it is a question of learning whether a male worries about castration or somehow equates vasectomy with castration.

In explicating some of their findings, Rodgers and Ziegler (1973)[a] offered an explanation that presents a wide diversity of theory. In our culture, especially around 1960, they suggested, men felt psychologically threatened by vasectomy. Such threat may lead to dissonance-reducing strategies of which the men are typically unconscious. For example, an increase in sexual activity may be a desperate attempt to prove that one is functioning properly, despite having undergone surgery. Similarly, an exaggerated and brittle masculinity or self-reports of satisfaction with vasectomy may be a defensive maneuver to contain one's unconscious anxiety.

Theory, of course, not only helps to explain research findings; in science, a good theory generates testable hypotheses. By way of illustration, one might take the limited area of motivation for contraceptive sterilization and its consequences for the relationship between husband and wife.

Among the "standard" hypotheses long held by some psychoanalytically oriented psychotherapists about vasectomy are: (1) People often view vasectomy as a sort of castration. (2) Therefore, some men want the surgery because of a

---

[a]This series of studies will be referenced hereafter as "Rodgers and Ziegler (1973)"; the chapter cited in the References lists many other publications in which either Ziegler or Rodgers was first author. A recent book (Ziegler et al., 1973) reprints several of the articles.

desire, usually unconscious, to be emasculated. (3) Neurotic wives may want their husbands to have vasectomies as a way of demasculinizing them and may thus subtly lead them into undergoing the procedure. (4) Some men and women may also regard female contraceptive surgery as de-sexing, though this influence is probably less strong than in the case of surgery for the male. (5) From other theoretical perspectives, it has been hypothesized that men who choose vasectomies are more considerate of women (or more favorable to women's liberation, or less dominant, or weaker personality types, etc.) than men in couples that elect for female contraceptive sterilization. (6) Some wish the definitive contraception of surgery so that they may be more free for premarital or extramarital relations. (7) Accordingly, some parents and/or spouses oppose the procedure to avoid the possibilities of such sexual behavior on the part of the candidate for surgery (Cf. Fitzgerald, 1972; Barnes and Johnson, 1964).

## Experimental Designs

### Ideal Experiments

It may be instructive to review some research designs that come close to being ideal for the study of the psychosocial effects of vasectomy. Among the desirable features of these designs are: (1) the use of control groups, (2) pre-post comparisons, and (3) the "double-blind" testing of hypotheses.

Imagine 300 men, constituting a strictly random sample from a known population of men who want a vasectomy ("vas"). After pretesting, the 300 men are divided into three matched sets of 100 Ss, each of whom is randomly assigned among three research treatments: (1) a real vas; (2) a "sham" vas, involving surgery of the scrotum, but with the vas deferens left intact; (3) a non-operation control. Both the true vas and the sham vas groups are led to believe that they have been vasectomized. They are both, in fact, unaware that any sham operations were performed. On some pretext, however, all three groups are induced to use traditional contraception for the whole duration of the study—designed as longitudinal, with follow-ups for ten years. Those who assess the effects of the three treatments—the Rorschach artists, psychiatrists, palm-readers, etc.—do not know which of the three treatments a man has had; indeed, they are ignorant of the three treatments and even of the purpose behind the research endeavor. This design is shown in Figure 7-1 as Design A.

By contrasting the true vas group with the other two groups, one tests for the effects of the *physiological* concomitants of vasectomy. Contrasting the two groups that *thought* they were being vasectomized with the no-operation control group could reveal the *psychological* effects of believing that one has undergone surgery.

(Incidentally, sham vasectomies on animals have been done as a routine

DESIGN A: Prospective, double-blind design with two control groups[a]

| | Group | | |
| Steps | X | Y | Z |
|---|---|---|---|
| 1) Pretest | Yes | Yes | Yes |
| 2) Experimental treatment | Vasectomy | "Sham" vasectomy | No surgery |
| 3) Posttest(s) | Yes | Yes | Yes |

DESIGN B: Prospective, double-blind design with one control group[a]

| | Group | |
| Steps | X | Z |
|---|---|---|
| 1) Pretest | Yes | Yes |
| 2) Experimental treatment | Vasectomy | No surgery |
| 3) Posttest(s) | Yes | Yes |

Adapted from Wells and Poffenberger, "Research Designs for Evaluating After-effects of Vasectomy," 1965.

[a]Men who choose *but do not have* vasectomy.

**Figure 7-1.** Two "Ideal" Experimental Designs for the Study of the Psychosocial Effects of Vasectomy.

control [for example, Phoenix, 1972; Sackler, Weltman, Pandhi, and Schwartz, 1973]. Phoenix [1972] compared vasectomized rhesus monkeys with sham-operated controls on a variety of measures of sexual performances, including rates of mounting, intromission, and ejaculation. No statistically significant differences were found in a one-month follow-up analysis; later follow-up work is still to be reported. The preliminary animal data are thus consistent with the interpretation that if there are postsurgical changes in sex behavior among humans, they are the result of learned psychological factors rather than of physiological alterations *per se*.)

Making the sham vas group believe they had had contraceptive surgery would be ethically repugnant to most researchers, governments, and funding agencies. Aside from ethics, it would be difficult to persuade the operated groups to continue using condoms or other methods of birth control throughout the years entailed by the study; even the offer of free abortions would scarcely solve many problems.

For the idea of these three groups, I am in debt to Wells and Poffenberger (1965). Their original suggestion sounded less drastic than mine and was also less scientifically pure: they would secure (in advance) from all participants their permission to be assigned to one of the three groups. Ss would be warned that some operations would be sham. This foreknowledge, of course, compromises the research somewhat. To the extent that a man doubted that his was a "real" vasectomy, one intended independent variable—the belief that one had had effective surgery—would be weakened.

Wells and Poffenberger also advanced a second experimental design which dropped the sham operation group, leaving only a two-group comparison between vasectomized men and men who wanted the surgery but were somehow persuaded or kept from having it (see Figure 7-1, Design B). With or without the sham vas group, in such a study men would sign up with the realization that they might not get the vasectomy for several years. An unknown but probably high proportion would refuse to participate; differences might be sharp between those netted for the research and those who refused. Were the researchers to offer large sums of money in an attempt to guarantee near 100 percent cooperation, the payment itself would make the participants different from men having vasectomy under the usual conditions.

Whatever their practical or methodological problems, the two designs outlined in Figure 7-1 have much to commend them. They share the following features (which, as we shall see, are far from prevalent in the vasectomy research so far conducted):

1.  All Ss want "true" vas, but some are assigned at random to groups where they do not get it.
2.  The studies are "double-blind" as much as possible, with those making pretest and posttest judgments not aware of which group is which—and, if possible, ignorant of the focus of the study or the existence of the various subsamples.
3.  The designs are equally applicable to research with women on tubal ligation.
4.  Spouses of Ss can also be studied (wives of vasectomized men or husbands of ligated women).

One should not reject out-of-hand the possibilities of experiments involving sham vas or at least control groups who want contraceptive surgery as soon as possible but are not allowed to have it. If population limitation were sufficiently important to national goals and national survival, if contraceptive sterilization were sufficiently important to population limitation, and if uncertainties about its psychological effects were a sufficient obstacle to acceptance of the procedures, some might feel that studies like those in Figure 7-1 were justified. Admittedly, for the present such designs seem all but impossible to allow practical application.

*Other Research Designs*

Barring the kinds of strategies outlined in Figure 7-1, *there are no true experimental controls* for people who choose contraceptive sterilization. For comparison, one must usually resort to sampling those who did not choose the method. Even if matched perfectly on demographic variables and no measurable personality characteristics, the two groups differ in a self-selected manner on whether to undergo surgery—a factor possibly associated with other uncontrolled psychological differences. In essence, the experimental and "control" groups are divergent on two confounded variables: (1) having had the surgery, as well as (2) *choosing* to have it. Interesting comparisons can be made between those who, after considering contraceptive surgery, do or do not proceed to have it; once again, however, for the reasons indicated, this involves a study without true controls. In practice, then, the researcher has had to be content with *comparison* groups, not perfect control groups. The attempt must simply be to make the comparison groups as similar as possible to those Ss who have undergone surgery.

Given the inherent inadequacy of any comparison group, let us examine briefly the experimental designs of the studies available in the literature on the psychosocial effects of vasectomy. In essence, investigators have chosen one of the following four approaches: (1) retrospective psychiatric or clinical interviews of vasectomized men, using no comparison groups whatsoever (e.g. Johnson [1964]); (2) more focused and detailed retrospective studies—usually direct, transparent questionnaire items—of men who had undergone the surgery, also without controls (Dandekar, 1963; Ferber et al., 1967; Garrison and Gamble, 1950; Grindstaff and Ebanks, 1971; Landis and Poffenberger, 1965; Lee, 1966; Poffenberger and Sheth, 1963; Poffenberger and Poffenberger, 1963; Rodgers et al., 1965; Simon Population Trust, 1969; Ziegler, Rodgers, and Prentiss, 1966); (3) "quasi-experimental" design (see Campbell and Stanley [1963]), as exemplified in the work of Janke and Wiest (1973); and (4) the use of longitudinal follow-up, together with comparison groups, a strategy almost synonymous with the pioneering studies of Rodgers and Ziegler (1973) and now being pursued by our group in California. Figure 7-2 diagrams the various investigative approaches, except for that of the quasi-experimental design. The first two strategies are combined under the rubric of Design C, since both are retrospective and make no claims for having comparisons to nonvasectomized controls; Design D is the longitudinal approach using quasi-controls. It is interesting that the different research strategies appear to have yielded findings at variance with one another. To oversimplify greatly, studies using designs (2) and (3) have tended to find a positive picture and minimize any negative effects of vasectomy; those using designs (1) and (4) have raised the possibility of some negative effects resulting from the procedure. Before attempting to reconcile the findings, some more detailed description of the studies and their designs is in order.

DESIGN C:   Retrospective self-report (e.g., clinical interview, questionnaire)
            without controls

| Steps | Group $X$ |
|---|---|
| 1) Pretest | No |
| 2) Treatment | Vasectomy |
| 3) Posttest | Yes |

DESIGN D:  Prospective studies, comparison group (quasi-control)[a]

| | Group | |
|---|---|---|
| Steps | $X$ | ($Z$) |
| 1) Pretest | Yes | Yes |
| 2) Experimental treatment | Vasectomy | No surgery |
| 3) Posttest(s) | Yes | Yes |

[a]Men who *neither choose nor have* surgery.

**Figure 7-2.** Two Designs Available in the Literature for the Study of the Psychosocial Effects of Vasectomy

**Retrospective Studies.**   In its more pervasive variant (the second research strategy
mentioned earlier), people are asked, usually through transparent questions on
questionnaires, how they feel about a vasectomy that has already occurred.  In response to such questions, men (and their wives, when they are studied) typically
report satisfaction with the surgery, that they would do it again, that they would
recommend it to others, and that their sex life is better after the vasectomy or
at least no worse than it was before they underwent the procedure.  Typically,
90 percent or more report positive reactions, while only a minority state some
degree of dissatisfaction.

Further research of this type will probably contribute little, except when
done (1) among cultures or subgroups not already studied extensively (most of
the work is based on samples from the United States, Canada, Great Britain, and
India) or (2) after the passage of at least a few years, when sufficient time will
have elapsed to warrant speculation about possible changes in the attitudes of the
population toward contraceptive sterilization, thereby creating a need for replica-
tions of the earlier research.

The retrospective clinical interview (the first design noted above) shares the
logic and methodological flaws of the survey and questionnaire approach.  In
practice, this design has been used primarily by psychotherapists who began
their study with a group of emotionally disturbed people and asked how many
of them had previously undergone contraceptive surgery.  Typically, some of

the disturbed people had indeed been subjected to the procedure and some believed there to be a cause-effect relationship between the surgery and their emotional problems; the investigators tend to agree. No controls are used to tell us who had surgery but did not become disturbed or who did not have surgery but became disturbed anyway. As a means of generating hypotheses, the retrospective clinical study has merits; it is a dubious enterprise, however, for testing assumptions.

**Quasi-Experimental Design.** This research strategy has been applied by Janke and Wiest (1973) in a study recently begun in Portland, Oregon. The problem of finding adequate controls for vasectomized $S$s was handled rather ingeniously through drawing and matching samples postsurgery by a computerized search through the extensive and detailed membership records of the Portland Kaiser Foundation group health plan. As will be discussed later at length, this approach eliminates the conceivable biases of conducting prevasectomy interviews and psychological testing which could unduly sensitize $S$s to the possibly deleterious effects of the surgery. The samples of Janke and Wiest had supplied pretest data to the Kaiser Foundation well before vasectomy was the issue under investigation.

According to Janke and Wiest, at any rate, their data show no negative psychological impact to be consequent to contraceptive sterilization. We shall examine this conclusion more closely later in this chapter.

**Prospective, Longitudinal Design with Quasi-controls.** This research approach is closely identified with the Scripps Foundation studies carried out by Rodgers and Ziegler (1973). Summarized in Figure 7-2 as Design D, the strategy in the work of Rodgers and Ziegler has involved a prospective sequence, control groups, and standardized psychological tests administered before and at one or more times after the experimental group underwent surgery.

Rodgers and Ziegler have inferred from their data that vasectomy may have certain negative psychological effects for some individuals, particularly given a culture and historical period when the procedure is somewhat negatively regarded by the larger society as a whole or the person's smaller reference group. Because these investigators have also studied male surgical contraception by using retrospective questionnaires, they were in the position to report a curious finding: they very same individuals who give favorable self-reports about vasectomy (Figure 7-2, Design C) may also experience negative psychological reactions as measured objectively by pre- to posttreatment changes on standardized instruments (Figure 7-2, Design D).

This apparent contradiction, as has been noted, emerges in the literature as a whole. Most retrospective studies show great satisfaction with vasectomy; the thrust of the Scripps Foundation prospective work is not as salutary. Logically, there are two broad paths to resolving the discrepancy. One is to suggest

that the retrospective questionnaires present at best an incomplete picture, reflecting only superficial and conscious views that are in conflict with deeper
patterns and may indeed be a defensive cover-up for them.  Rodgers and Ziegler
entertain this hypothesis seriously.  An alternative solution is to suggest that
Rodgers and Ziegler have arrived at unjustified conclusions and that the positive
reports men give should be taken just about at face value.  Which view is correct
can best be decided by waiting for further research (among which our own
group's is to be numbered).

The work of Ziegler, Rodgers, and their colleagues represents the outstanding—
indeed, the towering—contribution to date among empirical studies of the psychological effects of contraceptive sterilization.  Precisely because of this, there is a
danger of elevating the resulting publications into a Talmud, to be made the subject of endless commentaries on this or that twist of the data or of interpretation.
Instead, I believe we should forge ahead with new  studies—investigations that
would not have been possible without the pioneering efforts of Rodgers and
Ziegler but that will answer our questions much better than fruitless speculation
about what is admittedly only limited evidence.  The conclusion drawn by these
investigators from their data have been severely challenged (Wiest and Janke,
1974), as we shall review later in some detail.  For the moment, suffice it to say
that the Rodgers and Ziegler studies were based on small and nonrandomly selected
middle class, white samples.  And, since the research was conducted about 1960,
it may not be relevant to a later period's conditions and concerns.


*Some Other Problems of Experimental Design*

Among the many factors that threaten to confound research designs in this area,
four may be singled out:

1. The very process of studying individuals before surgery may somehow
influence them.  Giving them psychological tests, for example, may make them
believe that the surgery must entail a psychological risk—or else why would
psychologists be studying them?  Some of the quasi-experimental designs of
Campbell and Stanley (1963) get around this problem (see the previous discussion
of the work of Janke and Wiest [1973]).  In our own study, a subgroup of men
is being studied *only*  after vasectomy so as to measure the prejudicial effects, if
any, of pretesting.

2. When interviews are conducted or there is extensive personal contact between Ss and the research staff, these contacts can unwittingly soften the otherwise negative psychological effects of contraceptive sterilization.  This was
suggested *post hoc* by Rodgers and Ziegler as a possible explanation for some of
their data.  We are testing this hypothesis more systematically by comparing the
postsurgery status of interviewed and noninterviewed subjects.

3. When candidates for surgery are briefed systematically about the

operations, the kinds of information given and the biases (pro or con) of the in-formation-givers can affect outcomes. If a health educator implies or suggests to a group, for example, that vasectomy will produce psychological or sexual problems in a certain proportion of them, there may be a self-fulfilling prophecy effect. Fortunately, our data permit some systematic comparison among different information-giving patterns and staff biases.

4. People studied shortly before contraceptive surgery or after they have decided on the step may already be changed from their modal predecision personality and marital relationship patterns. One physician has speculated, for example, that if pre-post comparisons show a decline in psychological adjustment, this is not because the surgery makes a person worse. The "post-" measure may merely reflect a return to drab average adjustment after a period of unusual well-being associated with the decision to undergo the surgery. For some people, the decision may be a focus of expectancy and hope, even representing perhaps the magic solution to all sexual, marital, and interpersonal problems (Ziegler, personal communication). (Inconsistent with this hypothesis is the finding of Ziegler and Rodgers that certain negative differences between pretest and two-year follow-up disappeared when the four-year follow-up was made.)

To investigate longer-range patterns of stability or shift, at any rate, ideally one needs a longitudinal study with a very long time perspective. In some geographical or agency settings, it may be possible to gain access to personality measures that were administered routinely some years before the decision for surgery was contemplated. In our study, we are asking subjects whether they recall having taken any psychological tests previously (in the military, college, for employment, etc.). We then seek subjects' legal permission to request the test-giving agency for reports of the results.

## A Critique of Previous Research

Before describing the design of our own study on the psychosocial consequences of contraceptive surgery—an investigation undertaken to address questions we consider far from answered—it seems appropriate to review some of the relevant literature critically and in some detail. In this manner, we shall be recapitulating for the reader some of the thinking that led to our current study; it is in this section, as well, that we articulate some of the challenges to previous studies that were only relatively implicit in the earlier discussion of research design. In this review, we draw heavily on the work of Wiest and Janke (1974).

### Retrospective Questionnaire Studies

As noted earlier, most investigators using retrospective reports gathered by questionnaire have found vasectomized men to be quite satisfied with the outcome of surgery. The following objections, however, raise serious doubts as to the scientific standing of conclusions based on the retrospective questionnaire strategy:

1. Subtleties of questionnaire wording may lead respondents to produce the positive answers the investigator wants to hear.
2. Questionnaires have always been given in a context such that respondents knew the investigators were studying vasectomy. Perhaps this led them to "put on a good show." If men could be asked postsurgery about their sex lives or marital happiness, but in a context not revealing the investigator's focus on vasectomy, results might perhaps be different.
3. Deep commitment to anything, whether to having a vasectomy, purchasing a rotary-engine Japanese car, or joining ZPG or the Buddhist church, may influence people toward saying that the action has improved their lives, perhaps just as a matter of cognitive consonance.
4. Favorable questionnaire responses may be a defensive overreaction, as hypothesized by Rodgers and Ziegler (1973).
5. The kinds of couples drawn to choose vasectomies as a contraceptive method might also tend to be people with personality characteristics that lead them into giving favorable responses on questionnaires.
6. The typical questionnaire study does not include Ss who either refuse or neglect to participate. These nonrespondents might include high proportions of dissatisfied individuals.

## Retrospective "Clinical" Studies

Men in several cultures have stated their satisfaction with and even enthusiasm over having had a vasectomy; the rule of parsimony would indicate that these statements should be taken at face value unless there are convincing reasons to doubt them and plunge underground, mole-like, into a maze of speculations about unconscious factors and defensive distortion. Many clinical studies, unfortunately, seem bent on "proving" their hunches valid on the basis of completely inadequate research.

Johnson (1964), for example, interviewed eighty-three men who became psychiatric patients after having had a vasectomy; in a later study, Johnson and Miller (1970) interviewed forty-one wives of these eighty-three men. Of the wives, seven said they would not recommend the surgery. Of the eighty-three men, eleven had been hospitalized within one year of their vasectomy. Johnson believed that the surgery had helped precipitate some psychiatric and marital problems.

This study was utterly lacking in controls; it gives no indication of the proportions of men who had vasectomies but were not hospitalized or who were hospitalized without ever having had the surgery. A sample of psychiatric hospital patients, in any event, cannot be used to generalize to nonpatient men considering vasectomy. Had Johnson started studying the connection between drinking root-beer and hospitalization, his manner and approach might well have suggested to patients that the two were connected. He might have found eighty-three patients who had drunk root-beer before hospitalization, with a certain proportion of them convinced of a causal connection. Among their wives, at least seven would probably have recommended against root-beer drinking.

In general, one must be quite cautious about extrapolating findings to people who may not have been adequately interviewed or surveyed. A case in point is a British survey of 1,012 vasectomized men (Simon Population Trust, 1969). To the question, "Would you recommend vasoligation to others placed like yourself?" 99 percent answered affirmatively. Of the remaining 1 percent, none expressed regret over having had the surgery; instead, they gave as reasons for not recommending the procedure to others the fact that they were shy or did not consider themselves authorities on vasectomy. Skeptical of this totally glowing picture, Wolfers (1970) sent questionnaires to ninety-five of the men, asking if they thought any sexual or marital problems had resulted from the vasectomy. If they had, they were offered an appointment with a visiting psychologist. Of the ninety-five men, eighty-two answered and seven requested interviews. Of the seven, four gave retrospective evidence of some psychological, sexual, or marital instability even before surgery. The striking feature of Wolfers's study was that in a population where apparently 100 percent had had favorable reactions to surgery as judged by one retrospective survey, some 8 percent (seven of eighty-two) reported problems when asked a seemingly similar question by a different, quasi-clinical route.

Although Wolfers's study is provocative, it cannot lead us to any rigorous conclusions as to the proportions of men who have favorable or unfavorable outcomes after vasectomy. Had some people with psychological, marital, or sexual problems been miraculously *cured* by vasectomy, for example, her design would not have revealed this. Hypothetically, eighty-eight of the ninety-five men to whom Wolfers sent questionnaires might have been thus cured without her having learned of it.

*Quasi-Experimental Designs: The Work of Janke and Wiest (1973)*

Wiest and Janke's (1974) frank criticisms of the Ziegler-Rodgers investigations makes us less hesitant to submit their own study (Janke and Wiest, 1973) to equally vigorous examination. Their research compared thirty-three Kaiser Hospital (Portland, Oregon) men, studied only after vasectomy, with a group studied only before vasectomy and with several other groups who had not chosen vasectomy, including thirty-three men matched by computer with elegant precision from among hundreds who were members of the group health plan. Their hypothesis was that vasectomy leads to better psychosocial adjustment.

Janke and Wiest reported that the only significant differences they found were in the levels of the Psychosocial Adjustment Index (PAI). The crux, then, is this instrument, the PAI. The appendix to the article lists the questions from which the PAI was assembled—self-report items developed for practical hospital screening. Some of the questions are obviously psychological in import, others are straight medical, while yet others provide information about problems that are often psychosomatic in origin (such as dizziness, persistent coughs, backaches). Obviously psychosocial items include (1) the kinds of activities the man has done with his wife in recent weeks, (2) spouse decision-making patterns, (3) ratings of one's marital happiness, (4) feelings about whether one is the kind of husband one should be, (5) time spent with children, and (6) satisfaction with parenthood. This collection, singly and as a whole, is of interest. Unfortunately, the authors have not provided any citations to the work of others with the PAI nor have they demonstrated its validity as a psychological test.

By studying men who had already been interviewed for other purposes, the authors escaped the usual pattern in which both men and interviewers know that the study relates to vasectomy. Even so, if the Rodgers and Ziegler (1973) hypotheses are correct, men after vasectomy might have been defensively overstating their psychosocial health to themselves and their interviewers. The PAI, even "double-blind," is no substitute for a validated psychological inventory which could get beneath the possible defensiveness.

Janke and Wiest did not find any negative correlates of vasectomy, either on the PAI or in terms of the "masculinity and rigidity" hypothesized by Rodgers and Ziegler. But "not rejecting the null hypothesis" (in either direction) can occur because of having had small sample sizes, imprecise measures, or having studied the wrong variables. With only thirty-three men in the vasectomized group, the results are not convincing. Since a key feature of the Rodgers-Ziegler hypotheses was the contrast between generally favorable postvasectomy self-reports and the less sanguine psychological inventory scores, any study offering to do battle with the hypotheses should ideally have used psychological inventories. The flavor of the Janke-Wiest report and the Wiest-Janke literature review somehow led one to expect from them more substantial refutations of the conclusions of the Scripps Foundation research group.

Other criticisms that could be raised regarding the study of Janke and Wiest include the lack of any data gathered directly from wives or any "triangulation" from several sources of psychosocial information—for instance, one or more other measures—and the absence of any before-and-after longitudinal comparisons.

The authors justify this last omission by reference to Campbell and Stanley's (1963) work on quasi-experimental designs, which warns against the possible contamination of subjects when before-and-after studies are made. Nonetheless, Janke and Wiest could safely have followed the group of men already studied

prevasectomy and seen them again after surgery. It appears that the lack of longitudinal contacts was a necessity of time limitations (which was then rationalized
into a virtue) and that the choice of variables was not made in advance but was
an opportunistic decision about data already gathered by the hospital. This is all
to the good, provided one is aware of the limitations of the study. It does add
to knowledge, serves as a model of matching procedures, and is a warning against
glib acceptance of any "antivasectomy" doctrine. But the study just raises questions and provides hypotheses; it does not test them substantially.

*The Longitudinal Studies of Rodgers and Ziegler (1973)*

One cannot think of research on the psychosocial effects of vasectomy without
immediately invoking the studies of Rodgers and Ziegler (1973) and their
colleagues—valuable, pioneering, and creative. Reviewing criticisms of their
investigations—points about which these researchers are themselves keenly aware,
incidentally—in no way detracts from the importance of these early efforts.

The Ziegler-Rodgers group actually did two separate longitudinal studies.
The first (supposedly a pilot study) used MMPI (Minnesota Multiphasic Personality Inventory) scales and no interviews; the second (the "full" study) began
with CPI (California Psychological Inventory) scales and interviews. The CPI
was given as the pretest in the full study, but was later judged inadequate to the
task. In an attempt to return to the MMPI, MMPI scale scores were *estimated*
from those of the pretest CPI to permit comparisons between prevasectomy
(CPI-based) *estimates* and postsurgery MMPI *measures.* This procedure has
obvious drawbacks.

What was supposed to have been the pilot effort involved roughly the same
$N$'s as the later study of vasectomized men and their wives. The first study
showed more of the deleterious effects of vasectomy than did the second. The
authors suggested that the interviewing and related contacts in the full study
may have somewhat decreased the negative psychological outcomes of vasectomy.
Although this is plausible, it is a *post hoc* invention, not a hypothesis stated in
advance and tested systematically. A more parsimonious explanation for the full
study having failed to give strong support for some hypotheses emerging from the
pilot might attribute the original findings to sampling quirks in a small sample.

Wiest and Janke (1974) have provided a detailed critique of the Rodgers-
Ziegler studies. Among their more cogent observations is that the alleged differences between the vasectomized couples and the controls may well be a chance
finding. The argument of Wiest and Janke runs as follows: at the two-year
follow-up, nine statistically significant differences were observed between the
vasectomy couples and the controls; seven of the nine were unfavorable to the
couples that had had the surgery. But, Wiest and Janke noted, ninety-three comparisons must have been made in analyzing the data—figuring thirteen MMPI

scales and eighteen CPI scales (13 + 18 = 31), with each comparison made three times (for men, women, and both spouses together). There is no impressive difference between nine significant findings out of ninety-three and the five out of 100 to be expected under the null hypothesis, using the .05 level and two-tail tests. Running comparisons on husband and wife scores together, when this group is not independent of husbands separately and wives separately, is also questionable. When the findings failed to be replicated at the four-year follow-up, Wiest and Janke saw this as possibly springing from unreliability of measurement or of supposed patterns, rather than from the intricate psychological processes hypothesized by Ziegler and Rodgers.

On another aspect of data analysis, Wiest and Janke (1974) have stressed that, on both the personality inventories and the interviewer judgments, Ziegler and Rodgers compared the *number* of vasectomized subjects shifting their scores in a positive or negative direction with the *number* of controls who did the same. The existence of significant differences in these numbers does *not* in itself show, however, that the *mean score change* for the two groups is significantly different nor that any *individual* made a significant change. Take, for example, MMPI Scale 7, which can be said to measure anxiety. Significantly more vasectomized men and their wives had increases of at least five T-score units on Scale 7 than did control men and wives. This does *not* necessarily mean either that (1) mean posttest anxiety scale scores or mean increases in these scores were higher among experimentals; (2) the vasectomy group scores were elevated to a degree that has clinical significance; or (3) particular individuals had statistically significant changes. A change of five T-score units on this scale is not statistically significant and can be produced by changing responses on only one or two items.

The negative inferences made by Ziegler and Rodgers from psychological inventory data involved some very intricate patterns of interpretation. The inferences to be drawn from the inventory profiles do not simply stand out glaringly for the untrained observer, familiar though he might be with statistics and research generally. The proper interpretation of such inventories as the CPI and MMPI is a business for the trained expert, and not for mere score-readers. (Dr. Rodgers' article on the MMPI in the Buros Mental Measurements Yearbook [Rodgers, 1972] —the "bible" of testing—and his authorship of the CPI-MMPI combined test [Rodgers, 1966] are additional indications that the Rodgers-Ziegler team had special expertise in this area.) Our point here is that to the extent that profile interpretations depend on clinical skill rather than cold statistical comparisons, the judgment is an expert matter and, hence, somewhat private, subjective, and debatable.

Certain interview ratings made in the Ziegler-Rodgers full study followed the same general pattern observed in the personality inventory data; that is, findings that held true in the two-year follow-up did not persist at four years postsurgery. Two years after the vasectomy, differences between the experimental group and controls were found in interview ratings of marital satisfaction, as well as in sexual and overall psychiatric adjustment. No such differences were found later. Even the differences found in the first follow-up are somewhat weakened, however, because these ratings were not made "blind"; the rater was aware which were the surgery couples and which were controls. Admittedly, "blind" ratings might have been extremely difficult or even impossible to make; nonetheless, nonblind ratings are in fact suspect.

The cynical reader of the Scripps Foundation studies might be willing to ascribe the authors' inferences from their data to the familiar pattern described by Festinger (1957) in his book *"When Prophecy Fails."* Having generated hypotheses and made "prophecies" from analysis of the pilot study data, the researchers were then prepared to cling to these interpretations and defend themselves against the obvious message of the full study, which did not bear out the pilot. Similarly, since the two-year follow-up in the full study showed traces of support for their theses, the investigators failed to accept the implication of the nonconfirmatory four-year follow-up.

This *ad hominem* attack would gain respectability were it the case that Rodgers and Ziegler had started whole series of studies with an antivasectomy bias. Some have assumed this, but the assertion is unwarranted. Ziegler (1973, personal communication) has reported that his group had originally supposed vasectomy to be probably innocuous for healthy men and had hoped that research would demonstrate this to be true and thereby dispel some of the cloud of error surrounding the procedure. Their data, rather than their preconceptions, Ziegler held, led to greater reservations about the effects of the surgery.

A final point concerning the Rodgers and Ziegler studies: their inferences are based on small and nonrandom samples, primarily middle class whites. The urologists from whom referrals were secured sent some of their vasectomy patients along as subjects but not others. Some patients agreed to participate and others did not; the authors did not report the proportions who did and did not get into the study from among those eligible for the sample. The possible consequences of nonrandomness cannot be gauged; conceivably, the way in which the sample constructed itself may have enhanced the chances for negative outcomes.

Ziegler (1973, personal communication) does not think so. It is his opinion that the most psychologically healthy individuals, those least likely to be negatively affected by vasectomy, got into the study; if anything, then, the nonrandomness of the sample would have played *down* the likelihood of the research finding psychologically harmful consequences from the surgery.

Ziegler continues to feel, moreover, that the chances for negative sequelae of vasectomy are not to be casually dismissed. Although he has no formal statistics, in his psychiatric practice he reports having seen a disproportionately large number of patients with marital dissolution, extramarital sexual "affairs," and sexual and personality problems that started shortly after a vasectomy. As one possible explanation, Ziegler has wondered if a woman's finding her partner truly stimulating sexually must be predicated on her belief that she runs some risk of impregnation.

These are clinically-based speculations, with all their associated limitations, of course. They demand rigorous testing.

## Outline of a Longitudinal Study in Progress

Throughout the preceding pages, reference has been made to a study of my own. It is one of several recently initiated or completed North American projects on the psychosocial effects of contraceptive surgery.[b] Supported by a three-year grant from the Center for Population Research, the research program is in many ways patterned after the work of Rodgers and Ziegler (1973), both of whom are among our consultants. The study addresses itself to both male and female contraceptive surgery; our subjects include a group of couples where the woman has undergone the surgery (usually by laparoscopic procedures). In many cases, both members of the couple are being seen. There is also a no-surgery comparison group.

Subjects are being gathered for the study from agencies in Stockton, Sacramento, and Oakland, California; most of these do a large volume of contraceptive surgery. All the different social classes are represented in our sample; most subjects are white, but some are black. As of this writing, we are still collecting pretest data. The general research design (with only approximate $N$'s) is shown in Figure 7-3. Note the similarity to Design "D" in Figure 7-2.

| | | | | Group | |
| *Steps* | | *Vasectomy* | *Laparoscopic Tubal Ligation* | *No Surgery* |
|---|---|---|---|---|
| 1) Pretest (1972—1973) | Men | Yes (N = 300) | Yes (N = 80) | Yes (N = 120) |
| | Women | Yes (N = 180) | Yes (N = 120) | Yes (N = 120) |
| 2) Experimental treatment | Men | Male has | Female has | No |
| | Women | vasectomy | tubal ligation | No |
| 3) Posttest (1973—1974) | Men | Yes | Yes | Yes |
| | Women | Yes | Yes | Yes |

Note: N's only approximate, with some shrinkage expected in posttest. The "men" and "women" included in the study are legal spouses or living with one another.

**Figure 7-3.** Outline of Research Design for Prospective Longitudinal Study Currently in Progress.

---

[b]Grindstaff and Ebanks (1971) in Canada, Janke and Wiest (1973) in Portland, Oregon, and Zaltman, Klein, and Ratnow in Chicago (see Ratnow, 1974) are among others investigating the problem.

Fortuitously, it seems that we may be able to use some of our "experimental" subjects as additional "controls." Some of the agencies have a backlog of cases and have delayed surgery for a substantial time. If these delays continue long enough, it may be possible to test some couples a second time before they have vasectomies, resulting in the useful research design shown in Figure 7-4.

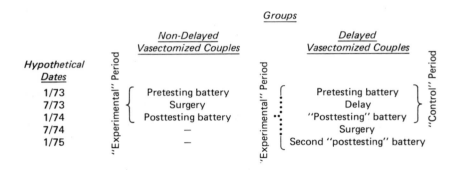

**Figure 7-4.** Delay of Surgery as an Additional Source of Control Groups

The "Delayed Vasectomized Couples" group in Figure 7-4 has two functions. During the first year it serves as a *control* group; during the second, it is an *experimental* group. As a control group, it can be compared not only to the experimental, nondelayed group, but also to itself in its second role. This design has distinct advantages because there is no more closely matched group than that of "own control." However, such presumably minor factors as changes with age and with taking the same tests three times are not controlled.

Figure 7-4 shows what may be possible by unexpected coincidence. This design might also be achieved deliberately by collaboration between researcher and agency or physician, although we have no plans for such skullduggery. As noted earlier in connection with the ideal designs shown in Figure 7-1, there are clear practical and ethical constraints on the kinds of studies that social scientists are permitted to conduct.

### The Development of a Short-Form Predictor Instrument

One goal of our study is to find a brief set of items that can, in a stable and valid way, predict those individuals—if any—most likely to be upset by contraceptive sterilization. Such a set of items might be used in various ways, depending on the judgment of particular agencies and gate-keeper personnel. Individuals beyond a cut-off point on the scale (a cut-off that could itself be varied) might be required to have individual counseling, endure a waiting period to be sure they were not going to change their minds, or might even be denied surgery altogether. Whether such a scale can be developed is not known; if it can be, it should be further refined, tested, and adapted in multinational research. (We shall have more to say in the concluding section of this chapter about cross-cultural comparability in designs and instrumentation.) The search for a valid predictor scale and for answers about which individuals react in which ways to their operation constitutes a research effort more sophisticated than that which asks only whether individuals who have surgery are healthier or less healthy than controls.

Standard technical procedures for the development of the instrument require cross-validation. It is for this reason (as Figure 7-3 indicates) that we have a disproportionately large number of experimental subjects in comparison to the number of controls. The cross-validational strategy demands that should we have 200 vasectomized men, for example, tested before and after surgery, this number be split into two groups of 100. Each group, in turn, would be halved according to worst or best adjustment on the criterion measure—resulting in four groups of fifty.

### Limits on the Generalizability of Findings

In the foregoing pages, we have outlined research designs, described methodological pitfalls, criticized the major studies of the psychosocial effects of contraceptive sterilization, and presented briefly an account of our study. In the final section of this chapter, we suggest that future research should attempt to overcome some of the limits inherent in the conceptualizations that have shaped the bulk of studies in this area.

### *The Need for Periodic Replications*

For the sake of argument, let us assume that the Rodgers-Ziegler group were perfectly correct in all the inferences they made about their samples and that their sampling was perfectly representative of U.S. couples who obtained vasectomies circa 1960. Even if this were the case, data and conclusions might now be out of date to an unknown and possibly large extent because the population from which they drew was importantly different from that of couples currently having vasectomies, for at least three reasons:

1. The U.S. population as a whole may have changed.
2. The population of couples electing for male contraceptive surgery is never a random sample of the entire U.S. population; the selective factors were probably very different around 1960 from what they are today. Only a few

couples were then getting vasectomies. The much larger numbers now undergoing the procedure suggest it to have become almost fashionable or even faddish. The population who had vasectomies when it was relatively uncommon may be avant-garde pioneers, brave souls, possibly either especially emotionally healthy or especially confused or in other ways psychologically "different."

Because findings are, in any case, somewhat specific to the populations of men getting vasectomy, it is worth emphasizing how rather special have been the samples on which is based much of our current knowledge of the effects of vasectomy. In the past, most vasectomized men in the United States, Canada, and England seem to have been thirty to forty years of age, white Protestants, with three or four children, and disproportionately from the higher socioeconomic levels. As reasons for choosing the surgery, they report dissatisfaction with other methods and contraceptive failure; the proportion with unwanted children appears high. (Documentation for these points is found in the review by Wiest and Janke [1974].) With the increasing popularity of vasectomy, as well as the possibility of selecting other successful means of birth control, it is altogether likely that today's vasectomized man is, in fact, not typical of the sort who had the surgery fifteen years ago.

3. The social environment to which vasectomized couples are exposed has changed. A vasectomized man's self-perceptions—specifically his perceptions of how having had the surgery has changed him—respond to the opinions of family, peers, and the general public. If significant others regard it as shameful, insane, or immoral to have abortions, use condoms, swim naked, have group sex, deliberately remain childless, or wear a beard or crewcut, then those who do these odd things may suffer psychological upset from violating group norms. If these same activities become acceptable or even become the norm, the individual who does them may be less upset, if at all. If a vasectomy is a "queer" thing, it will *per se* be more upsetting than if it were widely accepted. Taking the sheer numbers of vasectomies performed as one crude measure of social acceptability, we must admit that the man who underwent the surgery circa 1960 was doing something more off-beat—and hence more socially risky and disturbing—than if he were to elect vasectomy today.

Social change has not ceased; the current population of vasectomized couples is not necessarily predictive of those five or ten years hence. Conceivably, the procedure may become even more acceptable; or it could become a thalidomide-type horror or the subject of backlash. New biomedical procedures might radically change the image of vasectomy. Should easily reversible vasectomy—100 percent reversible—be developed, psychological reactions to the surgery may be quite different from those encountered around current procedures. Given the pace of technological and social evolution in this country, we need comparable studies repeated every five or ten years.

## The Need for Internationally Comparable Studies

Studies are now being designed in many countries on the psychological effects of contraceptive sterilization. It seems, therefore, the opportune moment to cry out for greater comparability in study designs, sampling procedures, the instruments used, and the like, and to emphasize the gains to be made for theory and practice from mounting research efforts in different parts of the world whose findings could readily be compared and contrasted. The notion of internationally comparable investigations may raise the specter of monolithic conformity to an inflexible, bureaucratic guideline. The real danger, however, is quite the opposite—a rag-tag series of expensive studies using completely different measuring instruments and generating disgracefully noncomparable data. Every investigator naturally has pet ideas about these matters, but it seems doubtful if the incremental improvements from using personality test X instead of test Y, for example, are sufficient to offset the losses for knowledge that accrue with noncomparability in instruments. It is wasteful to use the Rorschach and 16-PF with lower class couples in Tennessee when the woman has undergone surgery, while someone else studies middle class vasectomized couples in Ontario with the MMPI and the Hand Test.

Much of the responsibility for generating comparable studies lies with psychologists. It is therefore gratifying that at the American Psychological Association convention in August 1973, a workshop on contraceptive sterilization research was held. With the procedures suddenly a big business in the United States and in the world, it is hard to think of more important psychosocial research questions, more important to mental health, than those about the psychosocial effects of contraceptive sterilization. A sane allocation of funds, which can realistically be demanded and expected, can support a large-scale and coordinated effort yielding internationally comparable data. Built into plans for such research should be a plan for systematically and repeatedly sampling the various populations over time.

## The Need for Similar Measuring Instruments

Among the most pressing necessities for studies in the psychosocial implications of contraceptive sterilization—both intranationally and internationally—is the agreement of investigators to use similar instruments, as has already been mentioned. In future studies, two basic types of core measuring instruments seem advisable: (1) some standardized personality inventory and (2) a set of tailor-made questions focusing on the surgery and related concerns. Eventually these questions, as well, could be standardized. Ideally, the same personality inventory and the same set of questions should be used in various studies, with other supplemental material being added to suit investigator's individual tastes.

To promote comparability among studies, we need to select objective measures that can be used in a standardized way, in contrast to procedures relying heavily on the private insights of individual clinician-artists. For this reason and in view of past research (such as Knutson, 1972), I believe that such instruments as the Rorschach, TAT, or projective drawings should not bear the central burden of assessment, however useful they may be to some investigators for auxiliary data. If interviews are to be used, they should not displace standardized inventories and should include heavy doses of standardized questions asked in standardized ways, to minimize interviewer bias. Incidentally, it seems very important that, wherever possible, any judges and raters work blind, not knowing which are experimental and which are control groups. In some situations this can be done for perhaps the first two-thirds of an interview, before the interviewer finds out whether this is a surgery or a control subject. Where possible, interviewers should not even be aware that the focus of the research is on contraceptive sterilization.

An added reason for favoring standardized personality inventories over projective devices and unstructured interviews is that if there is any hope of finding valid predictors of outcome such predictors are much more easily built, psychometrically, from inventories or at least from standard-form, objective questions. (This is not to assert that it would be impossible to validate a screening procedure involving, say, a given card of the Rorschach or TAT.)

What instruments seem the most likely candidates for selection as part of the core battery? Among the personality inventories, criteria for choosing include (1) availability of translations and restandardizations in other languages and cultures, (2) the tradition of what has been used by past studies and those in progress, as well as (3) standard technical criteria. Building on the experience of Rodgers and Ziegler, our own group is using Rodgers's combined version of the MMPI and CPI (Rodgers, 1966), a published test but available only for research purposes and with special permission. The CPI has been translated and standardized in a number of languages and cultures; it has an appealing emphasis, as well, on personality strengths rather than weaknesses. Nonetheless, Rodgers and Ziegler concluded that the CPI by itself was insufficient and consequently had to scramble in mid-stream to change their plans to include the MMPI (Rodgers and Ziegler, 1973). This experience should be instructive to others.

Our own group's basic questionnaire, focused extensively on contraceptive sterilization and related personal and sexual matters, is available on request. We have devised, after item analysis, an 8-item scale of attitudes toward vasectomy, patterned after five 8-item scales Gough has developed to measure attitudes in five population-related areas (Gough, 1975).

We are also using a 50-item checklist of "Life Situations," events that our subjects may have recently experienced. The checklist is scored in two ways, producing two separate weighted totals. In keeping with the work of Rahe (1972), we are weighting these events on sheer change, whether positive or negative. In line with the opinion of Paykel and Uhlenhuth (1972), however, we are also weighting the same items on degree of associated upset. Both groups claim some predictive validity for such weighted scales.

We have subjects draw a man and draw a tree as an attempt to tap less conscious reactions to the surgery. Some research on men who had *non*voluntary vasectomies suggests that such a procedure may result in more trees drawn with lopped-off branches, for example (Hammer, 1953).

Finally, some of our subjects are also being interviewed according to a structured interview guide. On this small group, interviewers are required to complete Gough's 50-item Q-sort (Block, 1961), Gough's 300-item Adjective Check List (Gough and Heilbrun, 1965), some overall ratings, and a two-page character sketch.

## In Conclusion

The psychosocial effects of sterilization are subject to a wide variety of influences, such as the characteristics of the patient, his or her family and cultural setting, the ongoing life situation, the specific nature of the surgical procedure, and the characteristics of those delivering medical care. The plethora of variables indicate the advantages of conducting a coordinated group of studies with systematic coverage of contrasting cultures, using somewhat comparable research designs and instruments, and repeating the investigations every five or ten years. For the present, more communication and joint planning among investigators currently studying the effects of sterilization might increase the comparability and meaning of their results.

Most research to date has been spotty and fragmentary, often using inadequate research designs and noncomparable samples. Ideally, meaningful research on sterilization should include appropriate control groups. Not surprisingly, different studies have been interpreted as supporting opposite conclusions as to whether vasectomy has deleterious psychological effects.

Continuing arguments over interpretations of the Rodgers and Ziegler (1973) studies seem less important than forging ahead with new research. The author is conducting a longitudinal study, patterned somewhat after the designs of Rodgers and Ziegler (1973).

## References

Barnes, E. and Johnson, G.B. "Effects of Vasectomy on Marriage Relationships."
    Unpublished paper. Des Moines, Iowa: Family Service-Travelers Aid, 1964.
Block, J. *The Q-sort Method in Personality Assessment and Psychiatric Research.*
    Springfield, Il: Charles C. Thomas, 1961.

Campbell, D.J. and Stanley, J.S. *Experimental and Quasi-Experimental Designs for Research.* Chicago: Rand McNally, 1963.

Dandekar, K. "After-Effects of Vasectomy." *Artha Vijnana* 56 (1963): 212-24.

Ferber, A.S. Tietze, C., and Lewit, S. "Men with Vasectomies: A Study of Medical Sexual, and Psychosocial Changes." *Psychosomatic Medicine* 29 (1967): 354-66.

Festinger, L. *A Theory of Cognitive Dissonance.* Stanford, CA: Stanford University Press, 1957.

Fitzgerald, J.A. "The Female Response to Male Vas Ligation." *Medical Insight* 4 (1972): 23-27.

Garrison, P.L. and Gamble, C.J. "Sexual Effects of Vasectomy." *Journal of the American Medical Association* 144, 14 (1950): 293-95

Gough, H.G. An Attitude Profile for *Journal of Research in Personality* 9 (1975): 122-135. Studies of Population Psychology."

_____ and Heilbrun, A.B. *The Adjective Check List Manual.* Palo Alto, CA: Consulting Psychologists Press, 1965.

Grindstaff, C.F. and Ebanks, G.E. "Vasectomy as a Birth Control Method." In *Critical Issues in Canadian Society,* ed. C. Boydell, C. Grindstaff, and P. Whitehead, pp. 25-32. New York and Toronto: Holt, Rinehart, and Winston, 1971.

Hammer, E. "An Investigation of Sexual Symbolism: A Study of H-T-P's of Eugenically Sterilized Subjects." *Journal of Projective Techniques* 17 (1953): 401-413.

Janke, D.J. and Wiest, W.M. "Effects of Vasectomy on Psychological Adjustment and Medical Health in a Sample of Subscribers to the Kaiser Foundation Health Plan." Privately circulated paper. Portland, OR: Reed College, 1973.

Johnson, M.H. "Social and Psychological Effects of Vasectomy." *American Journal of Psychiatry* 121 (November 1964): 482-86.

Knutson, J.F. "Review of the Rorschach." In *The Seventh Mental Measurements Yearbook,* ed. O.K. Buros, pp. 435-40, Vol. 1. Highland Park, N.J.: Gryphon Press, 1972.

Landis, J.T. and Poffenberger, T. "The Marital and Sexual Adjustment of Three Hundred Thirty Couples Who Chose Vasectomy as a Form of Birth Control." *Journal of Marriage and the Family* 27 (1965): 57-58.

Lee, H.Y. "Clinical Studies on the Influences of Vasectomy." *Korean Journal of Urology* 7 (1966): 11-29.

Parker, J.B., Jr. "Psychiatric Aspects of Sterilization." In *Psychological Aspects of Surgery,* ed. H.S. Abrams, pp. 105-113. Series No. 4 of *International Psychiatry Clinics,* 1967 (Whole No. 2).

Paykel, E.S. and Uhlenhuth, E.H. "Rating the Magnitude of Life Stress." *Canadian Psychiatric Association Journal* 17 (1972): 93-100.

Phoenix, C. "Sexual Behavior in Rhesus Monkeys After Vasectomy." *Science* 179, 4072 (February 2, 1972): 493-94.

Poffenberger, S. and Sheth, D.L. "Reactions of Urban Employees to Vasectomy
  Operations." *The Journal of Family Welfare* 10 (1963): 1-17.
Poffenberger, T. and Poffenberger, S. "A Comparison of Factors Influencing the
  Choice of Vasectomy in India and the U.S." *Indian Journal of Social Work*
  25 (1965): 339-51.
Poffenberger, T. and Poffenberger, S. "Vasectomy as a Preferred Method of
  Birth Control: A Preliminary Investigation." *Marriage and Family Living*
  25 (August 1963): 326-30.
Rahe, R.H. "Subjects' Recent Life Changes and Their Near-Future Illness
  Reports." *Annals of Clinical Research* 4 (October 1972): 250-65.
Ratnow, S.M. "Social and Psychological Correlates of the Selection or Rejection
  of Vasectomy." Ph.D. dissertation, Loyola University of Chicago, 1974.
  *Dissertation Abstracts International* 35: 1894-1895 (4-B). No. 74-22, 444.
Rodgers, D.A. "Review of the Minnesota Multiphasic Personality Inventory."
  In *The Seventh Mental Measurements Yearbook,* ed. O.K. Buros, Vol. 1,
  pp. 243-250. Highland Park, N.J.: Gryphon Press, 1972.
_____. *Rodgers' Condensed CPI-MMPI.* Palo Alto, CA: Consulting Psychologists
  Press, 1966.
_____ and Ziegler, F.J. "Psychological Reactions to Surgical Contraception."
  In *Psychological Perspectives on Population,* ed. J.T. Fawcett. New York:
  Basic Books, 1973.
_____, Ziegler, F.J., Prentiss, R.J., and Martin, P.L. "Comparisons of Nine
  Contraceptive Procedures by Couples Changing to Vasectomy or Ovulation
  Suppression Medication." *The Journal of Sex Research,* 1 (1965): 87-96.
Rosario, F.Z. "A Survey of Social-Psychological Variables Used in Studies of
  Family Planning." *Working Papers of the East-West Population Institute,*
  No. 11 (1971).
Sackler, A.M., Weltman, A.S., Pandhi, V., and Schwartz, R. "Gonadal Effects
  of Vasectomy and Vasoligation." *Science* 179 (January 19, 1973): 293-95.
Simon Population Trust Report. *Vasectomy: Follow-up of 1,000 Cases.*
  Cambridge, England, 1969.
Wells, H.B. and Poffenberger, T. "Research Designs for Evaluating After-effects
  of Vasectomy." Unpublished paper presented at the Seminar on Steriliza-
  tion, Gokhale Institute of Politics and Economics, Poona, India, November
  1965.
Wiest, W.M. and Janke, L.D. "A Methodological Critique of Research on
  Psychological Effects of Vasectomy." *Psychosomatic Medicine* 36 (1974):
  438-49.
Wolfers, H. "Psychological Aspects of Vasectomy." *British Medical Journal*
  4 (1970): 297-300.
Ziegler, F.J. et al. *Vasectomy: Current Research in Male Sterilization.*
  New York: MSS Information Corporation, 1973.
_____, Rodgers, D.A., and Kriegsman, S.A. "Effects of Vasectomy on Psychological

Functioning." *Psychosomatic Medicine* 28 (1966): 50-63.

———, Rodgers, D.A. and Prentiss, R.J. "Psychosocial Response to Vasectomy." *Archives of General Psychiatry* 21 (1969): 46-54.

# 8 Psychosocial Aspects of Contraceptive Sterilization in Women
*Warren B. Miller*

## Introduction

The story goes that as Gertrude Stein lay on her death bed and appeared to be staring into the Great Beyond, her close friend, Alice B. Toklas, asked her, "Gertrude, Gertrude, what is the answer?" Miss Stein turned her head toward her friend and replied, "Alice, Alice, what is the question?" We are in a similar quandary regarding the psychosocial aspects of contraceptive sterilization in women. Before providing answers, we must carefully sort out the many relevant questions.

Three broad questions emerge immediately: (1) What are the psychological characteristics of those choosing female contraceptive sterilization; that is, who selects the procedure? (2) What is the nature of the decision-making process behind the choice; that is, how do individuals and couples make the selection? and, (3) What are the psychological outcomes following female contraceptive sterilization? To these three basic questions, a fourth and superordinate query may be added: (4) What are the interaction effects among these three groups of variables, especially between psychological antecedents and decision-making processes on the one hand and psychological outcomes on the other? Although it is much too early to offer many answers, this chapter considers material relevant to all four questions.

As used here, *female contraceptive sterilization* refers to the interruption of fallopian tube patency through surgery and, to a lesser extent, to the surgical removal of the internal organs of reproduction. The term does not include contraception involving only minor surgical procedures, such as IUD insertion or the implantation of a slow-release, antiovulatory or abortifacient capsule in the gluteal fat. Both of these procedures are reversible, while the methods that are the subject of this discussion are, for all practical purposes, permanently effective.

This chapter emerges from interest in and experience with the field, both its research and clinical aspects. The writer has conducted extensive interviews with women who were either seeking contraceptive sterilization or had already undergone the procedure, with contraceptive counselors and physicians offering surgical services, and with colleagues involved in studies of the area. The normative view was gained through a recently completed survey of a random sample of 100 unmarried women regarding their attitudes toward both male and female contraceptive sterilization. The writer's review of the literature

119

on tubal ligation and hysterectomy, concentrating on the work since the early 1960s has provided the context within which the clinical interview data find their meaning.

## The Previous Literature

Recently, at least five general reviews of the literature have dealt directly with psychosocial aspects of contraceptive sterilization and tubal ligation, more specifically (Woodruff and Pauerstein, 1969; Presser, 1970; Borland, 1972; Rodgers and Ziegler, 1973; Schwyhart and Kutner, 1973). Regarding respondent satisfaction and adjustment, most follow-up studies, including those done in non-Western cultures, report satisfaction with the decision among 90 to 95 percent of those surveyed. In occasional investigations, however, overall dissatisfaction was found in 15 to 20 percent of the cases; in some instances, the percentage experiencing negative sexual effects or negative menstrual changes ran as high as 30 or 40 percent. These overall results echo the findings of earlier literature reviews (Adams, 1964; Barglow and Eisner, 1966).

Unfortunately, all previous investigations of female contraceptive sterilization have been subject to many major research limitations which severely compromise their impact. These limitations may be organized into five categories: conceptualization, design, methods of assessment, sampling, and data analysis and interpretation.

The original *conceptualization* behind research on contraceptive sterilization has been unrefined and without theoretical underpinnings. With regard to psychological antecedents, for example, it has frequently been said that emotional instability or psychopathology tends to interfere with a successful outcome (Woodruff and Pauerstein, 1969; Baudry, Herzig, and Weiner, 1971; Schwyhart and Kutner, 1973). While this may well be generally true, a great many women with "psychopathology" do exceedingly well following surgical intervention, while many "normal" women do not. Greater specificity is required concerning the kinds of psychopathology and aspects of emotional instability that lead to dissatisfaction, with a view to increasing the understanding of the psychological mechanisms involved. Conceptual vagueness appears also with regard to decision-making variables, when a voluntary choice is seen as more likely than an involuntary one to lead to postintervention satisfaction (Barnes and Zuspan, 1958; Thompson and Baird, 1968). A more sophisticated model of the internal and external constraints on decision-making is needed, as well as a testing of this model with respect to the psychological consequences of contraceptive sterilization.

Superficiality in conceptualization is especially evident in discussions of psychological outcome variables. Concepts such as "sexual deteriorization" (Thompson and Baird, 1968; Whitehouse, 1971), "unfulfilled maternal desire"

(Schwyhart and Kutner, 1973), and "satisfaction" (Presser, 1970) provide, it is true, a useful general measure of postintervention response. However, the over-simplifications may actually be quite misleading for understanding the complexities of sexual behavior or maternal feelings, which, once again, remain to be specified and considered dynamically. As used in most studies, the concept of "satisfaction" has its own special difficulties. When applied to the decision to be sterilized, it is retrospective over long time-intervals and thus is subject both to the adaptive reconstructions of memory and to the effect of cognitive dissonance on self-evaluation. The writer's clinical experience, furthermore, has shown contraceptive sterilization to be an emotionally-laden event which later tends to become an organizing point of reference used by the patient to explain much of the good and bad that has occurred in her life following the procedure. Other investigators have made similar observations (Barglow and Eisner, 1966). When this tendency for the event to become emotionally over-invested is reinforced by the interviewer's (or the questionnaire's) clear concern with the effects of contraceptive sterilization, it can hardly be doubted that the diffuse, evaluative character of "satisfaction" makes the concept of questionable value in research.

Investigations of female contraceptive sterilization also suffer from major problems of *design*. First of all, almost all such investigations are retrospective, in the sense that data were gathered following the surgical procedure (for example, Adams, 1964; Paniagua, Tayback, Janer, and Vásquez, 1964; Barglow and Eisner, 1966), with a few notable exceptions (Barglow, Gunther, Johnson, and Meltzer, 1965; Thompson and Baird, 1968; Brody, Meikle, and Gerritse, 1971). The distortions in self-report as a function of retrospective inquiry have already been mentioned. Second, the follow-up time period after surgical intervention varies greatly, not only among studies (for example, Barglow, Gunther, Johnson, and Meltzer, 1965; Barglow and Eisner, 1966), but also within a given study (for instance, Paniagua, Tayback, Janer, and Vasquez, 1964; Thompson and Baird, 1968). Third, most investigations have no adequate control or comparison groups (for example, Whitehouse, 1971; Schneider, 1972) —again, with a few exceptions (Barglow, Gunther, Johnson and Meltzer, 1965; Brody, Meikle, and Gerritse, 1971). A fourth design problem is inadequate attention to potentially important sources of variance like the effect of the physician and his attitudes, the type of surgical procedure, the indications for the surgical intervention, and the timing of the surgery with respect to the last pregnancy. With regard to the latter, with the prevalent medical distinction between puerperal and interval tubal ligation, it is surprising that no investigators have addressed themselves systematically to the psychological differences between contraceptive sterilization immediately following childbirth and contraceptive sterilization at some other point in time unrelated to childbirth. Considering the prevalence of simultaneous therapeutic abortion and tubal ligation, it is similarly puzzling that so little attention has been given to the study of psychological outcomes with and without concomitant therapeutic abortion or other concurrent procedures (Brody, Meikle, and Gerritse, 1971; Schwyhart and Kutner, 1973). A fifth and final design problem has been the neglect of research interest in the impact of the social field upon the patient. Social norms governing a course of action significantly influence not only the way the decision is made to pursue it but the types of feelings that develop later regarding the decision. As with the public change regarding therapeutic abortion, the current liberal trend in attitude about tubal ligation can be expected to result in more open decision-making and less guilt and shame on follow-up. To date, most studies have not taken this phenomenon into account, much less studied it in its own right.

Besides the problems of conceptualization and design, the *assessment* methods used in research on female contraceptive sterilization have generally been superficial, with little or no attention given to their validity, reliability, or standardization (Schwyhart and Kutner, 1973). A simple illustration of these problems can be found by returning to the issue of measuring post-procedural "satisfaction." No one has considered the validity of instruments assessing satisfaction through, for example, concurrent measurement by questionnaire, interview, and observer ratings. The reliability of the measurements has not been determined by seeing, for instance, how the response varies when repeated after a short interval of time or when using a different instrument or interviewer. Purporting to be using the same measure, finally, some investigators ask, "Are you satisfied?", some ask, "Do you regret?", and some ask, "Would you do it again?" Obviously, more carefully developed and standardized psychological inventories and interview schedules would permit better measurement of the psychological variables in question and greater cross-study comparability.

*Sampling* problems constitute an additional major limitation of previous investigations. The size of the sample in some studies is relatively large and reasonably representative of the universe from which it has been drawn (Paniagua, Tayback, Janer, and Vásquez, 1964; Barglow and Eisner, 1966). In most studies, however, samples have been unsystematically collected (for example, Thompson and Baird, 1968), drawn from very special populations (for example, Barglow, Gunther, Johnson, and Meltzer, 1965), or subject to very large attrition (for example, Sacks and LaCroix, 1962; Norris, 1964). According to a recent analysis of pooled data from the available literature (Schwyhart and Kutner, 1973), the latter factor has proved to be a likely source of bias for follow-up results because respondent satisfaction increased as study attrition increased.

The final major limitation of the research on female contraceptive sterilization involves *data analysis and interpretation.* The frequent lack of comparison groups has already been cited. Another important shortcoming of many studies is the failure to use even elementary statistical methods (for instance, Adams, 1964; Ellison, 1964) or, when appropriate, the more sophisticated techniques such as multivariate analysis (for example, Norris, 1964; Barglow, Gunther, Johnson, and Meltzer, 1965). As a result, some investigators have interpreted their own data in a way that leads them to unjustified conclusions (for instance, Ellison, 1964).

## Future Directions

The remainder of this chapter focuses on potentially useful future research, concentrating on the three areas previously discussed: psychological antecedents, the decision-making processes, and psychological outcomes. In this treatment, individual psychology will be emphasized, but, to the extent that space permits, concepts relative to couples and couple interaction shall also be developed.

### Psychological Antecedents

What are the psychological antecedents to female contraceptive sterilization? Which women select this procedure and what are their psychological characteristics? In this context, *psychological antecedents* mean motivations, either situationally derived or developing out of enduring personality traits, which move the woman in her actions, disposing her, if you will, toward or away from the selection of female contraceptive sterilization.

Findings from the literature and the writer's own clinical observations suggest that women who select contraceptive sterilization:

1. have relatively satisfied their maternal aspirations in terms of both the number and the quality of their children;
2. have a relatively high sense of urgency to avoid any further pregnancies;
3. have relative confidence in the persistence of their current childbearing desires into the future and in their ability to know their future childbearing needs;
4. have relative comfort about making procreational decisions independently and taking procreational initiative;
5. have a relative lack of confidence in their ability to contracept effectively by any other method;
6. have a relative skepticism regarding the reliability or applicability to them of other effective methods of contraception;
7. are relatively accepting of themselves as sexual beings and of sexual pleasure as a legitimate goal in itself;
8. are relatively devoted to female role-activities other than the traditional domestic ones; and

9.  are relatively free from bodily fears and from anxieties with regard to
    surgical manipulation and subsequent pain.

These characteristics have been expressed in terms of their *relative* strength
in order to emphasize their dimensionality.  In other words, the traits are con-
ceived to be present to a greater or lesser degree in each individual and should
be measurable by methods assessing an individual's procreative, contraceptive,
and sexual dispositions.  By way of illustration, in the writer's own research,
a group of self-report inventories has been developed which taps psychological
dimensions related to motivation.  The instruments include a Sexual Attitude
Questionnaire, a Contraceptive Attitude Questionnaire, a Feminine Interest
Questionnaire, and a Maternal Attitude Questionnaire, each of which measures
two or more empirically-derived behavior dimensions.

The relative importance of these hypothesized dimensions may vary with
certain subsidiary factors, such as parity (for instance, the nulliparous woman
selecting contraceptive sterilization), age (the woman under twenty-five, for
example), or marital status (the unmarried or formerly married woman, for
instance).

One subsidiary question deserves special consideration.  What psychological
characteristics of women are related to the choice among the different available
surgical procedures, all of which result in permanent infertility?  Hysterectomy,
for example, is currently receiving more general consideration for use in female
contraceptive sterilization (Hibbard, 1972; Roach, Krolak, Powell, Llorens, and
Deubler, 1972; Schulmann, 1972).  The few studies on the psychological consequences of hysterectomy for medical purposes (Lindemann, 1941; Drellich
and Bieber, 1958; Ackner, 1961; Melody, 1962; Barglow, Gunther, Johnson,
and Meltzer, 1965) offer little information about the psychological antecedents
to the selection of hysterectomy for contraceptive purposes.  Primarily on the
basis of clinical interviewing, the writer would hypothesize that women who
do or would select hysterectomy:

1.  are relatively negative in their feelings about the future experience and
    meaning of menstruation; and
2.  are relatively inclined toward a masculine identification and toward
    traditional male role activities.

Several other surgical procedures are currently available which prevent
conception by obstructing the fallopian tube (Calderone, 1970; Duncan, Falb,
and Speidel, 1972).  At present, since women have little or no say about which
of these procedures they undergo, discussion of the psychological antecedents
to the various procedures can only be speculative.  Should the selection of a
procedure rest with the patient, it seems possible that there will be motivational
and personality trait differences between women who choose culdoscopy—

involving a transvaginal approach, no abdominal scar, and minimal postoperative interference with the patient's activities, including sexual intercourse—and those selecting laparotomy, a procedure that requires hospitalization but is less likely to fail.

Discussion to this point has been focused upon the psychological dimensions of the individual. Of equal importance is the analysis of the decision as a function of the qualities of both members of the couple. Two separate questions can be discerned: (1) What are the psychological characteristics of couples who decide to terminate their reproductive careers by means of an irreversible surgical intervention and, more specifically, (2) What are the characteristics of couples who elect tubal ligation as compared with those choosing vasectomy?

With respect to the first of these questions, the psychological dimension already discussed can also be applied to couples if the characteristics are adequately extended and elaborated to take into account the man's procreative, contraceptive, and sexual perceptions and desires. With respect to the second, which member of a couple undergoes contraceptive sterilization depends upon the relative salience to each of them of the various procreational, contraceptive, and sexual issues, especially as these interact with other concurrent problems and decisions. Thus, reformulating the individual psychological dimensions previously outlined, it may be hypothesized that the member of the couple most likely to have contraceptive sterilization:

1. is the more antagonistic to the possibility of (additional) childbearing and the more concerned about the uncertainties of reproductive control;
2. is typically assigned responsibility for contraception by the couple themselves;
3. is perceived as being less in jeopardy both psychologically and physically as a result of contraceptive sterilization;
4. is less apprehensive about his (her) own sexual freedom and/or more apprehensive about his (her) spouse's sexual freedom as a result of contraceptive sterilization; and
5. is more secure about his (her) own reproductive and marital future.

It need hardly be said that these are highly simplified hypotheses and that such generalizations are subject to complications arising from the various tradeoffs and arrangements that take place during actual decision-making. For example, a woman who had assumed sole contraceptive responsibility may argue that her husband should now take his turn; similarly, a husband, sensing that his "sacrifice" can be used to his advantage in his sexual relationship with his wife, may agree to take the pain and inconvenience of the surgery upon himself. Which member of a couple has the surgery will, of course, also be influenced by local factors such as peer group influence, the availability of the different types (male versus female) of contraceptive sterilization, and the relative financial costs of the different procedures.

*Decision-making*

Discussion of marital negotiations leads naturally to the second set of variables outlined earlier, those involving the decision-making process. The model to be invoked for this discussion is fundamentally different from that which applies to other forms of effective contraception (Miller, 1973). In the latter instance, one may draw upon the paradigm of the ego integrating and expressing a rich variety of motivations throughout the fluctuations of time and situation. Such a dynamic model is appropriate when considering a relationship that involves multiple sexual contacts, many chances to use or not use contraception, and the variety of situations in which couples can develop and modify feelings about childbearing. Under such circumstances, decisions are being made, remade, and unmade with a high frequency across time; it is the ego that acts most importantly to integrate and give coherence to changes in behavior and attitude. In the case of contraceptive sterilization, however, the procedure is irreversible, practically speaking, and the decision to have surgery is made and carried through only once. What demands explanation, therefore, is not coherence over time, but the stages toward the choice, that is, decision-making. This model, developed from the relevant literature (Brim, Glass, Lavin, and Goodman, 1962; Hamburg, Coelho, and Adams, 1973) and from clinical interviews with women who were actually making a decision regarding contraceptive sterilization, is shown in Figure 8-1.

In the model, there are three stages—predecision, decision, and postintervention—through which an individual or couple moves in sequence. Each stage involves one or more psychological tasks which are influenced by certain environmental factors and psychological dimensions relevant to decision-making. Planning is the most important psychological task in the predecision stage. In the decision stage, there are four tasks which themselves occur in sequence: recognition, consideration, commitment, and action. Adaptation, finally, is the main psychological task in the postintervention stage.

Each of these six tasks has one or more psychological dimensions which significantly influence that step in the decision-making sequence. It should therefore be possible to measure an individual (or couple) on each of these dimensions and then construct a decision-making profile which would shed light upon an individual's probable response to a decision-making situation. The assessment of the process of the decision would complement any profile developed from the motivational dimensions discussed earlier.

Let us consider each step in the decision-making sequence, primarily as it applies to individuals. The *predecision* stage obtains just before a woman

| Stage | Predecision | Decision | | | | Postintervention |
|---|---|---|---|---|---|---|
| | | Recognition | Consideration | Commitment | Action | |
| Psychological Task | Planning | Recognition | Consideration | Commitment | Action | Adaptation |
| Environmental Factor | Information Critical Event | | Information Guidance | | Resources Surgery | Social Field Support |
| Decision-Making Dimension | Future Oriented–Present Oriented | Acknowledging–Denying | Unconstricted–Constricted | With Closure–Without Closure | Active–Passive | Adaptively Flexible–Rigid |

**Figure 8-1.** Model of the Decision-making Process Regarding Female Contraceptive Sterilization

has reached a point in her reproductive career when termination of childbearing by contraceptive sterilization is being considered. At this juncture in her thinking, she projects herself into some as-yet-undetermined future time and sees herself as unwilling to have (more) children. On the basis of the information available to her in her social environment and her own degree of future orientation, her attitude toward contraceptive sterilization can be placed into one of four categories: (1) tubal ligation is not known about; (2) tubal ligation is known about but has not been considered; (3) tubal ligation has been considered but is not planned; and (4) tubal ligation is intended and planned.

At some point, a woman will realize that she wishes or is ready to terminate childbearing; with this *recognition*, she enters the *decision* stage. Clinical experience has shown that women are often moved into the decision stage by the occurrence of a particular life-event. Numbered among these events are those related to pregnancy (her own pregnancy, a pregnancy scare, or the awareness of an unwanted pregnancy in someone else), to birth control (a physician's suggestion that she stop her regular method of contraception; for example, discontinue the pill for awhile) to menstruation (the development of menstrual irregularity, especially excessive bleeding), and to contraceptive sterilization itself (hearing about tubal ligation from a friend who has had one). Other important life-events probably precipitate decision-making as well. A job opportunity, geographic mobility, the youngest child's entering school, or a major health change in the family, for example, could easily prompt one into making the choice against conceiving any (more) children. What life-event or personal experience it takes to move an individual to consider an irreversible and potentially threatening course of action will be influenced by that person's tendency to acknowledge or deny threat or conflict. Thus, there is an interaction of both environmental (life-event) and personality factors that influences the woman's entry into the decision stage.

Recognition leads to *consideration*—both in fantasy and in interpersonal discussion. In fantasy, the woman applies to herself her notions of what tubal ligation entails and its implications for the future. Simultaneously, she considers the various alternatives to tubal ligation. The interpersonal form of consideration occurs through the seeking of information, the discussion of possible courses of action, the securing of opinions, and the sounding-out of strategies. Interpersonal consideration is influenced by the information and guidance available in the environment and by two general characteristics of the woman's decision-making: the degree of its independence and the extent to which it is based on a serious review of the other options.

Once consideration has been completed and the decision is made, psychological *commitment* takes place, with or without closure. The latter is the case with people who continue to fantasize and discuss alternative courses of action. This apparent ambivalence may be based on motivational conflict; it may, however, simply be stylistic—a characterologically-based tendency to achieve or not to achieve closure in decision-making.

The final step in decision-making is *action,* that is, action that effectively accomplishes what has been decided. How and when action occurs are influenced both by the availability of community resources and the woman's characteristic way of responding to situations that require initiative. The latter personal quality is indicated in the decision-making model by the psychological dimension of activity-passivity.

After surgery, the woman's main task relevant to her procreative and contraceptive decision is adaptation to the changes which the surgery has brought into her life. This adaptation will clearly be facilitated by support from her social network and by her own degree of flexibility in the face of change and stress.

The overall decision-making model has thus far been applied to the stages of the individual woman's movement toward contraceptive sterilization. The different stages, the psychological tasks, and, to a large extent, the specific decision-making dimensions can be applied equally well to a couple, with perhaps some elaboration of the consideration stage to include a dominance-submissiveness dimension related to the couple's negotiations. An additional analytic feature of the model when applied to couples is the possibility of predicting which of the two spouses will ultimately have the contraceptive sterilization. By investigating the respective activities of each member of the pair concerning a given decision-making task, one could establish, for example, whether husband or wife was first to recognize the problem, which one gathered the information, and which one was most committed.

How is decision-making related to the other general areas outlined at the beginning of this chapter—the characteristics of adopters, the psychological outcomes of surgery, and their interaction? Only some of the decision-making factors appear relevant to determining which women will select female contraceptive sterilization. Thus, it is likely that such women:

1. are relatively high on future orientation;
2. have a relatively greater tendency to acknowledge threat and conflict;
3. are relatively unconstricted when considering solutions to a problem; and
4. are relatively active in putting their decision into effect.

The decision-making variables probably have greater bearing for the psychological outcomes of contraceptive sterilization. Before developing a set of specific hypotheses in this regard, let us turn to a general discussion of these outcomes.

## Psychological Outcomes

The psychological outcome variables relevant to female contraceptive sterilization embrace three distinct levels: the biological, the intrapsychic, and the social (that is, the woman's relation to her own body, to herself [her "self"], and to her social field).

In considering the topic of "body image," Kolb has distinguished between "body percept" and "body concept" (Kolb, 1973); body percept refers to sensations arising from within the body, while body concept refers to the cognitive understanding of these sensations and of bodily function in general. We know relatively little about the effect of contraceptive sterilization upon either. It is quite possible that bodily sensations (body percept), especially in the genital-reproductive area, are relatively unchanged following tubal ligation. An unaltered body percept is consistent with the simplicity of the surgical approaches and the minimal anatomical and physiological changes that contraceptive surgery is believed to provoke. The rudimentary available research evidence also suggests that pelvic consciousness is unchanged following tubal ligation (Sacks and LaCroix, 1962). It is much more doubtful that bodily perceptions are similarly unaffected following hysterectomy (Barglow, Gunther, Johnson, and Meltzer, 1965; Drellich and Bieber, 1958).

Changes in body concept are quite another matter. Clinical experience shows an impressive frequency in the number and variety of distorted fantasies held by women—both before and after surgery—concerning the effects of tubal ligation. These fantasies concern their pelvic anatomy, their menstrual function, their hormonal status, their susceptibility to illness, especially cancer, and their overall energy level and physical attractiveness. Some investigators have reported a very high incidence of perceived menstrual change following tubal ligation (Adams, 1964). Others have described postsurgical changes suggestive of important psychosomatic effects, such as the occurrence of significant weight changes in a large proportion of their sample (Thompson and Baird, 1968). The actual effects of the surgery, as well as the patients' preoccupation concerning such effects, demand a full, careful explanation of the impact of contraceptive sterilization on the body concept. Somewhat in the manner of Drellich and Bieber (1958) regarding hysterectomy, we must develop a natural history account of how women feel, think, and fantasize about their bodies, especially the genital-reproductive areas, following contraceptive sterilization. Studies of this type could use and extend concepts and instruments such as those derived from Fisher's work on body boundary (Fisher, 1963; Fisher, 1966).

At the intrapsychic level, as well, several outcome variables suggest themselves for investigation. These include the status of the woman's procreative desires and how she evaluates her procreative accomplishments, her level of sexual satisfaction and how she feels about herself as a sexual being, and her general feelings about herself as a woman—particularly her self-respect and self-confidence. Careful specification and measurement of these variables should allow a test of the frequent observation in the literature that some women feel defeminized and empty (Ekblad, 1961) or perceive themselves as devalued by their spouses after contraceptive sterilization (Whitehouse, 1971).

The third area in which outcome must be assessed is the interpersonal and social. In considering the family, it is useful to distinguish between the impact of surgery on the spouse and on the children. Of primary interest with regard to the spouse are the subsequent patterns of sexual behavior and the modes of interaction around issues of affection, respect, dependency, power, and trust. Relative to the children, it may be that female contraceptive sterilization will have effects upon the woman's degree of involvement with them, on her ability to nurture and discipline them, and on her differential attitudes toward and handling of boys and girls. Potentially important variables at the social level include the woman's ongoing relationship with her parents, especially her mother, her pattern of friendships with other men and women, and her work activities.

It should be noted that the passage of time is a crucial element when assessing the outcome of female contraceptive sterilization; outcomes can be expected to vary according to the point in time after surgery chosen for study. It is quite possible, for instance, that the sexual effects of tubal ligation will be considerable at six months postsurgery but minimal at six years. The opposite may be true regarding the effects of tubal ligation on reproductive sentiments. These variations in outcome variables along the trajectory of the postintervention stage also depend on the woman's age when the surgery was undergone. Other things—such as parity—being equal, postsurgical changes in the self-esteem of a twenty-year-old woman may follow quite a different course from that of a woman of thirty-five.

It has frequently been claimed that the woman's mental health prior to surgery is the best predictor of psychological outcome (Woodruff and Pauerstein, 1969). This is not necessarily the case. An analogy may be drawn to the field of plastic surgery, with which contraceptive sterilization has a number of significant similarities; both involve the use of physicians and medical technology for the pursuit of personal goals frequently unrelated to a disease state or disability. The experience of the plastic surgeons has refuted the intuitive notion that psychiatrically disturbed individuals are generally bad risks (Edgerton, 1960; Meyer, 1964). Greater experience with contraceptive sterilization may well do the same. In addition, it must be kept in mind that — as with therapeutic abortion for the psychiatrically disturbed—inaction on the part of physicians may be as risky as granting the request. In other words, since the risk runs both ways, the chances of a bad outcome may be increased when the procedure is *not* carried through.

How a woman's mental health prior to surgery affects her psychological outcome is, of course, only a special instance of the more general problem of risk following female contraceptive sterilization. The question is complex. Many different types of outcomes must be considered, each manifesting itself according to a different post surgical time schedule. Without trying to do justice to these subtleties, let us turn to a consideration of psychological outcomes, making use of the motivational and decision-making variables that have already been considered.

First of all, with regard to the motivational dimensions listed on p. 123-124, a woman with a high level of any given motivation may be expected to have a better psychological outcome than someone less motivated, the optimum outcome occuring when most or all of the nine motivations for surgery were high. Second, with regard to the decision-making variables, the best psychological outcomes should occur among women who:

1.   are more future-oriented;
2.   more readily acknowledge the social and psychological problems that confront them;
3.   are more unconstricted in their problem-solving;
4.   are more independent in their problem-solving.

With regard to couples, it was noted earlier that the dominance-submissiveness dimension may be important during the consideration phase of decision-making. Supporting this hypothesis is the conclusion of Ziegler, Rodgers, and Prentiss (1969) that female contraceptive methods will be highly satisfactory for the couple when the woman is not subordinate to her husband, whereas the male forms will be more satisfactory when she is more subordinate. Thus, in predicting couple satisfaction, it may be hypothesized that the best outcome following female surgical contraception will occur in couples when the women are relatively high on dominance.

There are two additional noteworthy observations in the literature about women at risk following contraceptive sterilization. Adams (1964) provides some suggestive evidence that the imposition of a waiting period between the application for surgery and the procedure itself successfully decreases the incidence of dissatisfaction on follow-up. While the enforced hiatus is, of course, only a crude way of helping patients make an appropriate final choice, Adams's finding highlights the fact the the decision-making process is an important variable in the outcome. In the future, rather than imposing a waiting period, it should be possible to counsel applicants, using knowledge gained from further studies of the decision-making process. A second observation is that of Barglow and his colleagues, who identified a "working-through" period following contraceptive sterilization which involved the patient's use of certain adaptive, compensatory mechanisms, such as a fantasy restitution of fertility (Barglow, Gunther, Johnson, and Meltzer, 1965). Such adaptation and coping mechanisms are certain to influence the postsurgical course and to differentiate among the types of individuals at risk for an undesirable outcome. The processes of adaptation, especially the more successful ones, must be described and studied more fully to facilitate anticipatory guidance at the time of decision-making and to improve the effectiveness of psychological intervention following surgery when adaptive difficulty has developed.

## Final Comments

The preceding remarks have concentrated on those variables, concepts, and hypotheses which appear to be most useful in future research. However, several other methodological issues of equal importance also deserve careful thought and attention. Special consideration, first of all, must enter into the selection of comparison groups in studies of contraceptive sterilization. A true control group is, in practice, impossible to obtain. Comparison may be made between women seeking contraceptive sterilization and a random community sample; to the degree that the contraceptive group is highly self-selected, however, such a comparison would be rather misleading in any outcome study. For research on outcome, it would seem better to compare the female contraceptive sterilization group to other homogeneous groups of women at an equivalent decision point in their lives who select a course of action other than surgery; such as couples where the wife selects a non-permanent method of contraception or where the husband obtains a vasectomy. Again, to avoid misleading comparisons, at least two such groups should be included.

A second methodological issue regards the development of research instruments. There is a pressing need at this time for intermediate and large-scale studies (with $N$s from 100 up to several thousand) which can comfortably be paired with and complement detailed, in-depth, "clinical" studies. For the larger investigations, relatively short assessment instruments must be developed. These instruments can best be validated through an in-depth approach, but should be designed so that they may be applied readily with large samples and under the pressures of a clinical situation.

Finally, the importance of the cultural context of future investigations demands reemphasis. Most of what has been said in this chapter applies reasonably well to middle-class America. The hypotheses are conceivably applicable beyond this population, one that on a world scale must be considered a very definite minority, but it is impossible at this point in the development of our knowledge to know to what extent such an application will be useful. Whatever happens, it is clear that cultural factors will significantly influence the relationships between the variables that have been suggested here. Future work should take this into account by implementing cross-cultural investigations that allow systematic comparison of different samples, in two or more cultural settings, concerning the numerous questions about the psychosocial aspects of contraceptive sterilization in women which confront us.

## References

Ackner, B. "Emotional Aspects of Hysterectomy. A Follow-Up Study of

Fifty Patients Under the Age of 40," in A. Jores and H. Freyberger, eds., *Advances in Psychosomatic Medicine,* Symposium of the Fourth European Conference on Psychosomatic Research. New York: Robert Brunner, Inc., 1961.

Adams, T.W. "Female Sterilization." *Amer. J. Obstet. Gynec.* 89, 3 (June 1, 1964): 395-401.

Barglow, P. "Pseudocyesis and Psychiatric Sequelae of Sterilization." *Arch. Gen. Psychiat.* 11, 6 (December 1964): 571-80.

Barglow, P. and Eisner, M. "An Evaluation of Tubal Ligation in Switzerland." *Amer. J. Obstet. Gynec.* 95, 8 (August 15, 1966): 1083-94.

Barglow, P., Gunther, M.S., Johnson, A., and Meltzer, H.J. "Hysterectomy and Tubal Ligation: A Psychiatric Comparison." *Obstet. Gynec.* 25, 4 (April 1965): 520-27.

Barnes, A.C. and Zuspan, F. "Patient Reaction to Puerperal Surgical Sterilization." *Amer. J. Obstet. Gynec.* 75 (1958): 65.

Baudry, F., Herzig, N., and Wiener, A. "Assessment of Patients Seeking Tubal Sterilization on Psychological Ground." *Obstet. Gynec.* 38, 3 (September 1971): 411-15.

Borland, B.L. "Behavioral Factors in Non-Coital Methods of Contraception: A Review." *Soc. Sci. & Med.* 6 (1972): 163-78.

Brim, O.G., Jr., Glass, D.C., Lavin, D.E., and Goodman, N. *Personality and Decision Processes.* Stanford, Ca.: Stanford University Press, 1962.

Brody, H., Meikle, S., and Gerritse, R. "Therapeutic Abortion: A Prospective Study, 1," *Amer. J. Obstet. Gynec.* 109, 3 (February 1, 1971): 347-53.

Calderone, M.S. *Manual of Family Planning and Contraceptive Practice.* 2nd ed. Baltimore: The Williams & Wilkins Co., 1970.

Drellich, M.G. and Bieber, I. "The Psychologic Importance of the Uterus and Its Functions," *J. Nerv. & Men. Dis.* 126, 4 (April 1958): 322-36.

Duncan, G.W., Falb, R.D., and Speidel, J.J. *Female Sterilization: Prognosis for Simplified Outpatient Procedures.* New York: Academic Press, 1972.

Edgerton, M.T., Jacobson, W.E., and Meyer, E. "Surgical-Psychiatric Study of Patients Seeking Plastic (Cosmetic) Surgery: 98 Consecutive Patients with Minimal Deformities." *British J. Plastic Surgery* 13 (1960): 136-45.

Ekblad, M. "The Prognosis After Sterilization on Social-Psychiatric Grounds, A Follow-Up Study of 225 Women." *Acta Psychiatric Scandinavica.* Supplementum 161, (1961) Vol. 37.

Ellison, R.M. "Psychiatric Complications Following Sterilization of Women." *The Medical Journal of Australia* 2 (October 17, 1964).

Fisher, S. "A Further Appraisal of the Body Boundary Concept." *J. Consulting Psychol.* 27, 1 (1963): 62-74.

Fisher, S. "Body Attention Patterns and Personality Defenses." *Psychological Monographs* 80, 9, No. 617 (1966).

Hamburg, D.A., Coelho, G.V., and Adams, J.E., eds. *Coping and Adaptation.* New York: Basic Books, 1973.

Hibbard, L.T. "Sexual Sterilization by Elective Hysterectomy." *Amer. J. Obstet. Gynec.* 112 (1972): 1076.

Kolb, L.C. *Modern Clinical Psychiatry.* 8th ed. Philadelphia: W.B. Saunders, 1973.

Lindemann, E. "Observations on Psychiatric Sequelae to Surgical Operations in Women." *Amer. J. Psychiat.* 98 (July 1941): 132-39.

Melody, G.F. "Depressive Reactions Following Hysterectomy." *Amer. J. Obstet. Gynec.* 83 (Jan-Mar 1962): 410-13.

Meyer, E. "Psychiatric Aspects of Plastic Surgery," Ch. 15, in J.M. Converse, ed., *Reconstructive Plastic Surgery.* Philadelphia: W.B. Saunders, 1964, pp. 365-83.

Miller, W.B. "Conception Mastery: Ego Control of the Psychological and Behavioral Antecedents to Conception," *Comments on Contemporary Psychiatry,* 1 (1973): 157-77

Moore, D.W. "Sequelae of Tubal Ligation, Medical and Psychological." *Amer. J. Obstet. Gynec.* 101, 3 (June 1, 1968): 350-51.

Norris, A.S. "An Examination of the Effects of Tubal Ligation: Their Implications for Prediction." *Amer. J. Obstet. Gynec.* 90 (1964): 431.

Paniagua, M.E., Tayback, M., Janer, J.L., and Vázquez, J.L. "Medical and Psychological Sequelae of Surgical Sterilization of Women." *Amer. J. Obstet. Gynec.* 90, 4 (October 15, 1964): 421-30.

Presser, H.B. "Voluntary Sterilization: A World View." *Reports on Population/ Family Planning,* No. 5 (July 1970).

Roach, C.J., Krolak, J.D., Powell, J.L., Llorens, A.S., and Deubler, K.F. "Vaginal Hysterectomy for Sterilization." *Amer. J. Obstet. Gynec.* 114 (1972): 670.

Rodgers, D.A. and Ziegler, F.J. "Psychological Reactions to Surgical Contraception," in J.T. Fawcett, ed., *Psychological Perspectives on Population.* New York: Basic Books, 1973.

Sacks, S. and La Croix, G. "Gynecologic Sequelae of Postpartum Tubal Ligation," *Obstet. Gynec.* 19 (1962): 22.

Schneider, H.E. "Aussagen and Ergebnisse nach Tubensterilisation." *Geburtsh. u. Frauenheilk.* 32 (1972): 290-97.

Schulman, H. "Major Surgery for Abortion and Sterilization." Editorial, *Obstet. Gynec.* 40 (1972): 738.

Schwyhart, W.R. and Kutner, S.J. "A Reanalysis of Female Reaction to Contraceptive Sterilization." *J. Nerv. & Men. Dis.,* 56 (May, 1975): 354-70.

Thompson, B. and Baird, D. "Follow-Up of 186 Sterilised Women." *Lancet* 1 (7550) (May 11, 1968).

Whelpton, P.K. and Kiser, C.V. "Social and Psychological Factors Affecting Fertility." *The Eugenics Review* 51 (April 1959): 35-42.

Whitehouse, D.B. Letter. *Brit. Med. J.* 2 (June 1971): 707.

Woodruff, J.D. and Pauerstein, C.J. *The Fallopian Tube: Structure, Function, Pathology and Management.* Baltimore: The Williams & Wilkins Co., 1969.

Ziegler, F.J., Rodgers, D.A., and Prentiss, R.J. "Psychosocial Response to Vasectomy." *Arch. Gen. Psychiat.* 21 (July 1969): 46-54.

# 9

## The Incidence of Psychological Complications After Contraceptive Sterilization
### Helen Wolfers

Increasing research is being devoted to the psychological effects of sterilization. By identifying the characteristics of those who have proven to be psychologically unsuited to contraceptive sterilization, investigators ultimately aim for the pre-operative prediction of candidates with a high risk of bad psychological outcome. Two reasons inform this endeavor: patient welfare and the greater interest in the effectiveness of contraceptive sterilization for population control, which depends on widespread public faith.

The first duty of physicians to their patients is to do no harm. "Harm," however, is a relative concept. From the doctor's point of view, the situation may arise when contraceptive sterilization is medically indicated as the lesser of two evils even on persons likely to have negative psychological reactions. The public acceptability of contraceptive sterilization in the service of population control is threatened, however, by anyone who regrets having been sterilized and who remains for life an irremovable source of skepticism and fear to others. The effectiveness of contraceptive sterilization for population control is measured by the extent of its adoption by those who wish, definitively to end their reproduction, or by those whose families are large enough to indicate a need for sterilization. Widespread acceptance, in turn, depends on the growth of confidence in the method and in the integrity of those who advocate and administer contraceptive sterilization. Unless kept to a minimum, the likelihood of untoward psychological reactions would undoubtedly sap public confidence in contraceptive sterilization.

In 1957, Allan Guttmacher (1957, pp. 601-602) wrote, ". . . one may hazard the guess that nineteen patients in twenty will be happy and grateful for the permanent prevention of conception. . . . However, one patient in twenty will change her mind. . . can we pick out this twentieth patient? I think not."

Despite Guttmacher's misgivings, much effort has continued to be expended at least to reduce the incidence of this unfortunate occurrence. Public concern about postoperative psychological complications has also increased, especially since the advent of vasectomy as a large-scale contraceptive procedure. Today it is almost standard for doctors, clinics, and organized family planning programs to attempt some form of psychological screening and/or counseling before contraceptive sterilization.

As contraceptive sterilization has developed into a tool for population

137

control (as distinct from a method for individual family limitation), severe restriction of its use has given way to liberalization and, recently, to its active promotion. We do not know how the promotional changes have affected the incidence of postoperative psychological complications. With research in the area so unstandardized, simple comparison of currently reported complication rates with those of a decade ago are of little value. The definition of complication, the method of inquiry, and, above all, the bias of the researchers vary among studies to such an extent that reported psychological complication rates fluctuate widely even within the same culture at the same time.

A dilemma faces those interested in population research on contraceptive sterilization. It is unlikely that standardization of follow-up procedures will in practice be possible as long as contraceptive sterilization remains a controversial issue, for conflicting emotional motives are involved in the instigation of such research. Yet, because contraceptive sterilization remains a "hot" issue, there is urgency about assessing and reducing the incidence of negative psychological after-effects.

To evaluate the effects of contraceptive sterilization, it may be more productive to study each of several isolated variables, rather than the overall outcomes. Because institutions differ in their forms of preoperative counseling and screening, there is an opportunity for such a research approach.

The following five areas seem particularly worthy of consideration:

1. *Preoperative counseling*

It is universally accepted that a clear understanding by the patient of what is involved in the forthcoming operation reduces the incidence of postoperative regret. Important questions remain about preoperative counseling for contraceptive sterilization.

a. Does it convey information effectively? This question requires further research, but there appear to be indications that despite individualized preoperative counseling, some patients do not even realize after the operation that they are sterile.

b. Does counseling differ substantially between various large institutions— and if so, how? One dimension to examine might be that of activity-passivity in the interviews.

c. Could more effective counseling methods be devised, such as a requirement to pass a written or oral test before being accepted for contraceptive sterilization?

2. *Preoperative screening*

The elimination or dissuasion of applicants for contraceptive sterilization is based today on a number of fairly generally accepted criteria, some more widely used than others: age; parity; marital status; marital harmony; mental stability; and motivation.

Worthy of investigation are:

a. Comparison between several large clinical centers in the criteria they employ and in the strictness of implementation.

b. Comparison of the rejection rates among these institutions.

c. Follow-up of applicants who are accepted by one institution, but would ostensibly have failed to meet acceptance criteria set by others.

3.  *Fate of the patient refused contraceptive sterilization on first application*

a. What proportion of rejected applicants actually end up being sterilized? Some doctors, when refusing to carry out a contraceptive sterilization, refer the patient to other doctors or clinics where he or she may have better luck. It is therefore possible that the initial screening process has zero or near zero effect on one's chances to qualify somewhere for acceptance.

b. What is the outcome for patients who obtain a sterilizing operation after one or more refusals?

4.  *Effects of promotion*

Among doctors and clinics, there are those who *offer* contraceptive sterilization and those who *promote* the procedure. (The two categories are distinguished in the literature by the presence or absence of the adverb *only* in their reports of postoperative psychological complication rates.) The motivation of candidates for contraceptive sterilization coming to these two groups may differ significantly. The nature and intensity of preoperative counseling and screening may also be influenced by the orientation of the institution or physician, even to the extent of determining the side of the screen to which the patient is ultimately shunted.

It may be productive to compare promoting and nonpromoting institutions and doctors with respect to:

a. Screening and counseling procedures.

b. Rejection rates.

c. Initial (precounseled) motivation of the patient for seeking contraceptive sterilization.

d. Incidence of postoperative psychological complaints among patients (assessed by someone other than the agency or physician providing the contraceptive sterilization service).

5.  *Effects of incentives*

Few studies have addressed themselves to the incidence of postoperative complaints as a function of the payment of incentives. A Korean study by Lee (1966) found proportionately fewer nonsubsidized patients reporting a decrease in sexual desire or activity than did subsidized patients. Direct questioning of vasectomy patients in India as to their motives in undergoing the operation resulted in 43 percent of a sample of 297 men stating that money was "the sole motivating factor." In another follow-up study of 146 vasectomized men, 36 percent were found to have been sterilized, only or primarily for the money. Incentives have resulted in coercion, illegality, and illogicality in the practice of sterilization in India and it is not unreasonable to suspect that this has affected the psychological side effects of the procedure (Wolfers and Wolfers, 1973).[a]

These figures point to the need for controlled studies on the psychological outcome of subsidized contraceptive sterilization. In addition, even for those who seek the surgery primarily to render themselves sterile, the offering of an incentive (or subsidy) has complicated psychological overtones. Payment implies a buyer and a seller. Symbolically, it implies wanting something "of" the person, or "for" him. Alternatively, it could be viewed unconsciously by the recipient as a compensation, rather than an incentive; the next connection, even more dangerous at the unconscious level than at the conscious is, "To be compensated, I must have suffered some damage."

In the assessment of postoperative complication rates, the criterion of "bad" outcome urgently needs clarification. Once again, the eventual impact on public confidence must be considered. It is admittedly of importance, especially to the physician, to know whether the "bad" outcome is caused by the contraceptive sterilization. For the wider purposes of making contraceptive sterilization an effective population control method, however, the mere fact that the patient *attributes* his or her problem to the operation is the vital factor. Concern for the success of the program suggests the definition of bad outcomes as any believed by the patient to be bad and attributed by him or her to the contraceptive sterilization. It is irrelevant to argue whether the complication is "in fact" because of the operation or whether it would have occurred anyway as a result of some other life situation.

What is "good" and what is "bad," in any case, is not free of the impact of culture or time. In the assessment of reported postoperative sexual changes, for instance, increase in sexual desire and coital frequency is taken automatically as indicative of "good" outcome. This may be true for the permissive society characteristic of the latter half of the twentieth century in the West. However, it is frequently found that Indian men *complain* of increased sexual appetite after contraceptive sterilization and have even been known to offer this as a reason for seeking reanastomosis. Even in Western society, increase in coital frequency after contraceptive sterilization has been interpreted in some cases as a sign of psychological distress and a neurotic manifestation of anxiety about potency. The same reaction (heightened sexuality) can thus indicate either a "good" or "bad" psychological outcome.

A legitimate case can be made here for the adoption of a double standard. "Good" outcomes believed by the patient to be bad should be defined as bad

---

[a]In an as yet unpublished study of female sterilization in Singapore involving over 2,000 women, we have found no difference in the incidence of reported psychological ill-effects between those undergoing contraceptive sterilization with and without monetary reward. It would appear that no sweeping statement on the question of monetary inducement in this area is justified and that each program must be assessed in its own context.

outcomes by the investigators on the theory that the subjective evaluation will undermine public confidence in contraceptive surgery. Conversely, deleterious outcomes believed by the patient to be good must also be viewed by the investigators as unacceptable (on the same principle that one cannot go about performing lobotomies on people simply because they are unable to recognize their loss). Dual concern for both the patient and the effectiveness of the contraceptive sterilization program for population control points research toward maximizing "good" postoperative adjustment that is perceived as such both by the patient and by others.

## References

Guttmacher, A.F. "Puerperal Sterilization on the Private and Ward Services of a Large Metropolitan Hospital." *Fertility and Sterility* 8 (1957): 591-602.

Lee, H.Y. "Studies on Vasectomy: (3) Clinical Studies on the Influence of Vasectomy." *Korean Journal of Urology* 7 (1966): 11-29.

Wolfers, D. and Wolfers, H. *Vasectomy and Vasectomania.* London: Granada Publications, 1973.

# 10

## Acceptability of Contraceptive Sterilization: Psychosocial Research Approaches
### Henry P. David and Herbert L. Friedman

### Introduction

Throughout the world, psychosocial research on the acceptability of fertility-regulating methods and procedures is gradually attracting the interest of a wide spectrum of behavioral scientists and their colleagues in related fields of knowledge. Technical advances in contraception, abortion, or fertility termination, in family planning and population education, and in advertising and marketing concepts are but partial determinants of fertility behavior. The actual decision to have or not to have a child—or when to have another or how many—flows from complex couple interactions and choice behaviors, influenced by a universe of variables, many of which are culturally determined (David and Friedman, 1973). No doubt, a given characteristic of a particular fertility-regulating or fertility-terminating method may have an intrinsic "acceptability"; the importance of the feature, however, is subject to a much broader set of variables.

In considering contraceptive sterilization, for example, a couple faces a decision with psychological dimensions other than the sheer nature of the surgery. Should the man or the woman have the operation? Or both? How is the decision reached? To what degree does the virtual irreversibility of the procedure affect the choice among the two spouses, each a potential candidate for surgery? For contraceptive surgery what is the differential influence of the factors that commonly weigh for or against fertility termination, such as the fertility career stage of the couple, their ages and marital status, number of living children, and the lapse of time between the possible decision and acting upon it? To what extent are potential consequences taken into account? How will contraceptive sterilization affect sexual behavior and the subsequent relationships of the couple?

The contributions of many disciplines are needed to describe, study, and understand fertility-regulating behavior in diverse sociocultural milieux. Of paramount importance is the development of psychosocial methods to assess "acceptability"—and related components of individual and/or couple choice behavior. Ideally, research methods should grow in tandem with a theory of fertility behavior and testable hypotheses oriented to the interests of both social scientists and clinical investigators.

We are pleased to acknowledge the considerable contributions to this paper of our colleagues in the Cooperative Transnational Research Program in Fertility Behavior.

143

With an eye on needed research, this chapter surveys briefly some background considerations related to fertility termination, and outlines the investigative approach of the Transnational Family Research Institute and its associated Cooperative Transnational Research Program in Fertility Behavior. Other topics ripe for study are delineated in the concluding section.

### Fertility Termination (Contraceptive Sterilization)

In the whole spectrum of choices available for fertility limitation—from coitus interruptus and condom to diaphragm, pill, IUD, or abortion—contraceptive sterilization is the only method giving both the woman and the man equal opportunity for initiating action. Fertility termination (or contraceptive sterilization) is generally a one-time event, 100 percent effective if well done, and usually permanent. As noted in the introduction, little research has been reported on the couple's communication and decision-making process and on which partner should have the operation when the choice is viable for both.

A worldwide shift in fertility-regulating behavior appears in the making. In the United States, there is considerable evidence from the 1965 and 1970 National Fertility Surveys of a dynamic change in the fertility-regulating behavior of couples. Until the early 1960s, about 50 percent of American births were the result of accidental pregnancy (Bumpass and Westoff, 1970). At the time of conception some 20 percent were unwanted, often with subsequent psychosocial cost to the child, the family, and society (David, 1972). The growing incidence and prevalence of contraceptive sterilization in the United States—whether by female or male methods—is documented by Presser and Bumpass (1972a, 1972b); Bumpass and Presser (1972), and by Bumpass (1974). Similar trends internationally have been well summarized in a number of recent papers (Presser, 1970; Ross et al., 1972; Speidel, 1972a, 1972b; Potts, 1974).

During the past decade in the United States the rapid diffusion of modern contraceptive methods has greatly improved protection against accidental pregnancy. More recently, safe, legal abortion as a back-up procedure has become available in many major U.S. cities. Abortion has become even more accessible since the gradual implementation of the 1973 U.S. Supreme Court decision which makes the procedure during the first trimester only a matter of medical, not legal, judgment. With the recurrent questions about longer-term sequelae of oral contraceptives and intrauterine devices, couples wishing to avoid unwanted pregnancies are giving increasing consideration to fertility termination by male or female contraceptive sterilization. Presser and Bumpass (1972a), noting the rapid rise in the incidence of sterilization among older couples, concluded that "voluntary sterilization may well become the preferred contraceptive method among couples who desire no more children" (p. 18). Other available contraceptive techniques are simply not sufficiently reliable to control fertility throughout a fertile lifetime (Potts, 1974). Definitive fertility control is particularly important for less-developed countries, where age at marriage is low and desired family size is achieved early.

The provision of fertility-terminating methods is, of course, related to its legal status, which in much of the world is unclear. Except for a few jurisdictions, laws specifically covering voluntary sterilization are either nonexistent or outdated (Stepan and Kellogg, 1973). Where laws have been promulgated, they tend to be found in the criminal code, although restrictive legislation is usually disregarded and prosecutions are rare. There are some paradoxes in legal attitudes. The German Democratic Republic, for example, recently adopted very liberal abortion legislation (German Democratic Republic, 1972), but limits "irreversible contraception" to instances based on eugenic and medical reasons (Rothe, 1973). In liberal Sweden, similarly, vasectomy for contraceptive purposes is illegal; Swedish men fly to London for the operation (Potts, 1974). In view of radical changes in official attitudes toward fertility termination in the form of abortion, it seems possible that terminating fertility capability may eventually be deemed a basic human right in the United States and elsewhere.

An IPPF Panel of Experts recently recommended that both male and female contraceptive sterilization should be made available as part of a comprehensive family planning service (Potts, 1974). Medical/societal constraints continue to work against this recommendation, with physicians' prejudices and administrative barriers in many countries tending to limit contraceptive sterilization to women of advanced age and high parity. Again, there are curious paradoxes: witness the more favorable medical attitude in Puerto Rico compared to New York City or most Latin American countries. In recent years, however, the health professions have become more favorably disposed toward contraceptive sterilization. In the United States, many professional societies have dropped restrictive standards; a growing number of vasectomy clinics and voluntary and governmental family planning programs are providing fertility-terminating services; and hospital facilities have become more accessible (sometimes following lawsuits) (Presser and Bumpass, 1972b).

As more and more couples are able seriously to deliberate whether either partner or both should terminate fertility capability, the medical profession's major task may well become to determine when *not* to perform the operation. Disturbed individuals, who seek the procedure for self-destructive reasons or to hurt their partners, for example, may be legitimately refused (Potts, 1974). The personal fears of potential candidates may also have to be dealt with; see Pai (1974) on the experience of Indian physicians.

Psychosocial follow-up studies and behavioral sequelae of contraceptive sterilization are the subject of other chapters in this volume and have been extensively reviewed elsewhere (Rodgers and Ziegler, 1974, 1973; Wolfers, 1970). Only a comment on the issue will be made here.

Under optimal conditions, according to authorities on the matter (Rodgers and Ziegler, 1974), fertility-terminating procedures have "minimal psychological side effects" and allow for "highly effective separation of sexual pleasure from procreation" for couples who do not desire additional pregnancies. Under non-optimal conditions, these procedures "can precipitate mildly to severely disabling psychological mediated reactions." The primary basis for these appears to be "a misconception of (the) procedures as having demasculinizing or defeminizing potential" (p. 165). The IPPF Panel on Sterilization observed that "perhaps too much emphasis has been placed on the special nature of sterilization," a medical undertaking which could be considered not very different from other elective surgical procedures (Potts, 1974, p. 100). It appears desirable to launch studies of the antecedents, as well as the short-term or long-term consequences or mental health implications, of fertility-terminating procedures.

**Psychosocial Research**

Throughout their fertile years, individuals and couples are faced with many choice points and alternative courses of action which determine the success of their efforts to control their fertility if they so wish. The extent to which the choice points and alternatives are recognized, as well as the degree to which costs and consequences are realistically appraised, are cornerstones of healthy fertility and fertility-regulating behavior.

As noted earlier, the "acceptability" of a specific method of fertility termination is just one of a much broader set of variables ultimately determining the behavioral choice. The psychosocial assessment of intrinsic "acceptability," in this sense, is likely to be affected by other aspects of the situation. A comprehensive psychosocial model of fertility choice behavior has been outlined by Friedman (1972, 1973). Five major categories of variables — interacting for or against delaying or preventing pregnancy — constitute the model: (1) environmental factors; (2) individual characteristics; (3) perception and evaluation of the environment regarding fertility-regulating decisions; (4) available alternative courses of fertility behavior, with their associated psychosocial costs, beliefs, and evaluations of real or potential outcomes; and (5) couple relationship. Within each of the major categories the relative weight of a given variable may differ between cultures or couples.

The model assumes the importance of both the "objective" environmental facts and the "subjective" ways in which they are perceived by an individual and/or couple, in a choice situation in which alternatives are available. The *perceptions* of the user and the *expectations* of the potential user (or rejector) play a major role in the "acceptability" of a particular method.

Still another important relationship to be considered is the interaction between service users and service providers (Friedman, 1973). As in the psychosocial model just described, studies of user/system interaction involve the subjective assessment of events affecting individual behavior, as well as "objective" data about the same phenomena — the psychosocial costs. Of major interest are those aspects of the system that concern the acquisition of information, supplies, or services related to a method of birth prevention and its associated costs. Variables to be measured might include:

1. *Service costs.* How and where to get service, relative economic costs, and the time needed for and comfort of service.
2. *Product and/or method costs.* Timing of method, the physical attributes of and number of actions needed for use, who is the responsible partner, the degree and type of skill required in use, and the product efficiency.
3. *Perception of user(s).* The relative evaluation of alternative systems by each attribute of the service, the product, and/or the method, partner concordance, and the accuracy of mutual perception.

Data on user/system interaction would be drawn from the users of the system, the service providers, and objective measures of the service system itself.

After the service has already been delivered, it is important to observe what the user reports to other people about the operation. The role of the user as informant to potential adopters has been recognized in studies of continuing provision of fertility-*regulating* methods. Word of mouth concerning contraceptive sterilization procedures, however, could also greatly influence the acceptability of such a service, particularly in less-developed countries.

**Additional Research Suggestions**

Despite considerable educational efforts, there remain gross misconceptions about the nature of contraceptive sterilization and its consequences. A report from Belgium (Thiery et al., 1974), for example, has suggested that many laymen and even physicians in developed countries still associate sterilization with castration. Medical and paramedical personnel unconsciously resistant to the procedure may unintentionally provide incomplete or wrong information about it to inquiring patients.

Very little study has been devoted to the effects among the public and policy-makers in diverse cultures of the nomenclature or euphemisms used to describe fertility-terminating methods and the events surrounding them. Even those most interested in research on the procedures do not agree on what to call the general topic. What this volume calls *contraceptive sterilization* has also been titled *permanent contraception* (McLaren, 1973), *surgical contraception* (Rodgers and Ziegler, 1974), *irreversible contraception* (Rothe, 1973), and *fertility termination* (Bernard, 1973). Psychosocial researchers should be particularly attentive to language because they depend a great deal on verbal reports which may be especially vulnerable to the effects and/or unconscious resistances generated by certain terms. Several available research measures could be applied to the matter of nomenclature, including the semantic differential (with different names for the same phenomenon), response latency as an indicator of difficulty or affective ambivalence, and other well-established psycholinguistic techniques. Both medical and popular terms should be studied, especially in regard to their meanings in different sociocultural milieux.

The influence of marital roles is another fruitful area for study. Deys and Potts (1973) have suggested that vasectomy may appeal more to men assuming a dominant role in marriage and fertility regulation, whereas female contraceptive sterilization may be more acceptable when marital partners share decisions and tasks. In Latin societies, where men frequently dominate and fertility regulation is often deemed by both sexes to be the "man's business," several countries have reported increasing resort to vasectomy (although female contraceptive sterilization continues to be preferred). Conversely, in the United States, where women have an increasingly stronger voice in decision-making, vasectomy is more openly discussed and used as a viable alternative. Indeed, some clinics now offer vasectomy for the husband while the wife has an abortion. The effects of dominance or mutuality in the marriage, at any rate, deserve further study.

A research perspective should also be invoked in thinking about public persuasion to undergo fertility termination procedures and the concomitant ethical and social ramifications of this pressure. Should individual needs and individual/couple decisions override public needs? To what extent is indiscriminate and excessive public persuasion coercive or perceived as such? In India, for example, the introduction of cash incentives has generated extensive discussion of the program's ethical, social, behavioral, perceptual, and organizational aspects (George, 1973). Such concerns loom much larger with irreversible contraceptive sterilization than with fertility-regulating methods that can be discontinued or corrected.

Research is no luxury. At the February 1973 Geneva Conference on Voluntary Sterilization, it was recognized that systematic evaluation, adaptable transnationally, is becoming increasingly necessary for effective and efficient public health program planning and management. In addition to generating new knowledge, social research should also have something to communicate to program administrators, clinic directors, and policy-makers. Studies of the population at risk must supplement clinic records, which are seldom representative of the total community served. Investigators embarking on transnational studies must also resign themselves to constraints on their questions in certain cultures particularly sensitive on some issues and should expect some categories of responses not to be reliable.

### Summary and Conclusions

Contraceptive sterilization for men and women is becoming increasingly available throughout the world. As a method, it is in certain respects fundamentally different from other contraceptive approaches. It provides permanent and, as yet, virtually irreversible contraception. Its provision by government and public and private health facilities raises ethical questions, while its freely determined adoption by individuals or couples raises psychological ones.

Because contraceptive sterilization provides both a certain and a permanent limitation of birth, the method, in general, is especially attractive for governments seriously concerned about excessive population growth. Relatively simple and done only once, the necessary procedures may constitute the most effective of all contraceptive programs, on a cost-benefit basis. Ethical questions remain, however. The fundamental issue is, minimally, who shall be allowed to choose such methods for themselves and, maximally, who should be motivated or persuaded to select the procedures. In densely overpopulated countries, for example, the public pressures are very great for the widespread adoption of vasectomy or tubal ligation. Should the methods be restricted, however, to couples who are married and have already had as many children as they wish? Should the consent of both partners be required? Should there be an age limit? Should eligibility be predicated on some minimum number of children already born to the couple? What is the realm of free choice for the mentally retarded? The nature of the questions will, of course, have specific cultural determinants to some extent, but the ethics of public policy in general involve problems that must be raised and somehow resolved.

From the individual or couple point of view, contraceptive sterilization brings up other problems. For the couple no longer wishing to have children, the advantages of the procedure are undeniable. Free of the need for any other method of contraception or abortion, they avoid unwelcome potential side effects and long-range effects, costs, and stresses on their sexual relations. At the same time, contraceptive sterilization may create its own difficulties. Some individuals, especially men, react to the procedure with unfounded fears of impaired sexual potency. Both members of the couple may also have to live with the fear that their living children will be lost through some misfortune, leaving them unable to have others. In some societies, finally, the question looms as to which partner, the man or the woman, or both, ought to have the procedure. Individual dominance within the couple and the specter of the unbridled infidelity of the sterilized partner may then become issues for the man and wife considering the procedure for themselves.

The social variable of method taboo is another major factor influencing the acceptability of contraceptive sterilization. In some societies—Latin America, for example — many men and women tend to consider vasectomy undesirable. Contraceptive sterilization will encounter taboos related to masculinity/femininity, the religious objection to sexual activity without procreational possibility, and, in some areas, a negative attitude toward surgery of any kind.

Research on these social, psychological, and public health issues is only beginning, largely because the methods themselves have not been widely available for long. Some approaches have been described in this chapter, particularly on psychological aspects of choice behavior in fertility regulation. Attention must be given especially to the fertility career stage of the couple when making their decision and the need to evaluate alternatives, their psychosocial costs to each partner, the expected outcomes, and the values placed on those outcomes. By studying the dynamics of fertility-regulating choice behavior, the consequences to individuals and families may be better judged.

**References**

Bernard, R.P. "Recent Concepts and Findings: Sterilizees in India and Bangladesh: A Background Collection in Twelve Charts." Paper presented at the Second International Conference on Voluntary Sterilization, Geneva, Switzerland (February-March 1973).

Bumpass, L. "The Increasing Acceptance of Sterilization in the U.S." In *Advances in Voluntary Sterilization,* Proceedings of the Second International Conference, Geneva, 1973, edited by M.E. Schima, I. Lubell, J.E. Davis, and E. Connell, pp. 104-111. Princeton, N.J.: Excerpta Medica, American Elsevier Publishing Co., Inc., 1974.

Bumpass, L.L. and Presser, H.B. "Contraceptive Sterilization in the United States: 1965 and 1970." *Demography* 9 (1972): 531-48.

Bumpass, L.L. and Westoff, C.F. "The 'Perfect Contraceptive' Population." *Science* 196 (1970): 1177-82.

David, H.P. "Unwanted Pregnancies: Costs and Alternatives." In C.F. Westoff and P. Parke, Jr., eds., *Demographic and Social Aspects of Population Growth.* Vol. 1 of Report of the Commission on Population Growth and the American Future. Washington: United States Government Printing Office, 1972, Stock No. 5258-00005, pp. 439-66.

David, H.P. and Friedman, H.L. "Psychosocial Research in Abortion: A Transnational Perspective." In H.J. Osofsky and J.D. Osofsky, eds., *Abortion Experience in the United States.* New York: Harper & Row, 1973.

Deys, C.M. and Potts, M. "Condoms and Things." Unpublished paper, 1973.

Friedman, H.L. *An Approach to Psychosocial Research in Fertility Behavior.* Washington: AIR/Transnational Family Research Institute, TFRI Working Paper No. 3, 1972.

Friedman, H.L. "Acceptability of Fertility-Regulating Methods: The User/System Interaction." Paper prepared for presentation at the First Cross-Cultural Conference on Psychology convened at the University of Ibadan, Ibadan, Nigeria (April 1973).

George, E.I. "Massive Vasectomy Camps in India: An Evaluation." Unpublished paper, 1973.

German Democratic Republic. "Law on the Interruption of Pregnancy." March 9, 1973, reproduced in *Abortion Research Notes* 1, 2 (1972) Supplement 2.

Klein, Z.A. "Psychological and Sociological Aspects of Vasectomy." Unpublished bibliography, Department of Psychiatry, University of Chicago, 1972.

McLaren, H. "Laparoscopic Sterilization." *Family Planning* 22 (1973): 18-19.

Pai, D.N. "Keynote Address: Voluntary Sterilization as a Component of a Family Planning Program." In *Advances in Voluntary Sterilization*, Proceedings of the Second International Conference, Geneva, 1973, edited by M.E. Schima, I. Lubell, J.E. Daves, and E. Connell, pp. 12-20. Princeton, N.J.: Excerpta Medica, American Elsevier Publishing Co., Inc., 1974.

Potts, M. "Current Status of Sterilization in the World – Prevalence, Incidence, Who and Where." In *Advances in Voluntary Sterilization*, Proceedings of the Second International Conference, Geneva, 1973, edited by M.E. Schima, I. Lubell, J.E. Davis, and E. Connell, pp. 97-103. Princeton, N.J.: Excerpta Medica, American Elsevier Publishing Co., Inc., 1974.

Presser, H.B. "Voluntary Sterilization: A World View." *Reports on Population/ Family Planning* (July 1970) no. 5.

Presser, H.B. and Bumpass, L.L. "The Acceptability of Contraceptive Sterilization Among U.S. Couples: 1970. *Family Planning Perspectives* 4, 4 (1972): 18-26. (a)

Presser, H.B. and Bumpass, L.L. "Demographic and Social Aspects of Contraceptive Sterilization in the United States: 1965-1970. In C.F. Westoff and P. Parke, Jr., eds., *Demographic and Social Aspects of Population Growth.* Vol. 1 of Report of the Commission on Population Growth and the American Future. Washington: United States Government Printing Office, 1972, Stock No. 5258-00005. Pp. 507-68. (b)

Rodgers, D.A. and Ziegler, F.J. "Effects of Surgical Contraception on Sexual Behavior." In *Advances in Voluntary Sterilization*, Proceedings of the Second International Conference, Geneva, 1973, edited by M.E. Schima, I. Lubell, J.E. Davis, and E. Connell, pp. 161-66. Princeton, N.J.: Excerpta Medica, American Elsevier Publishing Co., Inc., 1974.

Rodgers, D.A. and Ziegler, F.J. "Psychological Reactions to Surgical Contraception." In J.T. Fawcett, ed., *Psychological Perspectives on Population.* New York: Basic Books, 1973. Pp. 306-328.

Ross, J.A., Germain, A., Forrest, J.E., and van Ginneken, J. "Findings from Family Planning Research." *Reports on Population/Family Planning* (October 1972), no. 12.

Rothe, J. "Irreversible Contraception in the German Democratic Republic." Paper presented at the Second International Conference on Voluntary Sterilization, Geneva, Switzerland (February-March 1973).

Speidel, J.J. "The Role of Female Sterilization in Family Planning Programs. In G.W. Duncan, R.D. Falb, and J.J. Speidel, eds., *Female Sterilization.* New York: Academic Press, 1972. Pp. 89-104. (a)

Speidel, J.J. "Male Sterilization and its Contribution to Solution of Population Problems. *Urology* 1 (1972): 277-85. (b)

Stepan, J., and Kellogg, E.H. "The World's Laws on Voluntary Sterilization for Family Planning Purposes. *Population Report* (April 1973), Series C-D, no. 2.

Thiery, M., Cliquet, R.L., Wauters, M., and Maele, C.V. "A Prospective Investigation of Voluntary Sterilization." In *Advanced in Voluntary Sterilization*, Proceedings of the Second International Conference, Geneva, 1973, edited by M.E. Schima, I. Lubell, J.E. Davis, and E. Connell, pp. 167-84. Princeton, N.J.: Excerpta Medica, American Elsevier Publishing Co., Inc., 1974.

Wolfers, H. "Psychological Aspects of Vasectomy." *British Medical Journal* 4 (1970): 297-300.

# 11 Barriers to the Diffusion of Contraceptive Sterilization
### Everett M. Rogers

Because contraceptive sterilization is a new idea to the individual who considers adopting it, the communication of this innovation is one important determinant of its rate of adoption. How an individual perceives such an innovation affects his or her decision about it.

This chapter describes some of the most important perceptions of contraceptive sterilization that act as barriers to its diffusion. After a brief description of the diffusion model, this framework is applied to the particular case of sterilization, with emphasis on taboo communication and the sociolinguistic aspects of contraceptive sterilization.

## The Diffusion Model

Diffusion research has its origin in the work of rural sociologists in the early 1940s who studied the diffusion of hybrid seed corn among Iowa farmers. The number of diffusion investigations increased rapidly, reaching to about 400 by 1962, 2,000 by 1973, and 3,000 by 1977. In the early 1960s the scholarly field of diffusion research began to emerge as a single, integrated body of concepts and generalizations, although it continued to receive the attention of researchers in a variety of the social sciences. It became internationalized and its importance to family planning research started to be recognized.

In the diffusion of new ideas, as modeled, the *innovation* is *communicated* through certain *channels* over *time* among the members of a *social system*. Each of these main elements deserves a brief definition.

An *innovation* is an idea, practice, or object perceived as new by an individual. The characteristics of an innovation, as perceived by the members of a social system, determine its rate of adoption. The attributes of innovations — relative advantage, compatibility, complexity, trialability, and observability — can be illustrated by the particular case of contraceptive sterilization.

The relative advantage of an innovation is the degree to which it is perceived to be superior to the idea or practice it replaces. Many adopters of contraceptive sterilization, it is known, have had previous experience with the IUD, oral contraceptives, and other fertility-regulating measures. Sterilization adopters,

---

Certain ideas in this chapter are adapted from Rogers (1973).

presumably, see the innovation as holding some greater value for preventing unwanted pregnancy.

Contraceptive sterilization may be incompatible with the values and beliefs of many individuals who perceive it as sexually threatening. The confusion of sterilization with castration furthermore, is widespread and is known to have interfered with population control programs in Thailand, North India, Pakistan, and elsewhere. (See the discussion of sociolinguistic factors towards the end of this chapter.)

Compared with other contraceptive methods, sterilization has less trialability, in part because fertility termination upon sterilization is irreversible. Because of its site, contraceptive sterilization also has a low degree of observability; in India, interestingly, sterilized men often show their surgical scars to potential adopters whom they are attempting to recruit (Repetto, 1969). In the United States, the issuance of lapel pins to adopters by the Association for Voluntary Sterilization is an attempt to make the innovation more visible.

*Communication channels* are the means by which a message gets from a source to a receiver. Mass media channels are more effective in creating knowledge of innovations, whereas interpersonal channels are more effective in forming and changing attitudes toward the new ideas.

*Time* is involved in the innovation-decision process, in innovativeness, and in an innovation's rate of adoption. The innovation-decision process is that through which an individual passes mentally over time from first knowledge of an innovation, via persuasion to a decision whether to adopt or reject, and to confirmation of this decision. The process can be extended into the phase of discontinuance, the decision to cease use of an innovation after previously adopting it. Because contraceptive sterilization cannot easily be discontinued, it represents a decision requiring a high degree of commitment by the potential adopter.

Innovativeness — the degree to which an individual is relatively earlier in adopting new ideas than other members of his or her social system — is also, therefore, a function of time. Depending on when an innovation is adopted, the individual is ranked with the innovators, early adopters, early majority, late majority, or the laggards. Rate of adoption is the relative speed with which an innovation is accepted by members of a social system.

A *social system*, finally, is a set of interrelated units that can be distinguished from their environment as a single entity and is engaged in reaching a shared goal. The system's social structure — norms, social statuses, and hierarchy — influences the behavior of individuals with respect to the spread of new ideas. The adoption rates of contraceptive sterilization, for instance, vary widely between various sociocultural-ethnic groups such as Pakistan versus India and Bangladesh, Puerto Rico versus Latin American nations, or blacks versus whites in the United States. Presumably, the culturally-determined conception of masculinity-femininity makes for differential adoption rates.

After a false start with a medical clinic model, most national family planning programs switched their intellectual basis to a classical diffusion model. This paradigm, however, may not be completely appropriate for innovations that are often taboo topics and deal with beliefs highly central to the receiver.

## Taboo Communication[a]

At least among villagers and urban poor in less-developed areas and certain other groups in more developed countries, the idea of contraceptive sterilization is not open to free-flowing, uninhibited interpersonal communication. Surgical sterilization diffuses so slowly in many settings in part because it is a taboo topic for communication.

*Taboo communication* is that category of message transfer in which messages are perceived as extremely private and personal in nature because they deal with proscribed behavior. There is a continuum of "highly taboo" to "highly nontaboo"; messages concerning family planning are perceived as occupying one end of this continuum. It is the perceptions of the source and receiver that determine whether a message is taboo or not. Many types of message-content are perceived by almost everyone as taboo because they deal with ideas or behavior that are illegal, immoral, or contrary to strongly-held norms, such as drug use, having an abortion or venereal disease, or being a homosexual, a swinger, or an exconvict. Nonetheless, the degree to which a message is taboo is never independent of the particulars of time, place, and participants. An abortion, for instance, is not a taboo topic between two women who know that each has had the experience. The acceptability of such a taboo message, however, might change drastically when others are present, especially if the others are men. Abortion is not considered taboo in Seoul, but it is in some places in the United States. Finally, an issue generally perceived to be taboo at one point in time may be much less so at another. Using marijuana is much less taboo in 1976 in the United States than even five years previously, although the legal hazards have not changed. Over this period, as well, sterilization has become much less taboo in the United States. Highly taboo topics are not completely forbidden to discuss; even the most taboo topics are usually discussed with at least someone.

*The high degree of homophily between individuals who engage in communication on a taboo topic acts as a barrier to rapid and widespread diffusion of taboo messages. This, in turn, perpetuates the taboo status of the topic.* This interrelationship is depicted in Figure 11-1.

---

[a]"Taboo" in this chapter is equivalent to "strongly forbidden," i.e., similar to its popular meanings, as distinguished from the anthropologists' "strongly forbidden behavior (that is) enforced by supernatural sanctions deeply embedded in the belief system" (Polgar, 1972).

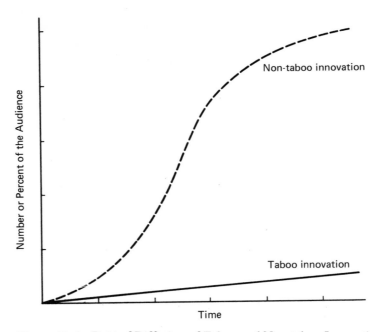

**Figure 11-1.** Rate of Diffusion of Taboo and Non-taboo Innovation.

Some communication programs seek to break this circle by making taboo messages more public. Thus, Paul Ehrlich, in *The Population Bomb* (1968), publicized the fact that he had had a vasectomy and urged other sterilized men to publicize their operations also, thereby diffusing the idea of vasectomy by breaking down its taboo status. A 1972 issue of the *New York Review of Books* carried an advertisement by twenty prominent women who professed to having had an abortion. Implied in these activities is the communication strategy of "Everybody's doing it," with the intent of changing public perceptions of the innovation messages to a lower degree of tabooness.

*Taboo communication is facilitated by encouraging more widespread communication about the taboo message, thus reducing its tabooness.* The use of this strategy is illustrated by the Ernakulam vasectomy campaign in India, where the taboo on vasectomy was overcome by creation of a festival spirit (for example, having groups of adopters parade through the streets of Cochin, singing and waving placards).

For the individual seeking taboo information, such as a woman trying to locate an abortionist in countries where it is forbidden, the high degree of homophily involved in taboo communication has the special disadvantage that those most readily available as sources of information are unlikely to know much more than the seeker already knows. Lee (1969) has found that most of her sample of North American women desiring abortion information went first to their best friends, with whom they were highly homophilous. Communication among them was facile, but unlikely to be instrumentally rewarding. Lee (1969) gave one example of a woman who canvassed several friends, her mother, and a family doctor; all provided information about the same abortionist (who, in fact, was no longer performing abortions).

The futility of information-seeking from extremely homophilous and intimate friends is due, in part, to the high degree of redundancy in homophilous friendship networks. A seeker's closest friends are themselves usually already friends of one another, thus constituting a relatively closed *interlocking network*. A *radial network*, in contrast, in which the seeker's friends are not themselves friends and are not engaged in interaction with each other, is open to its environment (Figure 11-2). *Taboo communication is more likely to occur in interlocking than in radial networks, thus restricting the flow of taboo messages.*

Taboo communication plays a role in retarding diffusion and change of a kind deemed undesirable by the broader social system. Certain topics are relatively more taboo because they are perceived to threaten important social values. Family planning ideas in India are a case in point. At least among the majority of the population that lives in villages, the messages are highly taboo, perhaps because the easy availability of contraceptive methods is seen as endangering premarital female virginity, on which extremely high value is placed. The diffusion of family planning methods is thus restricted by their taboo nature in (societal) hopes that the virginity value will be preserved.

In recent years, however, at least among national government officials in India, another value (population control) has called for the widespread

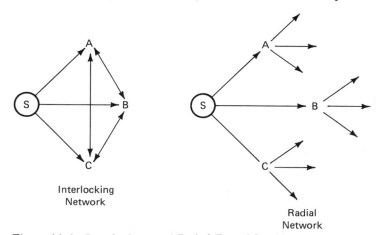

Interlocking
Network

Radial
Network

**Figure 11-2.** Interlocking and Radial Friendship Networks and their
Effect on the Accessibility of Taboo Messages
("S" is the Seeker of Information)

dissemination and use of family planning methods. A national family planning campaign aimed at villagers and urban poor has been launched, requiring an assault on the taboo nature of contraception. This program of directed social change has not been very successful. After about six years of intensive efforts, only about 8 million of the 100 million fertile couples in India were using family planning; to reach officially stated demographic goals in the near future, almost half the couples would have to use contraceptive methods. One reason for the program's lack of success is lack of official appreciation for just how taboo the family planning topic is among the target audience. In fact, only in the early 1970s did research evidence become available on this matter, from studies of scholars like Marshall (1971).

Research on the tabooness of family planning innovations such as sterilization should involve network analysis of interpersonal diffusion within a sample of villages, urban neighborhoods, and other local systems. Special emphasis should be given to determining why the idea of sterilization diffuses so slowly, while rumors about the side effects of sterilization spread so quickly.

### Sociolinguistic Aspects of the Innovation

The word-symbols used to refer to a taboo are of great importance in determining perceptions. "Abortion," "condom," and "venereal disease" have strong, negative meanings for most English-speaking audiences. *Taboo communication can be abetted by relabeling the taboo topic with different word-symbols.* This approach is exemplified in the relabeling of condoms in India as *Nirodh* and in Kenya as *Kinga.* The use of the term "tube tying" for female and male sterilization is yet another attempt to avoid the aversive connotations of the original labels.

As with other family planning methods, sterilization's rate of adoption is affected by the word-symbols for this innovation. In India and Pakistan, for example, vasectomy is called *nasbandi* ("tying a small vein") or the English words *male operation* are used to label the procedure. The perceptions of *nasbandi* versus *operation,* however, differ markedly—witness the story of the Indian peasant who asked the doctor to give him "a *nasbandi,* not an operation." Since many villagers perceive "operation" as a more fearful and serious experience, they are less likely to decide in favor of it. In Korea, on the other hand, vasectomy is known as *Chong won seesu* ("vas operation") in the native language, with apparently no negative connotations.

Unfortunately, in the minds of villagers there is often an association between vasectomy and castration. In India and Pakistan, vasectomy is occasionally referred to with the word used for the castration of bull calves. This confusion was important enough in West Pakistan for the government family planning program to publish a leaflet in 1970 distinguishing the two operations from one another.

Another instance of the confusion is that of Thailand, where the most commonly used Thai word for vasectomy (*torn*) also means "castration." Small wonder that very few men come forward for the operation even though about 22,000 Thai women have had tubectomies. (The Thai phrase *tam mun chai* ["to make the man infertile"] is popularly reserved for tubectomy, although, strictly speaking, the phrase is applicable to vasectomy, as well.)

The female operation that parallels vasectomy is known technically as "tubectomy," tubal ligation," or "salpingectomy." In India, it is commonly referred to as "operation" or "tubectomy," using English words, or "*aurat*" (woman's) *ka operation*." Although less popular than vasectomy in India and Bangladesh, the adoption rate for female sterilization began to increase in the early 1970s; perhaps, in these male-dominated cultures, husbands prefer that the wife have the operation. It has often been assumed by family planning programs that women are the crucial audience—the decision-makers—for tubectomy and men, for vasectomy. Such simplistic notions seem of doubtful validity. Research is needed on the nature and process of family decisions about contraceptive practices like sterilization.

Marshall (1971, p. 160) reported that in the Indian community he studied, the villagers called the female family planning worker *nasbandiwali* (literally, "the sterilizer"), a title that both reflects and helps create a popular conception of the procedure being advocated.

There have been no studies in the United States, unfortunately, on the sociolinguistic aspects of sterilization. Does the common man refer to sterilization by that name, as "vasectomy," or by other terms? The terminology and its associated meanings can tell us much about the perceptions of the innovations.

There is a widespread belief that sterilization, especially for males, interferes with sexual potency. Of the respondents in a 1965 fertility survey in the United States (Ryder and Westoff, 1971), for instance, 25 percent thought that sterilization would interfere with a man's ability to have intercourse. This figure decreased to 15 percent in a comparable study in 1970 (Westoff, 1972), but still included over one-third of all black women interviewed.

Such perceptions need to be studied much more carefully than they have been in the past. Sociolinquistic research must be focused on what sterilization is (and should be) called by the "man on the street" in various cultures, and on how the innovation is perceived, by the total fertile audience and by important subaudiences (like black men in the United States, for example, or Muslims in India). The semantic differential administered at the time of the adoption-decision could perhaps be useful as a measuring device.

**References**

Ehrlich, P. *The Population Bomb*. New York: Ballantine Books, 1968.

Rogers, E.M. *Communication Strategies for Family Planning.* New York: Free
      Press, 1973.
Lee, N.H. *The Search for an Abortionist,* Chicago, IL: University of Chicago
      Press, 1969.
Marshall, J.F. "Culture and Contraception: Response Determinants to a Family
      Planning Program in a North Indian Village." Ph.D. Thesis, Honolulu,
      University of Hawaii, 1971.
Polgar, S. "Anthropology and Population Problems." *Current Anthropology*
      13 (1972): 260-62.
Repetto, R. "India: The Vasectomy Campaign in Madras." *Studies in Family
      Planning* 1, 31 (1969): 8-16.
Ryder, N.B. and Westoff, C.F. *Reproduction in the United States, 1965.*
      Princeton: Princeton University Press, 1971.
Westoff, C.F. "The Modernization of U.S. Contraceptive Practice." *Family Plan-
      ning Perceptives* 4 (July 1972): 9-12.

# 12

## Sociological Aspects of Contraceptive Sterilization: The Role of Knowledge and Attitudes
### Duff G. Gillespie, William H. Spillane and Paul E. Ryser

## Introduction

This chapter examines the relationship between knowledge of and attitudes toward contraceptive sterilization in the United States, with particular emphasis on vasectomy, drawing on the results of a national survey conducted by the authors in the winter of 1971.[a] The chapter ventures, as well, into a presentation of two broad areas of needed research—not in terms of specific experimental designs but rather a discussion of issues with planning and policy implications for health programs. Special attention is focused upon persons who have no or insufficient knowledge of contraceptive sterilization but (1) desire to terminate their fertility or (2) are perceived by a second party, such as a physician or other health worker, to have a "need" for the procedures.

### Related Research

The popularity of voluntary contraceptive sterilization in the United States has been well documented by Presser and Bumpass ([1972a, 1972b] ; see also Bumpass and Presser [1972] ) and is adequately covered in other chapters in this volume. For our purposes, a brief summary will suffice.

Until recently, the number of people undergoing contraceptive sterilization in the United States was quite low, although steadily growing. The Growth of American Families studies (Freedman, Whelpton, and Campbell, 1959; Whelpton, Campbell and Patterson, 1966) and the National Fertility Survey (Ryder and Westoff, 1971; Westoff, 1972) show a constant increment in both male and female procedures since the mid-1950s. For the years 1955, 1960, and 1965, the proportion of white women eighteen to thirty-nine years of age who had this type of surgery was, respectively, 3, 4, and 5 percent. The figures for their husbands were

[a]The views expressed in this paper are the authors' and do not necessarily represent those of their organizations. The authors wish to acknowledge with special thanks the help provided by Mr. Denton Vaughan of OEO who unselfishly shared with them both the data he is currently analyzing and his valuable suggestions concerning this chapter.

161

1, 2, and 3 percent. Since 1965, there has been a substantial increase of both operations. Among married couples in which the wife was eighteen to forty-five years of age in 1970, 5.1 percent of the men and 5.5 percent of the women had had contraceptive sterilization. The dramatic change in prevalence was unanticipated before the 1970 National Fertility Survey data were available. By 1970, surgery had "become the most popular method of contraception currently used" by couples in which the wife was thirty to forty-four years of age (Westoff, 1972, p. 10).

Nevertheless, the overall prevalence of the method within the population at risk remains relatively low—a fact explained by some (for instance, Presser, 1970) as at least partially due to the presumed ignorance of and negative attitudes toward the procedures. One must say "presumed" since there were no national data concerning persons' knowledge of and attitudes toward contraceptive sterilization.

Small-scale studies do, however, suggest that the method is often viewed rather unfavorably. Rodgers, Ziegler, and Levy (1967), for example, had their Ss characterize two different hypothetical couples—one in which there was a vasectomized male, the other in which the wife was using oral contraceptives. The former couple was described in a clearly more derogatory manner. The authors suggested that the popular negative attitude, often considered the product of lack of information, might contribute to untoward reactions to vasectomy on the part of those who had chosen to undergo the surgery, since public disapproval makes for an adverse change in self-concept.

*The National Survey*

In the summer of 1971, we decided to undertake a survey of the public's knowledge of vasectomy and attitude towards it. Several forces converged upon restricting the survey to vasectomy. Like the counterpart female surgery, vasectomy was being selected by increasing numbers of couples as a method for fertility termination; little hard data were available on the subject of knowledge and attitudes—a question of some clinical value if negative societal attitudes provided a hostile environment for the vasectomized man and influenced his own response to the procedure. Male contraceptive sterilization, considering its simplicity and relative inexpensiveness, is also especially underutilized, hence more likely to show the influence of attitudinal and informational variables than would tubal ligation, which could be rejected for the supposedly more "practical" reasons of cost, health risk, or inconvenience.

Following a pretest, the field phase of the survey was begun in November 1971 and completed in January 1972. Part of a larger public opinion interview conducted by Opinion Research Corporation, the vasectomy questionnaire contained forty-four related questions. (That we were limited in the number of items we could include was yet another reason for restricting our research to vasectomy rather than asking about both male and female contraceptive sterilization.)

Unlike the main research instrument (where the interviewer read the questions and recorded the answers), the vasectomy questionnaire was completed solely by the interviewee. Pretests had shown the questions to be too "personal" for the interviewers to handle comfortably in face-to-face interaction. Most of the interviewers were middle-aged women without prior experience in surveys of fertility-related behavior.

Of the national probability sample of 2,003 men and women eighteen years and older living in private households, 72 percent (1,438) answered the vasectomy questions. Because all of the demographic questions were asked during the larger public opinion interview, we had a great deal of information on the 565 nonrespondents. The majority of nonrespondents tended to be fifty years of age and older with less than high school education who were either retired or unemployed and living on a low income. By simultaneously controlling for sex, religion, education, and age, nonrespondents were assigned for analytic purposes the responses obtained from their demographic counterparts in the respondent group.

## Knowledge and Attitudes

### Knowledge

Americans place a great deal of importance on having a knowledgeable population. We feel that many of our social problems can be resolved or alleviated if the populace is knowledgeable about the relevant issues. The Commission On Population Growth and the American Future (1972), for example, began its chapter on education by noting that, "One characteristic American response to social issues is to propose educational programs, and this Commission is no exception" (p. 79). Although we have great faith in "knowledge," what we mean by the term is not easy to define or operationalize exactly. Knowledge has a temporal quality which denotes its definition to be in flux. What is accepted as "knowledge" at one point in time is considered ignorance at another. People are also frequently confronted with competing and contradictory facts. Which set of facts one accepts is not necessarily based on objective truth. A decision can be influenced by such factors as the sources of the facts, how they fit into one's world view, and/or which set seems to offer the most personal benefits. Last, knowledge about a particular subject typically encompasses a large number of facts. Persons may know a great deal about one facet of the subject but be quite ignorant about the rest. The relative importance of these different facts is difficult to determine *a priori*. In other words, to have a working knowledge of a subject, some facts are probably more critical than others. The criticalness of facts will vary, of course, with the person's potential use of the knowledge.

For the purpose of this study, knowledge of vasectomy was operationalized by a series of eight true/false statements. Items were selected which we felt might be crucial for the formation of attitudes toward vasectomy and which would be considered important for the person deciding whether to undergo the procedure. We did not ask respondents, for example, if the operation entailed cutting of the vas deferens but did ask if the operation was difficult and required hospitalization. The eight items covered a wide spectrum of vasectomy characteristics—its popularity, difficulty, legality, reversibility, cost, and vasectomized persons' satisfaction with the procedure. A knowledge index was constructed from seven of these eight items. The item dealing with reversibility was not included in the index because its factor loading value was less than .50 (see Appendix 12B).[b]

For purposes of analysis, respondents were categorized as having "high" or "low" levels of knowledge about vasectomy. The procedure used to construct this index and the knowledge items are given in the appendixes to this chapter.

## Attitudes

Attitudes are as difficult to define and operationalize as is knowledge—if not even more difficult. Researchers are usually more sensitive to the methodological limitations on the measurement of attitudes than they are about those pertaining to knowledge. While we frequently impute an objectivity to knowledge (although this is not always justified), attitudes are clearly subjective phenomena. Perhaps the main difficulty in determining a person's attitudes through closed-ended questions is the hazard of prejudging the frame of reference. The researcher may unwittingly construct an instrument which reflects his own values and concerns rather than the framework of the respondents—if, indeed, they had ever even thought about the subject.

In this study, we attempted to go beyond measuring only the simple approval or disapproval of vasectomy. Although the reason persons have vasectomies is to terminate their fertility, there are usually conditions which prompt this desire. We therefore presented the interviewers with seven approve/disapprove rationales for why a man might have a vasectomy. The rationales included: no more children desired, protection of mother's health, financial reasons, potential child's health, previous birth control failure, and a doctor or the courts having decided that the couple was mentally unable to raise a child. As with the knowledge

---

[b]Approximately one-third (32 percent) of the respondents incorrectly considered it simple for the doctor to reverse a vasectomy so that the man may again have children. This important knowledge item has been treated in a separate analysis in another paper (Gillespie and Spillane, 1972).

items, a "high" or "low" approval index was constructed on the basis of the responses. The index is explained in the appendixes, where the attitude questions can also be found. All seven attitude questions are included in the index.

**Theoretical Model and Survey Findings**

Figure 12-1 is a heuristic model showing the route one must take to obtain a vasectomy. (Although this discussion concerns surgery for the male, the model is also appropriate for female contraceptive sterilization.) Each box can be considered as a potential source of attrition. The schema is oversimplified in that it deals only with the influence of knowledge of, attitudes toward, and desire for a vasectomy.

*The Relationship of Knowledge to Approval*

The first screening point is the person's knowledge of vasectomy (point A in Figure 12-1). Persons having relatively little or no knowledge of vasectomy, it can be argued, are less likely to hold positive attitudes toward the operation. This is based on the assumption that the characteristics of vasectomy are not inherently disagreeable; otherwise, knowledge would be directly related to negative attitudes.

Table 12-1 clearly suggests that knowledge is positively associated with favorable attitudes toward vasectomy. Approximately two-thirds (65.5 percent) of those scoring high on the knowledge index were also high approvers of vasectomy. Slightly more than two-thirds (67.5 percent) of the low vasectomy knowledge group were also low approvers. Thus, a person with high knowledge at point A in Figure 12-1 is much more likely to progress to point B1 than would a person with low knowledge, who would tend to be more indifferent or negative toward the procedure (B2).

**Table 12-1**
**Relationship of Vasectomy Knowledge to Vasectomy Approval**

| Vasectomy Knowledge Index | Vasectomy Approval Index | | | | | |
|---|---|---|---|---|---|---|
| | High Approval | | Low Approval | | Total | |
| | N | Percent | N | Percent | N | Percent |
| High Knowledge | 494 | 65.6 | 260 | 34.5 | 754 | 100 |
| Low Knowledge | 222 | 32.5 | 461 | 67.5 | 683 | 100 |

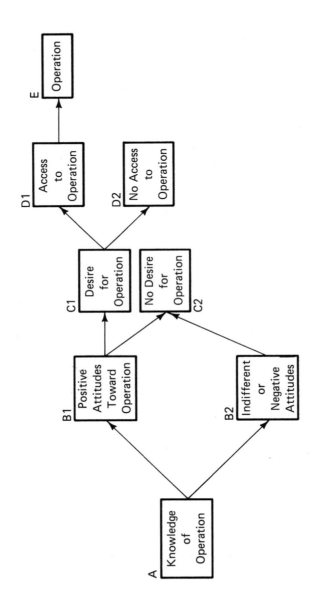

**Figure 12-1.** Heuristic Model for the Choice Points and Routes Toward Obtaining a Vasectomy

## The Relationship of Approval to Planning

Positive attitudes toward vasectomy do not necessarily mean that the respondent would ever personally consider having or her spouse having a vasectomy. The jump from B1 to C1 in Figure 12-1 (desire for the surgery) is substantial. Approval of vasectomy is frequently given in the abstract and need not reflect the person's wishes for action on the part of the male partner in the marriage.

To tap their degree of active interest in having a vasectomy, respondents were asked, "Do you believe you (your spouse) may have a vasectomy sometime in the future?" Table 12-2 shows that approval of vasectomy is, indeed, positively associated with planning to have a vasectomy. Of the high approvers, slightly more than one of ten respondents (10.7 percent), compared to fewer than one out of twenty low approvers (4.6 percent), indicated plans for a vasectomy. It should be further pointed out that over one-half of those not planning a vasectomy were also high approvers. It is probable that some of this group will ultimately seek the surgery when their life situation changes and their fertility is completed.

Table 12-2 shows the somewhat paradoxical finding that close to 5 percent of those actually planning a vasectomy were nonetheless low on approval of the procedure. Why, then, did they wish to undergo the surgery in the first place? It may be that certain reasons behind the decision (health, for example) do not involve the same degree of approval one expects in connection with vasectomies undergone only for contraceptive motives. In addition, we have no indication concerning the planners' strength of *commitment* to the operation. The group of planners with low approval are probably more likely, in fact, not to have a vasectomy than are the high approval planners. In this connection, it should be noted that the model in Figure 12-1 is a static one. For example, persons who hold negative attitudes (B2) may at a later time adopt positive attitudes (B1) toward the operation. In practice, no doubt a proportion of those desiring or planning a vasectomy (C1) actually change their minds.

**Table 12-2**
**Relationship of Vasectomy Approval to Desire for Vasectomy**

| Vasectomy Approval Index | Plan Vasectomy | | Do Not Plan | | Total | |
|---|---|---|---|---|---|---|
| | N | Percent | N | Percent | N | Percent |
| High Approval | 81 | 10.7 | 676 | 89.3 | 757 | 100 |
| Low Approval | 31 | 4.6 | 649 | 95.4 | 680 | 100 |

$X^2 = 18.61$

*The Relationship of Knowledge to Planning*

Table 12-3 shows that planners have considerably more vasectomy knowledge than do nonplanners. Although the majority of respondents are in the non-planner category, it is interesting to note that they are approximately evenly distributed with respect to having high and low vasectomy knowledge. Knowledge is a necessary but not a sufficient condition for planning. Planners will tend to have high vasectomy knowledge; the possession of vasectomy knowledge, however, does not mean that one will necessarily become a planner.

*The Relationship of Approval and Knowledge to Having Had a Vasectomy*

No matter how strong a person's desire for contraceptive sterilization, his or her wishes will remain frustrated if there is no access to the operation (see D1 and D2 in Figure 12-1). Access involves more than just having a medical facility in close geographical proximity; it also means that the potential client be aware of the facility and that there be no financial roadblocks or restrictive criteria, implicit or explicit. We have very little data concerning the prevelance of people who desire contraceptive sterilization but have no access in the broad sense, to the operation. That persons have been denied entry into the system is evident (Scrimshaw and Pasquariella, 1970), as is the fact that the growing demands for the surgery have created access (Presser and Bumpass, 1972b). The extent to which people are denied contraceptive sterilization is an area of needed research and will be discussed in another section of this chapter.

Our knowledge is somewhat weak concerning the process through which persons go once the issue of access is solved—that is, what transpires in the relationship of layman and professional before and after the operation (point E in

**Table 12-3**
**Relationship of Vasectomy Knowledge to Desire for Vasectomy**

| Vasectomy Knowledge Index | Plan Vasectomy | | Do Not Plan | |
|---|---|---|---|---|
| | *N* | *Percentage* | *N* | *Percentage* |
| High Knowledge | 93 | 83.0 | 623 | 47.0 |
| Low Knowledge | 19 | 17.0 | 702 | 53.0 |
| Total | 112 | 100 | 1325 | 100 |

$X^2$ = 52.15

Phi = .19

Figure 12-1). Although the surgical procedure for vasectomy is simple and that for female contraception is getting simpler, the social dynamics preceding the operations are rather complex. In a comparatively short period of time, there is intensive interaction between the client and medical personnel, including an exchange of information. We suspect that the effectiveness of this exchange varies from facility to facility, and that the programs discussed in the literature (for example, Sobrero and Edy, 1971; Sobrero and Kohli, 1975) are of disproportionately high quality in this regard. Client-medical interaction will be discussed in greater detail later in this chapter. At this point, suffice it to say that the nature of client management has great possible bearing on the individual's reaction to and satisfaction with the surgery.

It is difficult to compare reported satisfaction with vasectomy from one study to another because of differences in design and method. In five recent American investigations, the percents satisfied were 100, 100, 98, 80, and 99 (Presser, 1970). Although in our survey the number of vasectomized males or their wives was small (eighty-eight), our findings suggest that satisfaction with the operation may be lower than has been previously assumed. Since satisfaction with the surgery was not asked *per se*, our evidence is only indirect. It is drawn from examining the degree of approval of vasectomy among those who had undergone the procedure. (See Tables 12-4 and 12-5.)

In Table 12-4, we find that 27.3 percent of those having already had a vasectomy were low approvers. Although approving of vasectomy is not necessarily the same as satisfaction with it, one might have anticipated that those satisfied with the operation would also be approvers. Moreover, Table 12-5 shows that fully 19.5 percent of those having a vasectomy or their spouses had low knowledge of the method. Regarding one aspect that would appear crucial to decision-making, 18 percent of those already through with surgery incorrectly believed the operation to be easily reversible! These findings suggest that at least some individuals

**Table 12-4**
**Relationship of Vasectomy Approval to Having Undergone the Surgery**

| Vasectomy Approval Index | Vasectomized | | Not Vasectomized | |
|---|---|---|---|---|
| | N | Percentage | N | Percentage |
| High Approval | 64 | 72.7 | 688 | 51.0 |
| Low Approval | 24 | 27.3 | 661 | 49.0 |
| Total | 88 | 100 | 1,349 | 100 |

$X^2$ = 14.16

Phi = .10

**Table 12-5**
**Relationship of Vasectomy Knowledge to Having Undergone the Surgery**

| Vasectomy Knowledge Index | Vasectomized | | Not Vasectomized | |
|---|---|---|---|---|
| | N | Percentage | N | Percentage |
| High Knowledge | 70 | 79.5 | 648 | 48.0 |
| Low Knowledge | 18 | 19.5 | 701 | 52.0 |
| Total | 88 | 100 | 1,349 | 100 |

$X^2 = 31.86$

Phi = .15

are not receiving adequate information from the providers of vasectomy, or at least are not really absorbing the simple facts.

*Summary of Findings*

In sum, we found the public surprisingly knowledgeable about vasectomy. Sixty-eight percent had a relatively high amount of knowledge of the operation and 52 percent approved of it. Knowledge was statistically related to approval of the operation; approval, in turn, was related to planning to have a vasectomy. Our data suggest some concern about the relatively high proportion of vasectomized males or their spouses who had low approval and knowledge. (It should be mentioned that although all the relationships discussed were statistically significant, the strength of the association [Phi] is not impressively strong.) Last, a schema has been presented illustrating the possible role played by knowledge and attitudes in deciding upon and having a vasectomy.

**Needed Research**

For those who wish to terminate their fertility, the merits of contraceptive sterilization are well established. There are, however, large segments of the population who are not fully aware of vasectomy and, as a result, do not even consider it as a contraceptive alternative. While, as we have shown, the public as a whole is knowledgeable about vasectomy, under 30 percent of blacks and of persons with less than twelve years of education or less than $5,000 annual income have a high level of knowledge about the method. In short, it is the socially disadvantaged who are least aware of vasectomy. It is likely that this is also true for female contraceptive sterilization.

We are well aware of the relatively large percentage of tubal ligations among blacks who desired no more children and did not undergo surgery for noncontraceptive reasons. In 1970, the figures were 15 percent for black women under forty-five years of age; in the same age group for whites, only 6 percent had had tubal ligations. Here, we are discussing *knowledge* of the operation. It may well be that many of these black females were neither highly knowledgeable prior to their operation nor fully cognizant of the operation's implications after having it. (It is of interest to note, by the way, that although the proportion of tubal ligations among blacks is more than twice that for whites, the percent of blacks considering having the operation, according to Presser and Bumpass [1972b], is slightly *lower* than for whites [34 versus 36 percent]. There are a number of possible explanations for the seeming discrepancy. It may be, for instance, that blacks considering tubal ligation are more committed to the operation or have easier access to sterilization facilities.) The rest of this chapter, at any rate, proposes research addressed to the problem of engaging those individuals who would take advantage of the choice of contraceptive sterilization were the procedures genuinely accessible to them.

*The Availability of Information on Contraceptive Surgery*

Figure 12-2 presents a schema showing what may happen to persons who desire to terminate their fertility, have little knowledge of contraceptive sterilization, and come in contact with family planning services (point A). (The model omits the substantial numbers of people, especially in the lower socioeconomic strata of society, who never use professional family planning services.) Figure 12-2 attempts to show diagrammatically the process through which persons go in a family planning service. By "family planning service," we mean *any* professional facility that offers family planning services. Although our underlying emphasis is on private and public family planning clinics, the model also applies to physicians who offer family planning services. The model confines itself to discussing persons with little or no knowledge about contraceptive sterilization, but much of what will be said is also relevant to persons who are knowledgeable about the operation, for example, the later discussion on the availability of the operation.

Persons at point A in Figure 12-2 are unable to request surgery for themselves or their spouses because they are unaware of the method. Any information about the operation must, therefore, come from the family planning staff. The staff may consist of physicians, nurses, secretaries, or outreach workers. The type of information and advice given depends on a wide spectrum of variables, including the staff's previous experience with various methods of birth control, the kind of services offered by the facility, and the contraceptive history and family planning desires of the client. We know little of the type of interchange usually occurring between clients and staff except that there is probably a great deal of

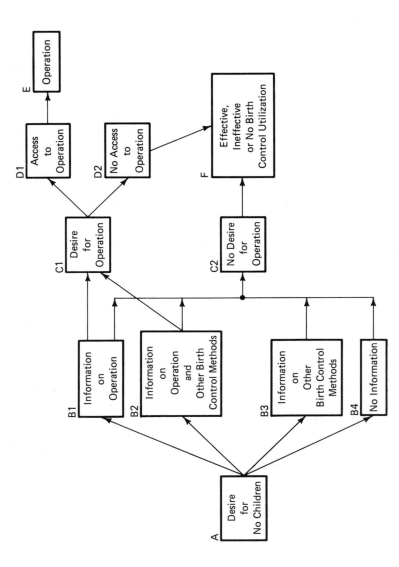

**Figure 12-2.** Heuristic Model for the Choice Points and Routes Toward Obtaining a Vasectomy in a Family Planning Service

variance among staff members and even more among clinics. For our purposes, it will be assumed that the staff elicits from the client that she/he wishes to have no (more) children. Let us also agree that the quality of the interaction is such that an effective exchange of contraceptive information occurs. (Later we will discuss problems associated with inadequate information flow between client and staff.) The information that particular clients receive at points B1, B2, and B3 in Figure 12-2 is thus both accurate and comprehensive. Finally, the model operates on the premise that clients will internalize this information and make a decision based on it. Although it is unlikely that the staff will give no information, for the sake of expository completeness that possibility is also indicated in the model (point B4).

Clients who are given information only about surgical procedures (B1) are more likely to have the operation than those who receive more or different information (points B2 or B3). Because they are given only one contraceptive alternative, B1 is the narrowest of the three sources of information. Furthermore, should they decide to have the operation (C1), it is unlikely that many will be denied access to the operation (D2) because the staff would probably not emphasize surgery were appropriate facilities not available. Persons who received only surgery information and do not desire the operation (C2) would progress to point F. These individuals would probably continue using whatever method they used at point A—which, since they sought family planning assistance, was probably not too effective. As a result, persons who go from A→B1→C2→F can be considered program failures.

The ideal family planning situation is found at B2. Here, the entire range of contraceptive alternatives is offered. Unlike those clients who went through B1 and decided not to have surgery, individuals exposed to B2 may very well upgrade the effectiveness of their contraception. Even if they decide against an operation, they have been given information on all forms of birth control. On the other hand, persons who receive only information on nonsurgical forms of contraception (B3) are at a distinct disadvantage: these individuals are denied the choice of what may be the most appropriate and effective method for persons in their situation. Unfortunately, B3 is the typical type of family planning service. In fact, evidence exists that suggest programs often restrict the kinds of contraceptive information services give clients.

Vaughan (1973) has analyzed 1972 data from OEO family planning programs that provided information to the National Reporting System for Family Planning Services. Of the 374 OEO programs, 63 percent participated in the System and accounted for about 80 percent of all 480,000 active OEO clients. Some of Vaughan's findings suggest that there are relatively few programs that offer information on contraceptive sterilization. Programs that do not offer such surgery, one may assume, are unlikely to give information about the procedure. Only 38 percent of the OEO programs reported one or more cases of contraceptive or noncontraceptive surgery having been performed in 1972. Furthermore,

of this 38 percent, one-fifth of the programs accounted for 85 percent of all surgery reported; that is, only nineteen OEO family programs had what could be
considered an active contraceptive sterilization program. It should also be noted
that from *all* family planning programs supported by the federal government and
Planned Parenthood, only 15,000 contraceptive operations were reported. This
suggests that most of the procedures take place outside organized family planning
programs.

Returning to Figure 12-2, the above data force us to conclude that services
like B1 and B2 are relatively rare alternatives. The surgical alternatives offered
by B1 and B2 are, in fact, even more limited than the reader has so far been led
to believe. Vaughan (1973) also found that programs offering surgery typically
offered either the male or the female procedures, but seldom both. Eighty-five
percent of all tubal ligations occurred in almost exclusively female-oriented surgical
programs, while 85 percent of the vasectomies were recorded in facilities that
offered virtually no surgery to women. In short, persons are likely to be given no
information at all about contraceptive sterilization; at best, they receive information only about the procedure suited to their own gender.

Why do not more family planning programs offer contraceptive sterilization?
Several explanations come to mind, such as lack of staff training or funds, inappropriate physical facilities, or community pressure against the method. It would
seem relatively simple to determine the answer empirically. One would expect
that in many instances the obstacle(s) in the path of surgery programs could be
rather easily removed. Whether the exercise is "research" depends on how one
goes about it. Whatever the label, the impact of the effort probably has more
potential for benefiting the public than much of the research that has been done
in this field.

*The Quality of Client-Professional Interaction*

Unlike Figure 12-2, which presumes objectively adequate and appropriate information of some type being given clients, the model presented in Figure 12-3 focuses
particularly on the original quality of client-professional interaction which influences the informational exchange. In addition, Figure 12-3 deals with an important type of client—the individual who is perceived by staff to have a *need* for
contraceptive sterilization. Because the definition of need is a value judgment of
the perceiver, no single criterion is possible. Among the factors that may be incorporated into such a perception are: ability to support more children, physical
and mental health, previous birth control experience, marital status, and race.
We will assume, furthermore, that the persons defined as "in need" have a low
level of knowledge of contraceptive sterilization. Their decision, therefore, depends solely on what transpires between them and the staff of the family planning
service.

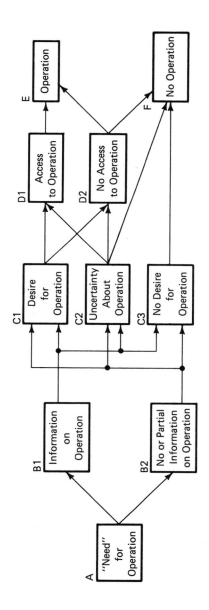

**Figure 12-3.** Heuristic Model for the Choice Points and Routes Toward Obtaining Contraceptive Surgery Where the Client Is Perceived as "In Need" of the Procedure

In Figure 12-3, we see that two types of information can be given. In B1, we would find staff who are well-versed in the surgical procedures and communicate information to the client who, in turn, successfully internalizes it. In other words, clients at B1 have had the operation fully explained to them, have been told why the staff feels it is an appropriate procedure for them, and thus have a knowledge base on which to make their decision concerning surgery. Clients going through B2, in contrast, do not emerge with adequately internalized information about the surgery and, to that extent, remain undisposed to a rational evaluation and decision.

Why clients at B2 do not get sufficient information can be due to one of the following four types of interaction:

1. Staff gives inadequate information, but is unaware of the failure.
2. Staff gives adequate information, but is unaware that the client does not understand it.
3. Staff gives adequate information and knows the client does not understand it.
4. Staff purposely gives inadequate information.

While the end product is the same in all four cases, the intentions of the staff obviously differ from instance to instance. In the first case, the problem is simply one of proper training. In the second example, one may also say that the staff member is inadequately trained, although what corrective learning is required is more difficult to determine. In cases (3) and (4), the staff member is aware that the client is not internalizing or getting adequate information. In these interactions, it is likely that the staff member is trying to exert subtle pressure on the decision to have the operation. In all cases, research is needed to identify these four types of interaction, the reasons they exist, and how their prevalence can be eliminated or reduced.

A client who receives adequate information (B1) may decide to have the operation (C1 in Figure 12-3), remain uncertain about the surgery (C2), or decide against it (C3). The important thing is that in all cases the decision is the client's. There is no way of knowing the relative prevalence of these three decisions. It should be added that with some individuals there will probably be an element of uncertainty concerning the operation (C2) no matter how qualified the family planning staff. For the type of family planning service diagrammed, the availability to the client of surgical procedures is presumed. Nevertheless, persons who desire an operation (C1 or C2) may be denied the procedure (D2) if someone in higher authority disagrees with the staff's initial definition of need.

With persons going through B2—who never absorb adequate information for whatever reason—none of the three possible outcomes is desirable. Persons who desire and obtain the operation (C1→D1→E) or are uncertain about the operation but still obtain if (C2→D1→E) are not fully aware of what the operation entails. They are therefore probably more likely to have negative psychological consequences from the operation. There are, of course, serious ethical questions concerning staff, no matter how good their motives, who knowingly deceive clients about the nature of contraceptive sterilization. Although it is quite possible that a client's life situation improves as a result of the operation, benevolent coercion is an unacceptable practice. Finally, clients who end with no desire for the operation (B2→C3→F) might have sought it had they received more complete and accurate information.

As was the case with Figure 12-2, the model presented in Figure 12-3 must be justified. Does it offer a reasonable facsimile of what takes place in the real world? Again we turn to the Vaughan (1973) data, although here we are on much shakier ground. Remembering that black females appear to have a disproportionately high number of tubal ligations, Vaughan found that among OEO projects that performed twenty or more contraceptive sterilization procedures per year and specialized in tubal ligations there were twice as many active black patients than were in other programs. Moreover, these facilities had two-and-a-half times as many clients on welfare than did the other OEO projects. While there is nothing inherently Orwellian about the data, they should prompt us to investigate whether blacks are being subjected to a contraceptive process of whose consequences they are unaware.

Research on the social processes in which persons participate en route to contraceptive sterilization can reduce the possibility that less knowledgeable persons will have the operation and experience later dissatisfaction with it. Such research should focus on the client-staff interaction and determine how it can be improved. From the point of view of family planning programs, it should be added that persons dissatisfied with the operation are potential sources of negative attitudes toward contraceptive sterilization. These attitudes may be communicated to friends and associates contemplating the choice of surgery who will, on the basis of the warning, decide against the operation.

## Summary

In the first part of this chapter, the contention was made that Americans place a great deal of faith in the problem-solving characteristics of knowledge. We share that faith and believe that many of the problems we have discussed would be resolved were the public knowledgeable not only about contraceptive sterilization but about all forms of birth control. Provided with knowledge, individuals have a great deal of latitude in planning their families. Not everyone, however, can be expected to become sufficiently knowledgeable to make effective family planning decisions without the assistance of organized family planning services. It is therefore essential that such programs be designed to explain and offer to clients all contraceptive alternatives.

Concerning needed research, we think it crucial to examine why different kinds of services exist among family planning programs. Of equal importance is the investigation into the social dynamics of the client-staff transaction in family planning services. All too often, social scientists evaluate or analyze subjects in terms of their ascribed and achieved characteristics. When an organization intervenes in an individual life, it is critical that the character and effect of the intervention be examined. In the case of contraceptive sterilization, the intervention consists of more than just the operation. The surgery must be viewed as the product of a complex social process which may be as important or more important than the actual operation itself.

# Appendix 12A:
## Survey Instruments

### Knowledge

For each of the statements below, please indicate whether you think the statement is True or False by placing an "X" in the appropriate column. If you are not sure, guess.

A. Once a man undergoes a vasectomy operation, it will decrease his sexual pleasure.

1 ( ) TRUE
2 ( ) FALSE

B. Vasectomy is a difficult operation which normally requires one or more days in the hospital.

1 ( ) TRUE
2 ( ) FALSE

C. The vast majority of men who have vasectomies are satisfied with their operations.

1 ( ) TRUE
2 ( ) FALSE

D. It is legal for the doctor to perform vasectomies in most states.

1 ( ) TRUE
2 ( ) FALSE

E. Once a man has had a vasectomy, it is a simple procedure for the doctor to reverse the condition so that he may again have children.

1 ( ) TRUE
2 ( ) FALSE

F. It is less costly for a woman to be sterilized than it is for a man.

1 ( ) TRUE
2 ( ) FALSE

G. The popularity of vasectomies is increasing, and more and more men are having them.

1 ( ) TRUE
2 ( ) FALSE

H. Men having vasectomies become less of a man as a result of the operation.

1 ( ) TRUE
2 ( ) FALSE

### Attitude

Would you approve or disapprove of a man having a vasectomy for any of the following reasons?

179

A. If his female sexual partner was in poor health and she could not safely bear another child.

1 ( ) APPROVE
2 ( ) DISAPPROVE

B. If a doctor informed a couple that they were mentally unable to raise a child.

1 ( ) APPROVE
2 ( ) DISAPPROVE

C. If the parents were unable to support any more children.

1 ( ) APPROVE
2 ( ) DISAPPROVE

D. If the husband or wife had a hereditary disease or illness which could be passed on to the child.

1 ( ) APPROVE
2 ( ) DISAPPROVE

E. If a couple does not want any more children.

1 ( ) APPROVE
2 ( ) DISAPPROVE

F. If the courts decided a couple was mentally unable to raise a child.

1 ( ) APPROVE
2 ( ) DISAPPROVE

G. If other birth control methods used by the couple failed.

1 ( ) APPROVE
2 ( ) DISAPPROVE

# Appendix 12B:
# Factor Analyses and Indices

To present the data parsimoniously, we decided to use factor analysis to construct the indices presented in this chapter. Factor analysis, as used here, provided a simple structural solution which identified those items that clustered together.

Each of the correlation matrices presented in Tables 12B-1 and 12B-2 was submitted to separate factor analysis. In both instances, a single factor emerged. These factor solutions revealed, in each of the analyses, that the items were clustered together. The factor loadings presented in the tables indicate the correlation of each item with the factor. As a rule of thumb, if an item does not correlate .50 with the factor, it is not included as an index item (note Item E in Table 12B-1).

### Vasectomy Knowledge Index

The knowledge index comprises six of the seven surgery items. Correct responses were assigned a value of one which was multiplied by the factor loading value

Table 12B-1.
Vasectomy Knowledge: Correlation and Factor Matrices

| Factor Loading Value | | A -.71 | B -.74 | C -.73 | D -.60 | E -.46 | F -.69 | G -.69 | H -.80 |
|---|---|---|---|---|---|---|---|---|---|
| *Items* | | | | | | | | | |
| A. | Decreases sexual pleasure | — | | | | | | | |
| B. | Difficult operation requiring one or more days in hospital | .52 | — | | | | | | |
| C. | Majority of vasectomized men satisfied | .52 | .55 | — | | | | | |
| D. | Legalized in most states | .39 | .39 | .46 | — | | | | |
| E. | Reversible | .31 | .33 | .30 | .31 | — | | | |
| F. | More costly than operation to sterilize the female | .49 | .54 | .46 | .44 | .35 | — | | |
| G. | Popularity increasing | .46 | .55 | .55 | .47 | .27 | .45 | — | |
| H. | Men having vasectomies become less of a man as result of operation | .63 | .59 | .57 | .45 | .41 | .54 | .51 | — |

(see Table 12B-1). Zero value was assigned to those knowledge items answered incorrectly. For each respondent, the scores on individual items were summed [e.g. (A × .71) + (B × .74) + (C × .73) + (D × .60), etc.] The higher the score, the greater the knowledge of vasectomy. Item E, which deals with reversibility, was not included in the vasectomy knowledge index because the item's factor loading value was less than .50. The range for the knowledge factor loading value was 0 to 4.96, with a median value of 4.47. Low vasectomy knowledge was 4.48 through 4.96 (i.e., above the fiftieth percentile).

**Vasectomy Approval Index**

This index consists of seven items. Table 12B-2 shows the factor matrix and a correlation matrix of attitude items pertaining to rationales for approving vasectomy. All of the correlations in the matrix are significant at the .01 level. If a respondent approved a specific item, this item was assigned a value of one which was multiplied by the factor loading value. The value of zero was assigned to the items that the respondent disapproved. The sum of the products of the seven items constitutes the approval score. For the 1,438 respondents, scores ranged from 0 to 5.36, with a median value of 4.68. As with the Knowledge Index, the median was used as the cutting point for "high" and "low" vasectomy approval.

**Table 12B-2**
**Vasectomy Approval: Correlation and Factor Matrices**

| *Factor*<br>*Loading Value* | *A*<br>-.78 | *B*<br>-.78 | *C*<br>-.81 | *D*<br>-.78 | *E*<br>-.68 | *F*<br>-.76 | *G*<br>-.77 |
|---|---|---|---|---|---|---|---|
| *Items* | | | | | | | |
| A.  Wife in poor health | — | | | | | | |
| B.  Doctor informed couple they were mentally unable to rear a child | .63 | — | | | | | |
| C.  Lack of financial resources to support another child | .64 | .61 | — | | | | |
| D.  For hereditary reasons of passing disease on to child | .64 | .64 | .65 | — | | | |
| E.  Court decided couple mentally unable to rear a child | .50 | .63 | .54 | .56 | — | | |
| F.  If birth control method failed | .59 | .54 | .62 | .58 | .49 | — | |
| G.  Couple does not want children | .60 | .54 | .67 | .54 | .71 | .48 | — |

## References

Bumpass, L.L. and Presser, H.B. "Contraceptive Sterilization in the U.S.: 1965 and 1970." *Demography* 9 (1972): 531-48.

Freedman, R., Whelpton, P.K., and Campbell, A.A. *Family Planning, Sterility and Population Growth.* New York: McGraw-Hill, 1959.

Gillespie, D.G. and Spillane, W.H. "Vasectomy in the United States, 1971." Paper presented at Session on Maternal and Child Health, Annual Meeting of the American Public Health Association, Atlantic City, N.J., November 12-16, 1972.

Presser, H.B. "Voluntary Sterilization: A World View." Reports on Population/Family Planning 5 (July 1970): 1-36.

Presser, H.B. and Bumpass, L.L. "The Acceptability of Contraceptive Sterilization Among U.S. Couples: 1970." *Family Planning Perspectives* 4 (1972): 18-26. (a)

_____. "Demographic and Social Aspects of Contraceptive Sterilization in the United States: 1965-1970." In *Demographic and Social Aspects of Population Growth,* ed. C.F. Westoff and R. Parke, Jr. Vol. I of the Commission on Population Growth and the American Future, Research Reports. Washington, D.C.: U.S. Government Printing Office, 1972. (b)

Rodgers, D.A., Ziegler, F.J., and Levy, N. "Prevailing Cultural Attitudes about Vasectomy: A Possible Explanation of Postoperative Psychological Response." *Psychosomatic Medicine* 29 (July-August 1967): 367-75.

Ryder, N.B. and Westoff, C.F. *Reproduction in the United States, 1965.* Princeton, N.J.: Princeton University Press, 1971.

Scrimshaw, S.C. and Pasquariella, B. "Obstacles to Sterilization in One Community." *Family Planning Perspectives* 2 (October 1970): 40-42.

Sobrero, A.J. and Kohli, K.L. "Two Years' Experience of An Outpatient Vasectomy Service." *American Journal of Public Health* 65, 10 (October 1975): 1091-94.

_____, Edy, H. "A Vasectomy Service Within a Planned Parenthood Clinic." In *Advances in Planned Parenthood,* ed. A.J. Sobrero and R.N. Harvey, Vol. 6, pp. 130-32. Amsterdam: Excerpta Medica, 1971.

U.S. Commission on Population Growth and the American Future, Report of the Commission. *Population and the American Future.* Washington, D.C.: Government Printing Office, 1972.

Vaughan, D. "Demographic Characteristics of Persons Sterilized in OEO Planning Services in 1972." A Working Paper, 1973.

Westoff, C.F. "The Modernization of U.S. Contraceptive Practice." *Family Planning Perspectives* 4, 3 (July 1972): 9-12.

Whelpton, P.K., Campbell, A.A., and Patterson, J.E. *Fertility and Family Planning in the United States.* Princeton: Princeton University Press, 1966.

**Part IV
Economic Aspects of
Contraceptive Sterilization**

# 13 Economic Determinants, Consequences, and Policy Implications of Contraceptive Sterilization
*George B. Simmons*

In countries around the world, contraceptive sterilization has achieved wide acceptance from men and women seeking to limit family size and has been adopted by many governments as a means of achieving national population goals. Economic factors are important determinants and consequences of contraceptive sterilization. Moreover, many of the important policy implications of contraceptive sterilization are primarily economic in nature.

The economics of contraceptive sterilization differs in degree and not in kind from that of other forms of contraceptive use. The economic determinants of the use of contraceptive sterilization are basically the economics of fertility control; the economic consequences that flow from contraceptive sterilization are best described as a particular instance of those related to any form of birth restriction. A very broad literature thus serves as our point of departure.

This chapter focuses on some of the economic determinants, consequences, and policy implications of contraceptive sterilization, including discussions of the general theoretical background, suggested hypotheses, and past research.

## The Economic Determinants of Contraceptive Sterilization

Economic factors are clearly central for couples in their reproductive years in deciding on the number and spacing of the children that they want. When questioned concerning their reasons for limiting family size, parents in many countries cite the economic factors compelling them to restrict the number of children they have. Children are the source of major financial demands upon the family. Costs are incurred with the child's delivery, with feeding, maintaining, and educating it throughout its development, and with related changes in the behavior of other family members, such as withdrawal of the wife from the labor force.

Microeconomic theory provides a framework for the study of the choices involved in family planning in general and the selection of one method of contraception over other alternatives. It is postulated that the individual (and by extension, the family unit) possesses a set of tastes (whose origin is not spelled out) in reference to which a universe of alternative states can be ranked.

Highly preferred states are said to provide high "utility"; low utility is attached
to those states that are given low preference. Scarcity constrains the individual
from achieving any state simply on the basis of his preferences. The best the
individual can do is to seek the highest level of utility consistent with a given set
of prices and the limited amount of income and time available to the family.
Economic theory predicts that individuals choose the highest level of utility
consistent with their budget constraints. Thus, when the tastes of the family
remain constant, it is possible to predict the effects of changes in the budget con-
straint on family size.

## The Economics of Fertility

Some of the costs of raising children have already been mentioned. On the basis
of a number of studies,[a] one may verify what every parent knows, that the total
costs are indeed substantial. The U.S. Commission on Population Growth and
the American Future (1972a), to take an extreme example, estimated an outlay
on the order of $60,000 to raise the first child to maturity (including the loss of
wages from the wife). Raising later children is, of course, less costly, but still of
significantly high economic importance to the family.

The constraints on family resources play an important role in determining
fertility behavior. In his original article on the subject, Becker hypothesized
that, contrary to popular opinion, with proper controls there should be a positive relationship between income and the number of children chosen by a family
(Becker, 1960). Later writers and critics have suggested alternative formulations
and extensions of the argument. Much of the extensive literature on the economics of fertility is concerned with the appropriate definition of the costs and the
income constraints relevant to family size decisions.[b]  Many recent commentators, most notably Willis (1973), take as their point of departure an economic
model of the consumption of consumer durables. Children are considered to
have many of the properties of durables in that they cost money but yield
utility over long periods of time. Families are assumed to maximize their total
utility from children and all other sources, subject to economic and biological
constraints.

This literature introduces a level of theoretical rigor which was hitherto
lacking in the study of a demographic behavior. Unfortunately, empirical
studies based on the economic models have not been able to explain variations
in fertility behavior to the extent research successfully handles other aspects

---

[a]The methodologies involved in these estimates have been reviewed by Espenshade (1972).

[b]The April 1973 supplement to the *Journal of Political Economy* contains an extensive
bibliography and a description of the current state of the art (Schultz, 1973).

of consumer behavior. In general, nonetheless, the economic models do about as well as those developed by other disciplines, insofar as the very different methodologies are comparable.

Many problems are associated with the literature on the economics of fertility. One obstacle to prediction, clearly defined in the literature, relates to the quality-quantity choice facing parents. The same total amount of money can be spent by having many children with relatively small expenditures per child or by having few children with relatively large expenditures per child. It is hard to know how a particular family will opt.

A more fundamental problem arises from the assumption by economic models that consumer tastes are fixed. For normal consumer choices, this formulation may be appropriate. For choices around fertility over a long time period (the years between marriage and menopause), this specification of the problem is highly restrictive; learning and change are, after all, an integral part of the process of family formation. At least in empirical applications of the models, the time span for fertility behavior also increases the likelihood that surveys are subject to the particular economic constraints operating on parents at the point of any one observation; these constraints change markedly over the course of a marriage. It may be inappropriate to construct a profile, for example, by combining retrospective fertility information provided by a forty-year-old woman with current data on the income or general economic situation of her family; the woman may have experienced a quite different set of economic circumstances when she was twenty-five or thirty, the years when most of her children were born. Knowledge concerning the economics of fertility will be considerably strengthened, therefore, by longitudinal studies.

The accuracy of predictions may also be enhanced through more use of data on expectations and perceptions rather than the hard economic information of the more traditional variety. In fact, the general use of interdisciplinary data may be the area of sharpest debate among economic scholars who work in the area. On one side is a group concerned with a straightforward application of economic models of fertility (for instance, Schultz, 1973). An opposing group, much more diffused and less well organized, is more interested in the integration of different social science approaches to the study of fertility (Easterlin, 1969; Mueller, 1972; Namboodiri, 1972; Arnold and Fawcett, 1973; Anker, 1973, Turchi, 1975). The differences in approach will only be resolved through more theoretical and empirical work.


*The Economics of Contraceptive Sterilization*

Application of economic principles to the choice of contraceptive sterilization is based on the assumption that this particular decision and its timing, as well, are dictated in part by economic considerations. Rational decision-makers, according to economic theory, attempt to minimize the cost of achieving any particular end—in this case, the prevention of further pregnancies. (There are, of course, considerations other than cost which are at least as important, if not more important. Any couple willing to adopt voluntary sterilization for contraceptive purposes must be content with the number of children that it already has; sterilization cannot be used for spacing.) For that subset of couples contemplating sterilization as a method of contraception, the economics of the choice may be an important consideration. The central issue is the definition of "cost."

Basically, there are a number of different costs that affect the decision, some strictly economic, some more social or psychological in nature (Simmons, 1974). The great advantage of sterilization rests in its once-and-for-all application, its long life, and its relatively low annual cost when the costs are spread over the years of fertility that would otherwise remain. In its disfavor are the high initial expense of surgery and the psychological costs which some persons may experience in undertaking such an operation. It is difficult to know how these costs are weighed against one another in decision-making, and this problem is worth investigating.

Table 13-1 gives some estimates of the direct and indirect costs for sterilization and other contraceptive methods in the United States and India. The numbers contained in the table are highly tentative. A problem with great research potential is the investigation of the costs of different types of contraception and a further investigation of the role played by different costs in determining the choices of contraceptors.

### The Economic Consequences of Contraceptive Sterilization

Contraceptive sterilization has important consequences both for the adopting couple and for the wider society, depending upon the circumstances of the individuals electing sterilization and the general conditions prevailing in the society at the time.

The principal immediate effect of contraceptive sterilization, of course, is to reduce fertility to an extent that varies with age of the parents, the alternative fertility they would have experienced, and a number of other factors. The reduced fertility, in turn, induces a series of changes in work habits, consumption, investment, government welfare expenditures, and other economic areas of choice. As in the case of the economic determinants, the primary consequences of contraceptive sterilization represent behavioral changes which are not unlike those resulting from almost any form of contraceptive behavior effectively lowering fertility.

The literature on the economic consequences of fertility decisions is

**Table 13-1**
**Estimated Costs[1] of Contraception (United States and India)**

| Contraceptive Method | Risks of Pregnancy | Convenience | Use | Direct Costs: India | Direct Costs: U.S. | Direct Costs for Five Years Protection: U.S. |
|---|---|---|---|---|---|---|
| Vasectomy | Very low | Fear | Final | Rs. 20-30 | $75-$150 | $75-$150 |
| Tubal Ligation | Very low | Fear | Final | Rs. 60-80 | $150-$500 | $150-$500 |
| Oral Contraceptives | Low | Side effects | Continuing use | Rs. 35/yr. | $25-$40/yr. | $125-$200 |
| IUD | Low | Side effects | Infrequent applications | Rs. 10 | $20 per insertion | $70* |
| Conventional (Condoms) | Moderate | Inconvenient | | Rs. 10-20/yr. | $25-$35/yr. | $125-$175 |

Adapted from material originally published in Simmons, G.B. (1974) "The Economics of Voluntary Sterilization for the Parent and for the Nation" *Advances in Voluntary Sterilization*, p. 154, M.E. Schima, I. Lubell, J.E. Davis, E. Connell, editors. Excerpta Medica Amsterdam.

[1]Not including the costs of recruiting cases in an active program of family planning.

*Two insertions, three check-ups.

extensive.[c] It is important to distinguish the consequences of these fertility decisions as they take place in industrialized countries from those taking place in the less developed countries.

In developed countries, such as the United States, the economic consequences of reduced fertility have been described in *Population and the American Future* (U.S. Commission on Population and the American Future, 1972a) and in more detail in some of the background papers for that report (Spengler, 1971; U.S. Commission on Population and the American Future, 1972a, 1972b). Traditionally, there has been some concern that a reduced rate of population growth would have adverse effects on the country because of lower level of aggregate demand. This is considered unlikely by most modern scholars. Recent developments have led to improved methods of controlling economic fluctuations, methods that should avoid such untoward consequences of changing rates of population growth.

The other important impact of population growth in the developed countries is on the size of the labor force. Given lower fertility, women who would otherwise have remained at home engaging in child care would be free to seek and find employment. This is, however, a temporary phenomenon. Over the longer run, higher population growth has the greater impact since it induces a more rapid rate of growth of the labor force itself. Thus, in labor-scarce economies, the population growth has the positive effect of encouraging a larger labor supply for economic development. Whether such development is considered desirable or not depends upon the specification of policy objectives.

The impact of the population growth in the less developed countries (LDCs) has been the subject of much speculation. Because our knowledge of economic relations in the developing world is still relatively incomplete, the issues are more complicated and perhaps less understood. In most LDCs, the labor supply is already sufficiently large, thus more labor is not an immediate need or benefit. There are some indications, moreover, that the impact of population growth on personal savings may be adverse and that rapid population growth may demand a redirection of funds away from economically productive uses by government toward less productive welfare and social services expenditures. The ultimate effect in LDCs may thus be to reduce the growth capacity of the economy. More immediately, the high rate of population growth leads to a somewhat lower level of per capita income than would have been attained otherwise.

This short review of the economic consequences of reduced fertility does little justice to the rich literature which exists in the area. Many issues are

---

[c]It would be impossible to list all relevant sources in this area. For less developed countries, a list of basic references can be found in Jones (1971). See also the papers contained in *Rapid Population Growth: Consequences and Policy Implications* (National Academy of Sciences, 1971).

still unresolved, but as most of them relate to wider questions than contraceptive sterilization *per se*, they will not be pursued here. It need be said in summary only that reduced rates of population growth have major beneficial implications for LDCs. The economic impact on developed countries is not as harmful as has often been suggested.

In both the developed and developing countries, population growth also has more subtle and indirect effects. As the report of the U.S. Commission on Population and the American Future (1972a) has indicated, in the United States (and presumably in other developed countries) population growth has seriously undesirable consequences for the quality of political institutions, social structure, education, the environment, and other conditions affecting the lives of the entire population. Inevitably, these changes will indirectly influence demographic and economic behavior. The impact of the indirect influences on economic growth and alternative patterns of economic activity is not entirely clear, but it would be unwise to suggest that all the economic implications of different rates of population growth are fully understood. The consequences of population growth are subtle, pervasive, and long term, making for relationships that economists are not well adapted to examining.

These comments might also be applied to the indirect economic effects of population growth in LDCs. It is known that rapid population growth affects the form and development of social and economic institutions in these countries. The size of a family living together at any given time and the rapidity with which land is subdivided are demographically determined conditions with important economic implications. Moreover, there are important ecological effects associated with population growth in many of the less developed regions—witness recent famines in central Africa. Little is known thus far about the exact dynamics of these relationships. Contraceptive sterilization, to the extent that it has demographic effects, shares with other methods of contraception in determining important and as yet incompletely understood economic consequences for the individual adopters and society as a whole.

## The Policy Implications of Contraceptive Sterilization

Should contraceptive sterilization have a role in publicly sponsored population programs? If the answer to this central policy question is in the affirmative, the next issue is the specification of that role. The economic framework is important to the examination of policy alternatives. Specifically, the economic approach analyzes the costs of government-sponsored contraceptive sterilization programs, the potential benefits, and to whom the benefits accrue.

Once again, the economic implications of government provision of facilities for contraceptive sterilization can be evaluated in the manner applied to other government programs. Admittedly, contraceptive sterilization is not solely or primarily part of economic policy. To the extent that policies involving contraceptive sterilization set in motion a series of events with important economic implications, however, government policies may be, and indeed should be, considered in terms of their costs and benefits.

The evaluation of economic policies is a complex process involving three major steps: (1) specification of the objectives to be promoted by a given set of activities (projects or programs); (2) specification of the relationship among the suggested activities and those policy objectives; and (3) the choice of the optimum set of activities which might be undertaken. These various steps have been treated in great detail in a wide-ranging literature.[d]

The use of contraceptive sterilization as a means of furthering economic policy demands an analysis of the benefits and the costs of the contraceptive sterilization program. On the benefit side, the consequent reduction in the level of fertility has favorable implications for a number of widely accepted economic objectives, such as improved standard of living and maximization of employment opportunities for the population. On the cost side, programs of contraceptive sterilization involve the deployment of scarce medical manpower and other resources which have important alternative uses. Almost all estimates in this area indicate that the costs of such programs are considerably less than the benefits, particularly in the LDCs. To some extent, judgment on this matter hinges on the definition of external effects, that is, the extent to which the consequences of fertility are felt beyond the family.

In making choices, the policy-maker is faced with the difficult choice of defining the scale of his activities. He must distinguish between the average benefit and cost versus the marginal benefit and cost. To a very large extent, the marginal benefit depends on the nature of what may be called the "response function" of the population, which is the intended primary beneficiary of an active program of contraceptive sterilization.

Clearly related to the determinants discussed in the first section of this chapter, the "response function" attempts to isolate changes in the use of contraceptive sterilization when the level of inputs to a public program increases, holding other factors constant. It is hard to overemphasize the importance of the response function for policy. The responsiveness of the population determines the cost of running a program of contraceptive sterilization. If a large number of people are volunteering for this form of contraception, the program can be run relatively cheaply. If people are reluctant to volunteer, however, contraceptive sterilization (especially an active program of recruitment) may be one of the more expensive elements

---

[d]The literature on the economics of population policy has recently been reviewed in Simmons (1976). See also Enke (1960), Ohlin (1961), Leibenstein (1969), Robinson and Horlacher (1971), Simmons (1971), and Zaidan (1971).

in a family planning program. The response function itself is partly determined by the way in which contraceptive sterilization is offered and how well people's fears of the procedure are overcome. In many parts of the world, contraceptive sterilization is confused with castration or conjures up the prospects of serious medical complications.

Even with great justification for providing a given level of services, it is possible that additional demand would be insufficient to justify more expenditures. In India, for example, the last few years' experience would seem to indicate that little marginal benefit is to be gained from additional expenditures promoting contraceptive sterilization programs within the conventional family planning structure. Of course, large benefits might accrue by structural changes like the recent use of large-scale vasectomy camps.

In examining the costs and the benefits of programs of contraceptive sterilization, the contraceptive alternatives to sterilization must also be considered. It may be cheaper and easier to achieve the same demographic effect using a method or procedure different from contraceptive sterilization. Ideally, an active population policy attempts to maximize overall social gain as measured by the difference between the total benefits generated and the total costs. In practical terms, this objective is identical with the greatest possible impact of the population policy on the birth rate—a goal that may be reached through the use of any one or some mixture of a number of contraceptive strategies. Each of the alternatives, of course, involves its own costs and may involve, in fact, some mutual exclusion of choices. When a couple uses an IUD, for example, they are unlikely to resort simultaneously to contraceptive sterilization.

Earlier, we reviewed briefly the economic models of fertility. These have certain policy implications for the developing countries. If economic factors are indeed important for fertility decisions, the use of contraceptive sterilization could be encouraged through changes made in the economic environment or through incentives for couples who volunteer for sterilization or other methods of contraception.[e] Such incentives have been associated with government programs of contraceptive sterilization in India and Pakistan. There is no agreement on their impact, but the use of incentives is a subject that presents interesting opportunities for research.[f]

## Research Needs in the Area of Contraceptive Sterilization

Throughout this chapter, references have been made to topics and questions

[e]For one description of the way incentives may affect individual decisions, see Simmons (1971, Chapter 6).

[f]The incentives literature is vast. For a review of the literature by noneconomists, see Pohlman (1971) or Rogers (1973).

deserving of empirical investigation. In this concluding section, some of the more pressing research needs are listed.

1.  There is a need for increased theoretical and empirical investigation of the effects of economic variables on family decision-making concerning fertility regulation and termination.
2.  Further work should be done on the costs of contraceptive sterilization in systems in which it is used as part of a publicly sponsored program of fertility control.
3.  The determinants of what we have labeled the "response function" should be explicated. The further definition would, of necessity, involve field studies of both the administrative and social contexts in which contraceptive sterilization is offered and the other patterns of behavior which determine the individual's decision to use the method. The issues involved are not exclusively economic; medical, administrative, and psychological research will be necessary before we can fully respond to the economic questions.
4.  We need to know more about the general consequences of demographic behavior and how variations in it influence economic growth or other forms of economic change. This question is, of course, not specific to any one form of contraception, but understanding the consequences of demographic behavior would make for better implementation of all programs, including contraceptive sterilization.
5.  There should be more research on the use of incentives in recruiting adopters of contraceptive sterilization.

Economic research directly relating to the use of contraceptive sterilization is conspicuous in its absence. The review of the field by Presser (1970), for example, contains almost no references to materials prepared by economists. In large measure, the silence merely reflects the fact that most of the economic issues relevant to contraceptive sterilization apply in varying degrees to the use of all methods of contraception. On the wider set of issues the economic literature is extensive—so large, in fact, that this chapter has cited only some of the key bibliographic studies available. Perhaps because of the recent entry of economics into the area of demographic research, thus far economists have treated contraceptive sterilization as a particular example of the wider classes of human behavior designated as contraception and fertility.

### References

Anker, R. "Socio-Economic Determinants of Reproductive Behavior in Households of Rural Gujarat, India." Unpublished Ph.D. Dissertation, The University of Michigan, 1973.

Arnold, F.S. and Fawcett, J.T. "The Rewards and Costs of Children: A Comparison of Japanese, Filipinos, and Caucasians in Hawaii." Unpublished paper presented at the Population Association of America, New Orleans, April, 1973, prepared at the East-West Population Institute, Hawaii.

Becker, G.S. "An Economic Analysis of Fertility" In *Demographic and Economic Change in Developed Countries, Universities—National Bureau Conference.* Series II, Princeton, N.J.: Princeton University Press, 1960.

Easterlin, R. "Towards a Socioeconomic Theory of Fertility: Survey Research on Economic Factors in American Fertility." In *Fertility and Family Planning,* ed. S.J. Behrman, L. Corsa, and R. Freedman, pp. 127-57. Ann Arbor: University of Michigan Press, 1969.

Enke, S. "The Economics of Government Payments to Limit Population." *Economic Development and Cultural Change* 8, 2 (July 1960): 339-48.

Espenshade, T.J. "The Price of Children and Socio-Economic Theories of Fertility: A Survey of Alternative Methods of Estimating the Parental Cost of Raising Children." *Population Studies* 26, 2 (July 1972): 207-221.

Jones, G.W. "The Economic Effects of Declining Fertility in Less Developed Countries." *The Population Council Occasional Paper Series,* 1968.

Leibenstein, H. "Pitfalls in Benefit-Cost Analysis of Birth Prevention." *Population Studies* 23, 2 (July 1969): 161-70.

Mueller, E. "Economic Motives for Family Limitation: A Study Conducted in Taiwan." *Population Studies* 26, 3 (November 1972): 383-404.

Namboodiri, N. "Some Observations on the Economic Framework for Fertility Analysis." *Population Studies* 26, 2 (July, 1972).

National Academy of Sciences, *Rapid Population Growth: Consequences and Policy Implications.* Baltimore: The Johns Hopkins Press, 1971.

Ohlin, G. *Population Control and Economic Development.* Paris: Organization for Economic Co-operation and Development, 1961.

Pohlman, E. *Incentives and Compensations in Birth Planning.* Chapel Hill: University of North Carolina, Carolina Population Center, 1971.

Presser, H.B. "Voluntary Sterilization: A World View." *Reports on Population/Family Planning* 5 (July 1970): 1036.

Robinson, W.C. and Horlacher, D.E. "Population and Growth and Economic Welfare." *Reports on Family/Planning* 6 (February 1971).

Rogers, E.M. "Effects of Incentives on the Diffusion of Innovations: The Case of Family Planning in Asia." In *Process and Phenomena of Social Change,* ed. G. Zaltman. New York: John Wiley, 1973.

Schultz, T.W., ed. "New Economic Approaches to Fertility." *Journal of Political Economy* 81, 2 (March/April 1973).

Simmons, G.B. "The Economics of Voluntary Sterilization for the Parent and for the Nation." In *Advances in Voluntary Sterilization,* Proceedings of the Second International Conference, Geneva, 1973, p. 154, ed. M.E. Schima,

I. Lubell, J.E. Davis, and E. Connell. Princeton, N.J.: Excerpta Medica, American Elsevier Publishing Co., Inc., 1974.

_____. *The Indian Investment in Family Planning.* New York: The Population Council, 1971.

_____. "Public Expenditure Analysis and Family Planning Programs." In *Population Growth and Economic Development in the Third World,* ed. L. Tabah, Vol. 1, pp. 543-92. Ordina Editions: International Union for the Scientific Study of Population, 1976.

Spengler, J. *Declining Population Growth Revisited.* Monograph 14. Chapel Hill: University of North Carolina, Carolina Population Center, 1971.

Turchi, B. A. *The Demand for Children: The Economics of Fertility in the United States.* Cambridge, MA: Ballinger Publishing Co., 1975.

U.S. Commission on Population Growth and the American Future. Report of the Commission. *Population and the American Future.* Washington, D.C.: U.S. Government Printing Office, 1972a.

U.S. Commission on Population and the American Future, Research Reports Vol. II, "The Economic Aspects of Population Change," and Vol. III, "Resource and Environmental Consequences of Population Growth in the United States." Washington, D.C.: U.S. Government Printing Office, 1972b.

Willis, R.J. "A New Approach to the Economic Theory of Fertility Behavior." *Journal of Political Economy* 81, 2 (March/April 1973): S14-S69.

Zaidan, G. *The Costs and Benefits of Family Planning Programs.* World Bank Occasional Paper, No. 12. Baltimore: The Johns Hopkins Press, 1971.

**Part V
Survey Methodological Aspects of
Contraceptive Sterilization**

# 14

## Problems in Survey Methodology Relating to Contraceptive Sterilization
### Leonard A. LoSciuto and Nancy Cliff

### Introduction

Since the mid-1950s, social scientists have used survey research techniques to generate a great deal of information about population and fertility control. Knowledge about nonmedical aspects of contraceptive sterilization in the United States has been gained through four national fertility and population surveys conducted since 1955—the 1955 and 1960 Growth of America Family Studies (GAF) and the 1965 and 1970 National Fertility Studies (NFS). The national surveys have helped characterize the population currently practicing contraceptive sterilization and have enabled some assessment of the present and potential roles of contraceptive sterilization in preventing unwanted pregnancy. Data are available about the prevalence of sterilization by demographic, socioeconomic status (SES), and life cycle categories, the general trends in the prevalence and incidence of contraceptive sterilization over time, its acceptance among the general population and certain subpopulations as reflected by attitudinal data, and the extent of public knowledge of the effects of male sterilization on sexual performance.

A substantial number of smaller studies employing limited survey research techniques have also been conducted. For the most part, because these studies have been concerned with particular populations of sterilized individuals, their generalizability is severely restricted. These more modest investigations have attempted to describe sterilized populations by SES, life cycle characteristics, and motivations for surgery, as well as to determine the perceived effects of the operation on health and sexual desire and performance. The shortcomings and inconclusive nature of these studies have been pointed out by several authors, especially by Presser (1970).

### Major Methodological Questions Posed by Survey Research

The concern here is with large-scale, formal survey research, which entails the administration of a set of items in questionnaire format to a fairly large sample of individuals who are reasonably representative of the larger population of interest. Before any survey can be conducted, four major methodological issues must be addressed: (1) the nature of the questions asked; (2) the nature

201

of the target population; (3) the timing of data collection; and (4) the validity
of the information gathered.

This chapter deals in turn with each of these problems and how they bear
particularly on research regarding contraceptive sterilization. Illustrative
examples are drawn from the four large-scale surveys previously mentioned
which fit the present rather limited definition of survey research.

*What Are We Going to Ask, and How?*

Tables 14-1 and 14-2 present the items regarding contraceptive sterilization
which were used in the GAF and NFS surveys (Freedman, Whelpton, and
Campbell, 1959; Ryder and Westoff, 1971; Whelpton, Campbell, and Patterson,
1966).

An inspection of the tables shows that the number of questions on sterilization increased with the succeeding studies, reflecting a growing interest among
researchers in contraceptive sterilization. Much of this interest may be attributed
to the increasing sophistication of contraceptive sterilization technology, as
well as to the increasing availability and adoption of the methods. Because the
questions added dealt largely with attitudinal matters, however, they appear to
have been prompted also by a growing awareness among population researchers
that the efficacy of contraceptive sterilization in preventing unwanted pregnancy
depends to a great extent on its acceptance by the population at risk.

A second point of interest is that the questions asked in the surveys were
fairly consistent from study to study. The use of comparable items, the first
step toward the accumulation of data which may be examined for long-term
trends, is an important consideration if maximum value is to be gained from
survey data. (Though this point may seem obvious, it should be noted that only
recently have representatives of the country's major survey research institutions
attempted to standardize the way in which certain demographic data are collected.)

A third concern of survey researchers reflected in the questions is that their
language is clear and simple. Terms like "contraceptive sterilization" and
"surgical contraception," although easily understood by professionals, may be
meaningless to the population under study and should therefore be avoided in
general surveys.

Although the previous research has its positive points, much more could be
done to make the best use of survey data collected. For example, a major in-
efficiency of the questions is that they have usually been discrete items rather
than the product of scaling procedures. Using well-established methodologies
(such as Thurstone, Likert, Guttman, or multidimensional techniques), scales
could be developed to tap any number of parameters which may be related to
attitudes toward contraceptive sterilization. Once established, such scales

**Table 14-1**
**Questions on the Occurrence and Nature of Contraceptive Sterilization Procedures Asked in Four National Surveys**

| Study | Questions | | | | |
|---|---|---|---|---|---|
| 1955 GAF | Have you or your husband had an operation which makes pregnancy impossible? | | | | In what month and year was the (operation, injury)? |
| 1960 GAF | Have you or your husband had an operation or injury that makes it impossible to have (more) children? | (IF YES) What kind of operation or injury was it? | (IF OPERATION) Why did (you, he) have the operation? | (IF APPROPRIATE FOR THIS R) Was the operation done partly because you or your husband thought you shouldn't have (more) children or didn't want (more) children? | In what month and year was the (operation, injury)? |
| 1965 NFS | Have you or your (present) husband had an operation that makes it impossible to have any more children? | (IF YES) What kind of operation was it? | | Was the operation done at least partly so that you would not have any more children? | In what month and year did that take place? |
| 1970 NFS | Have you or your husband ever had an operation that makes it impossible for you to have any children? | (IF YES) What kind of operation? | | Was the operation done at least partly so that you would not have any more children? | When did that take place? |

**Table 14-2**
**Attitudinal Questions on Sterilization Asked in Four National Surveys**

| Study | Questions | | | | | |
|---|---|---|---|---|---|---|
| 1955 GAF | None | | | | | |
| 1960 GAF | None | | | | | |
| 1965 NFS | Some men get operated on to prevent further pregnancies. Do you strongly approve, approve, disapprove or strongly disapprove of those men doing this? | | Do you think such an operation would interfere with a man's physical ability to have intercourse? | Some women get operated on to prevent further pregnancies. Do you strongly approve, approve, disapprove, or strongly disapprove of those women doing this? | | |
| 1970 NFS | Some men get operated on to prevent further pregnancies. Do you strongly approve, approve, disapprove, or strongly disapprove of those men doing this? | Do you think your husband would seriously consider this as a way of preventing unwanted children? | Do you think such an operation would interfere with a man's physical ability to have intercourse? | Some women get operated on to prevent further pregnancies. Do you strongly approve, approve, disapprove, or strongly disapprove of those women doing this? | Would you seriously consider this as a way of preventing unwanted children? | If a couple decides on sterilization in order to prevent unwanted children, should it be the husband or the wife who gets sterilized? |

would be more reliable predictors of the different attitudinal postures. Established scales also offer the advantage of ease of statistical manipulation in data analysis.

A final element missing in these surveys is some measure of the reliability and validity of items used regarding contraceptive sterilization. Though appropriate methods exist to obtain such measures, they have not as yet been applied to research on contraceptive sterilization. It is therefore not known how well the items actually tap the phenomena being investigated or how much of the variance in the data may be attributable to, say, random responses or item position in the interview schedule.

## How Is the Target Population to be Defined and Found?

There is to date no efficient or feasible way of obtaining a representative sample of sterilized couples in the United States. The current prevalence of contraceptive sterilization in the United States is far too low to permit the use of traditional survey sampling techniques.

**Area Probability Sampling.**  Suppose that one wished to study a sample of 2,000 American couples who had been sterilized for contraceptive reasons. To make the example more realistic, let the sample be further defined by saying that couples must be married and living together, with the wife under forty-five years of age.

From census data, one could expect to find a married couple of the specified ages in about one house in 2.4 (roughly 42 percent). If the overall rate of contraceptive sterilization among such couples is 11 percent, a sterilized couple would be found in one house in 22.2 (that is, $.11 \times .42 = .046$, close to 5 percent). Finally, assuming the usual factors of nonresponse are operative, one could expect about 75 percent of those couples to cooperate—or, put another way, complete interviews could be expected from only one house in about thirty. To get 2,000 interviews, then, over 59,000 households would need to be contacted and screened.

Were such a study conducted, of course, efforts would also have to be made to oversample blacks, since most evidence indicates important differences among racial groups in attitudes toward and prevalence of contraceptive sterilization. Even with sample clustering, interviews with 2,000 white and 2,000 black couples might necessitate contacting upwards of 300,000 households. Those 4,000 interviews, moreover, would allow only comparisons within basic categories like race, region, age, and parity; to get detailed breakdowns, a much larger sample would be necessary. The expense of such an undertaking would obviously be great, perhaps prohibitively so. Unfortunately, other strategies for obtaining a representative sample of contraceptively sterilized couples are equally as impractical.

**Other Samplings Strategies.**  One might consider obtaining a representative sample of sterilized couples from the medical facilities in which the survey is performed.  This universe, however, even for a small geographic area, would be nearly impossible to define.  The operations may be performed, after all, in physicians' private offices, clinics, outpatient hospital facilities, and in almost every hospital in the country with obstetric facilities.  The varying accessibility of patient populations, as well as the tremendous collaborative network required to obtain them, renders this approach to sampling impossible on a national level and impractical even for a metropolitan area.  The situation might be different were any systematic way instituted for reporting operations for contraceptive sterilization.

**Control Groups.**  Thus far, only contraceptively sterilized populations have been discussed.  As has been pointed out by Presser (1970, pp. 23 ff), in obtaining data only from sterilized individuals, many unknown factors of self-selection may be operative.  To assess changes which the operation may effect on individuals' attitudes and behavior, demographically matched control groups are necessary.

**Identifying the Population at Risk.**  A final problem is worthy of mention regarding sampling frames of contraceptively sterilized individuals.  To estimate the number of births averted by contraceptive sterilization, some better determination must be made of whether sterilized couples would really have been among a population "at risk" for pregnancy had they not been sterilized.  There is evidence to support the notion that sterilized couples are more highly motivated contraceptors and might have chosen some other highly effective method of birth control had they not chosen contraceptive sterilization.  However, there are also indications that at least some couples choose sterilization as a last resort, having already experienced one or more unwanted preganancies.  It is important to distinguish between these two subgroups in research on contraceptive sterilization.

*When Do We Interview?*

Virtually all of the surveys to date concerning contraceptive sterilization have been retrospective in nature.  Data from the four major national fertility studies were also collected at only a single point in time.  It is important to stress again that attitudinal data on past events may be especially unreliable, as respondents may tend to exercise selective recall in reporting past expectations, attitudes, and motivations. In the family planning literature, retrospective information has often been considered suspect.

The concept of the "unwantedness" of a child, for example, has been used in analyses of both the 1965 and 1970 NFS data as a possible factor in explaining why some couples may resort to contraceptive sterilization as a terminal solution to unwanted pregnancy (Bumpass and Presser, 1972; Presser and Bumpass, 1972; Whelpton, Campbell, and Patterson, 1966). Higher proportions of contraceptive sterilizations have been found at least among couples reporting their last child as "unwanted" than among those reporting their last child as "wanted."

As Ryder and Westoff (1971) have noted, however,

The 1960 and 1965 studies [as well as the 1970 study] are forced to rely on the post factum answers of women of all parities to the question of how many children they want, whereas the longitudinal study [Princeton Study] permitted assessment of this preference (for women with two children) prior to additional exposure to child-bearing, and then followed their subsequent histories. This before and after measurement avoids the tendency of the number of children wanted to be adjusted to correspond with actual fertility (p. 134).

Even without a pre-post methodology, the effects of selective recall and similar factors can be reduced. For example, in a methodological study of measures of unwanted child-bearing (LoSciuto, 1970), it was possible to improve the validity of retrospective attitudinal measurement by selecting questionnaire items according to least social desirability.

Accuracy of recall, however, is not the only problem with cross-sectional data; they have limited generalizability to the future, as well as to the past. In the 1970 NFS, for instance, women were asked whether they or their husbands would "seriously consider" sterilization as a "way of preventing unwanted children." Presser and Bumpass (1972) have noted in their analyses of these data that such questions may be more interesting as "indicators of current acceptability of sterilization rather than as a predicator of eventual levels" (p. 19).

It is evident that data collected on a prospective basis would be more reliable in predicting future trends, as well as in assessing past motivations. The major drawback of prospective survey designs is, of course, their cost. In place of the ideal, methodological work is needed to improve retrospective attitudinal measures and to develop alternative sampling designs employing control groups.

### How Can the Accuracy of Data Collection Be Maximized?

The most important concerns regarding the accuracy of survey data on the topic of contraceptive sterilization are related to the general problems of interviewing on sensitive issues.

**Interviewer Selection and Training.** Interviewer selection and training have produced the major difficulties encountered at the Institute for Survey Research (ISR) in studying issues that might be sensitive—especially those relating to sexuality and fertility behavior. Interviewers must feel comfortable when asking the questions. If they hesitate, mispronounce terms, hurry the questions, or show other signs of discomfort, respondents tend to become uneasy; either terminations or biased replies may result. Perhaps even more serious a threat to the research venture is the finding that interviewers who are unsure of themselves with regard to the subject matter are less likely to obtain even initial cooperation at the door of the household.

Several steps should be taken to ensure against large-scale problems because of poor interviewer selection or training. First, in sending out availability notices to interviewers and in recruiting efforts in general, the nature of the subject matter of the study should be made clear. This helps to preclude the initial hiring of interviewers who will only drop out later. Second, during the hiring process, any obvious interviewer biases should be noted related to the subject matter of the research.

Thorough interviewer training is the most important step that can be taken to reduce interviewer bias. Interviewers should be trained, in particular, to be completely neutral in probing. If one interviewer probes with "*Why* do you want that many children?" while another asks, "Why do you want *that* many children?", the two are likely to collect data that are hardly comparable.

During training, finally, interviewers should be exposed to all the terminology contained in the questionnaire. They should role play at being both respondent and interviewer until they are comfortable with each question. As a final precaution, it is helpful to have interviewers conduct practice interviews with nonsample respondents before they are permitted to proceed to their actual assignments.

**Self-administered Questionnaires.** If certain issues seem especially sensitive, a self-administered questionnaire (SAQ) can be used for those portions of the interview which may otherwise cause trouble. At ISR, respondents have handed their SAQs back to interviewers in sealed envelopes. By including a "candor" scale on the SAQ, it is also possible to get some measure of the respondents' frankness and honesty throughout the entire interview. Respondents who complete and SAQ can then be compared with those who don't, to assess what differences may exist between the groups. On sexual issues, as one might expect, nonrespondents are often older and more conservative.

**Interviewer-Respondent Sex-Mix.** Thus far, the major fertility surveys have focused on the female as the source of information. When only the wife is questioned, it is difficult to assess the implications of some information, such as whether the couple would seriously consider male contraceptive sterilization. Likewise, though women's perceptions of the effects of vasectomy have been obtained, husbands have not as yet been questioned on the same issue. In general, many components of the decision-making processes regarding contraception and fertility control may be affected by the male partner. For better predictions from survey data, males, as well as their mates, must be interviewed.

This brings up another dilemma: the interviewing staffs maintained by most national survey research facilities are predominantly female. A typical interviewer would be a housewife with school-age children who wants to work, but only part-time. Thus far, with women the respondents in the large surveys, there has been little need to be concerned about the effects on the data of interviewer-respondent sex-mix.

Were males also to be interviewed, however, the candor of their responses might be affected by the presence of a female interviewer. Moreover, maintaining a male field force is problematic. Men are less likely to want part-time work, have a more difficult time being admitted to homes, and are generally less accurate in recording correct and complete answers. Turnover is also higher among men, thereby increasing the costs of staffing and training for a study employing male interviewers.

It should be noted, finally, that if data are to be obtained from both partners, precautions must be taken so that the responses of one partner are not contaminated by hearing or discussing the responses of the other spouse. It may be that with the use of male-female interviewing teams, as well as SAQs, some of these potential sources of bias can be reduced.

**Obtaining Data about a Medical Phenomenon.**   Still other problems are inherent in collecting accurate survey data relevant to contraceptive sterilization, though in many cases no viable solutions can be offered at the present time.

How does one obtain accurate information, for instance, about the exact nature of the operation performed? The difficulty is most obvious, of course, for surgery on the female. Respondents cannot reasonably be expected to report on the technical nature of their operations or which parts of the female reproductive system were involved. Currently, the difficulty of obtaining such data accurately on a national basis may only affect the adequacy of knowledge on the incidence and prevalence of contraceptive sterilization. However, as the reversibility of some operations becomes possible, distinguishing among both male and female operations will become more critical for assessing the effects of contraceptive sterilization on population growth.

A similar problem, again pertaining primarily to female operations, involves determining the reason(s) for the surgical procedure. To know accurately the number of unwanted births which may have been or might be prevented by contraceptive sterilization, it seems necessary to distinguish between operations performed at least partly for contraceptive reasons and those performed for strictly medical-remedial reasons. Among some populations, sterilization may be more acceptable if performed for medical indications. Some individuals may therefore report (and requently believe) that their operations were performed for medical reasons when, in fact, they were not. A possible example of this phenomenon is Puerto Rico, where the prevalence of female sterilization is relatively high, yet the population is largely Catholic.

Could some of these difficulties be relieved by obtaining the actual medical records of the respondents? ISR's experience with the American Women's Health Program[a] suggests that this is no simple solution. Medical opinion often varies widely and it is difficult to gather comparable medical data from different medical facilities.

### Needed Methodological Research

As suggested by the previous discussion, much could be done to sharpen survey research as a tool for investigators in the areas of fertility control and population. The five concerns listed below present themselves as most immediate:

1. Standardized sampling frames of contraceptively sterilized individuals should be developed, as well as sampling frames of individuals considered to be "at risk." A uniform system of reporting vital statistics and health statistics to some national data bank would be a boon to many frustrated researchers.

2. The extent to which *reported* sterilization-related attitudes and behavior reflect actual attitudes and behavior should be investigated. Major contributions would result from the development of scaling techniques which can be quantitatively evaluated in terms of reliability and validity. In a related area, the extent to which measurements of reported behavior and attitudes are differentially valid for various demographic groups should also be investigated.

3. Once valid items and scales have been established, a system should be developed for a thorough and expeditious interchange of information on the item pool. Consistent question phrasing and terminology are essential if an orderly body of knowledge is to accrue.

4. To obtain a complete picture of the dyadic decision-making process, increased data collection efforts should be undertaken with males. Effects of the interviewer-respondent sex-mix in collecting data on sexual issues should also be studied, as should the ways in which such effects can be minimized.

5. Of increasing concern to survey researchers is the growing nonresponse rate, with a concomitant increase in potential nonresponse bias. The optimal conditions under which individuals will cooperate in studies of sensitive issues—and will do so with candor—should be investigated.

---

[a]A study being conducted at ISR on the relationship between oral contraception and abnormal cervical cytology among 25,000 women (NICHD Contract NIH-NICHD-71-2299).

## References

Bumpass, L.L. and Presser, H.B. "Contraceptive Sterilization in the U.S.: 1965 and 1970. *Demography* 9, 4 (November 1972): 531-47.

Freedman, R., Whelpton, P.K., and Campbell, A.A. *Family Planning, Sterility, and Population Growth.* New York: McGraw-Hill Book Company, Inc. 1959.

LoSciuto, L. "A Report on a Methodological Study of Measures of Unwanted Childbearing." Unpublished report of research performed at the Institute for Survey Research for the National Institute of Child Health and Human Development under contract no. PH 43-68-435, November 1970.

Presser, H.B. and Bumpass, L.L. "The Acceptability of Contraceptive Sterilization Among U.S. Couples: 1970." *Family Planning Perspectives* 4, 4 (October 1972): 18-26.

Presser, H.B. "Voluntarily Sterilization: A World View. *Reports on Population/Family Planning* (July 1970) 5.

Ryder, N.B. and Westoff, C.F. *Reproduction in the United States—1965.* Princeton, N.J.: Princeton University Press, 1971.

Whelpton, P.K., Campbell, A.A., and Patterson, J.E. *Fertility and Family Planning in the United States.* Princeton, N.J.: Princeton University Press, 1966.

# 15

## Needed Research and Research Approaches: Overview
### Zanvel E. Klein and Sidney H. Newman

The purpose of this overview is to highlight major areas of needed research in the field of contraceptive sterilization and the ideas and investigative approaches that emerged from the workshop on which this volume is based. At the conclusion of the workshop, time was spent reviewing themes common to many of the papers and issues brought up by participants. This chapter serves to focus on some major points elicited in that final review:

1. The limited amount and quality of social-behavioral research are inappropriate to the social, psychological, political, and economic significance of the increasing popularity of contraceptive sterilization.

2. Investigators should attempt to develop and use broad theoretical-conceptual approaches that would serve to direct and illuminate research on contraceptive sterilization. As research develops, contraceptive sterilization should be perceived in the context of general fertility theory as one alternative method of birth control whose relation to the others needs to be determined. These considerations are, of course, long-term in character; they should not restrict more immediate research that concentrates on contraceptive sterilization in its own right.

3. More ambitious and broadly-gauged methods should be used to study the antecedents and consequences of contraceptive sterilization. When possible, research should be multidisciplinary, including representation of the psychological, economic, sociological, political, anthropological, and other behavioral-social points of view. *Comparability* across studies—both nationally and transnationally—is to be stressed. Such comparability need not straight-jacket research strategies or severely limit conceptual freedom; the development of a common core of theory, methods, and measuring instruments would still permit considerable investigative variation at the discretion of individual investigators. The *longitudinal/life cycle approach*, a valuable but infrequently applied framework, for research in the social sciences, should be given high priority because it enhances understanding of relationships over time.

4. Decision-making about fertility regulation and prevention, with particular reference to contraceptive sterilization, is an area especially deserving of research. To be considered are the kinds of fertility decisions (contraception/prevention) made at strategic points in the life process; psychological, economic, cultural, political, and other factors affecting the decision; and the nature of

213

couple interaction in the decision-making. Further studies are also needed on
the determinants of family size, including the motivations for having small
families.

More studies are required on the communication process involved in contraceptive sterilization (as well as other birth control practices) and barriers to
communication at the couple, village, community, national, and international
levels. A special facet of the problem is research on public persuasion in
relation to contraceptive sterilization in the context of prevailing ethical-social
values.

5. There is great need for understanding and improving delivery systems
and user-system interactions associated with contraceptive sterilization and
other aspects of individual, national, and international family planning programs.
This relatively unstudied area is especially relevant to population policy and
policy-makers. Investigators might consider the organizations and mechanisms
through which people can obtain contraceptive sterilizations, and the pathways
followed by those seeking sterilization. The availability of trained personnel
required for sterilization programs, particularly in developing countries, also
needs attention, as do the attitudes, activities, roles, and influences of physicians and paramedical personnel involved in contraceptive sterilization and
other facets of family planning programs. In countries such as India, such
studies should also focus on population program administrators and policy decision-makers.

6. The consequences of contraceptive sterilization (and other practices)
are as worthy of study as the antecedents and determinants. Research on the
consequences of contraceptive sterilization has generally been synonymous with
interest in the *psychological* sequelae. Despite a fairly sizeable number of studies
(more work has been done in this area than in other aspects of the consequences
of the practice), some basic questions remain unanswered. How does timing of
the sterilization in the life cycle of males or females relate to its psychological
effects? How do the attitudes, knowledge, motivation, and adjustment of the
sterilized individuals affect the psychological consequences? Relatively little
research has been done on the *long-term* consequences of sterilization, a contraceptive method which, after all, is permanent in its effects. There is a need for
development of brief, valid techniques for predicting the psychological effects
of contraceptive sterilization, especially for those individuals at high risk for
adverse outcome. The procedure, like all successful birth control strategies,
makes for smaller family sizes. This is a psychosocial factor, not yet completely
understood, with implications for individuals, families, communities, and
societies.

The *demographic and economic* implications of contraceptive sterilization
have received little attention. Such studies would have extremely important
implications for population planners, administrators, and policy-makers. How
can the effects of contraceptive sterilization on population growth and decline

be isolated and evaluated? One suggestion, admittedly exploratory, is to attempt to discover the contraceptive method(s) that sterilized couples would have used had one or both of them not been sterilized.

7. Sampling strategies and the identification of control groups are among the most difficult and important problems arising in research on contraceptive sterilization. The establishment of sampling frames should be considered of high priority. Also of high priority are the design and development of standardized instruments, such as interviews and inventories, for psychological assessments and the collection of other data pertinent to sterilization research. The scaling, standardizing, and culling of items—as elsewhere in the social sciences— must be careful and psychometrically sound. The gender of interviewers, because of interpersonal and cultural delicacy relating to contraceptive sterilization, is a factor to be kept in mind in the conduct of the investigations.

This overview has emphasized only the major areas and high priorities for research on contraceptive sterilization. The reader has probably already noted that the state of our knowledge forces us to remain interested in fundamental questions about family planning—questions that often could as easily be addressed regarding practices other than contraceptive sterilization. In the preceding chapters, each of the workshop participants has made his or her own suggestions for research, sought to design models, and brought forth investigative problems and tentative solutions. It is clear that we lack neither important questions nor social scientists with the imagination and persistence to work on them. Those of us active in the field of population planning need not be reminded of the saliency of contraceptive sterilization as a method of birth control or of the urgency of the demand for behavioral-social research. This book, we hope, will become part of the imperative under which we live as scientists and citizens of a crowded world—to increase our understanding of what has already occurred in the area of contraceptive sterilization and other forms of family planning, of what is happening at the present time, and of the future which human initiative (or indifference) will help shape.

# Bibliography

## I. Books and Monographs

Agarwala, S.N. *Family Planning Performance in India.* Bombay: International
Institute for Population Studies, January 1972.

——. *Family Planning Performance in India, 1967-70: A District-wide Study.*
Mimeographed. Bombay: International Institute for Population Studies,
1971.

Association for Voluntary Sterilization. *The Case for Voluntary Sterilization.*
New York, February 1971.

Balakrishna, S. *Vasectomy: A Follow-up Study in Andhra Pradesh.* Hyderabad:
National Institute of Community Development, 1936.

Barnes, E. and Johnson, G.B. *Effects of Vasectomy on Marriage Relationships.*
Des Moines, Iowa: Family Service — Travelers Aid, 1964.

Batiwalia, A.S. *Sterilization in the Male.* Bombay: Kohinoor Mills Family
Planning Center, 1970.

Bauer, K.H. and Mijulicz-Radecki. *Die Praxis der Sterilisierungsoperationen*
(Practice of Sterilization Operations). Leipzig: Verlag von Johann Barth,
1936.

Bellman, P.C. *Physicians' Attitudes and Behavior Toward Vasectomy.* Berkeley,
Calif.: University of California Press, 1970.

Bhende, A. *The Vasectomy Programme in Greater Bombay.* Bombay:
Demographic Training and Research Centre, 1968.

——. *The Vasectomy Programme in Greater Bombay.* Bombay: International
Institute for Population Studies, December 1970.

Bradshaw, L.E. *Vasectomy Reversibility: A Status Report.* Publication No. 3.
Washington, D.C.: George Washington University, Department of Medical
and Public Affairs, May 1976.

Burnight, R.G. et al. *Male Sterilization in Thailand: A Follow-up Study.*
Working Paper No. 5. Bangkok: Mahidol University, Institute for Population and Social Research, April 1974.

Chandrasekhar, A. *Final Population.* Paper 1 of 1972. Census of India 1971,
Series 1, India. Delhi: Government of India Press, 1972.

---

This comprehensive bibliography should be useful to those who wish to engage in research
on the behavioral-social aspects of contraceptive sterilization or to pursue the subject
matter in depth.

We wish to express our deep appreciation to Ms. Bates Buckner, Director, Technical Information Services, Carolina Population Center, University of North Carolina and her colleagues,
for invaluable aid in organizing the comprehensive bibliography and arranging it in its present format. We also wish to thank Ms. Susan Manners and Ms. Mary Berlin for their hard
work in the final preparation of the bibliography.

Chatterjee, B.B. *Decision for Vasectomy*. Rajghat, Varanasi, India: Gandhian Institute of Studies, 1969.

Chun, D. *Surgical Sterilization*. Mimeographed. Hong Kong: Family Planning Association, 1969.

Curt, J.N. *Evidence Relating to Acceptability of Sterilization: Individual, Social, Legal, Medical, Religious, and Professional (The Puerto Rican Experience)*. San Juan: The University of Puerto Rico, School of Public Health, 1973.

Darbari, B.S. *Sterilization Programme (Vasectomy)*. Mimeographed. New Delhi: Department of Family Planning, Ministry of Health and Family Planning, n.d.

Dodds, D.J. *Voluntary Male Sterilization*. Toronto: Damian Press, 1970.

Duncan, G.W., Falb, R.D., and Speidel, J.J. *Female Sterilization: Prognosis for Simplified Outpatient Procedures*. New York: Academic Press, 1972.

Ehrlich, P. *The Population Bomb*. New York: Ballantine Books, 1968.

Erikson, H.M. *Family Planning Programme in Punjab State: Survey and Field Studies*. Chandigarh, Punjab, India: Directorate of Health Services, 1967.

Fleishman, N. and Dixon, P.L. *Vasectomy, Sex and Parenthood*. Garden City, N.Y.: Doubleday, 1973.

Fletcher, J.F. *Morals and Medicine*. Princeton, N.J.: Princeton University Press, 1954.

Franda, M.F. *Mass Vasectomy Camps and Incentives in Indian Family Planning. Fieldstaff Reports of the American Universities. South Asia Series.* 16, 7, India, Hanover, American Universities Field Staff, 1972.

Freedman, R., Whelpton, P.K., and Campbell, A.A. *Family Planning, Sterility and Population Growth*. New York: McGraw-Hill Book Company, 1959.

Fried, J.J. *Vasectomy: The Truth and Consequences of the Newest Form of Birth Control*. New York: Saturday Review Press, 1972.

George Washington University Medical School. Department of Medical and Public Affairs. *Population Report: Sterilization,* Series C-D (Female and Male Sterilization). No. 1. February 1973.

Gillette, P.J. *Vasectomy: The Male Sterilization Operation*. New York: Paperback Library, 1972.

_____. *The Vasectomy Information Manual*. New York: Outerbridge and Lazard, 1972.

Greenfield, M. and Burrus, W.M. *Vasectomy: The Male Birth Control for Complete Sexual Freedom*. New York: Beach Publications, 1972.

Grindstaff, C.R. and Ebanks, G.E. *Personality Characteristics of Men Undergoing Vasectomy*. London and Ontario, Canada: University of Western Ontario, 1972.

Guttmacher, A.F., Best, W., and Jaffe, F.S. *Planning Your Family: The Complete Guide to Birth Control, Overcoming Infertility, Sterilization, With a Special Section on Abortion*. New York: Macmillan, 1964.

Hague, A. *Fertility Control Through Surgical Sterilization*. Lahore, Pakistan: District Family Planning Board, May 1968.

Hatt, P.K. *Backgrounds of Human Fertility in Puerto Rico.* Princeton, N.J.:
Princeton University Press, 1952.

Huang, T.T.Y. *Ways of Family Planning.* Taichung, Taiwan: Committee on
Family Planning, Provincial Health Department, 1968.

Hungar, S. *Schwangerschaftsunterbrechungen und Sterilisation von Frauen in
Hamburg: Analyse des Materials der Gutachtenstelle bei der Arztekammer
Hamburg der Janre 1964 und 1965.* Abortion and Sterilization of Women
in Hamburg: Analysis of Materials from Records of Decisions of the
Medical Board, Hamburg, 1964 and 1965. Sozialhygienische Forschungen,
Band 19. Bielefeld: W. Bertelsmann, 1968.

India, Kerala. Demographic Research Centre, Bureau of Economics and Statistics. *Demographic Particulars of Sterilised Persons, 1961-1962.* Trivandrum,
India, 1963.

———. Demographic Research Centre, Bureau of Economics and Statistics.
*Demographic Particulars of Sterilised Persons, 1962-1963.* Trivandrum,
India, 1963.

India, Ministry of Health and Family Planning. *Family Welfare Planning in
India: Year Book 1972-1973.* New Delhi: Government of India Press,
n.d.

India. Ministry of Health and Family Planning, Department of Family Planning.
*Family Planning in India: Programme Information 1970-71.* New Delhi,
1971.

India. Ministry of Health, Family Planning and Urban Development. *Sterilization
and IUCD insertions in the States and Union Territories, 1956 to March 1968.*
New Delhi: Government of India Press, 1968.

India. National Institute of Family Planning. *Vasectomy Camps – A Study.*
NIPF Report Series, No. 13. New Delhi: September 1973.

India. Planning Commission. Programme Evaluation Organization. Social
Development Division. *Family Planning Programme in India: An Evaluation.*
P.E.O. Publication No. 71. New Delhi, 1970.

India. Program Evaluation Organization. *Family Planning Programme in India:
An Evaluation.* New Delhi, Department of Family Planning, Ministry of
Health, Family Planning and Works, Housing and Urban Development:
Government of India Press, 1970.

India, Rajasthan. State Family Planning Bureau. *Family Planning Programme
in Rajasthan.* By B.L. Agrawal and K.M. Mathur. Jaipur, 1972.

Indian Chamber of Commerce, Family Planning Department. *Report on Beggar's
Camp.* Calcutta, 1971.

Intergovernmental Coordinating Committee. S.E. Asia Regional Cooperation in
Family and Population Planning; University of North Carolina. *Proceedings
of the Expert Meeting on Comparative Fertility Research, Sterilization and
Post-Conceptive Regulation.* Singapore: Eurasia Press, 1975.

International Planned Parenthood Federation. Middle East and North Africa
Region. *Islam and Family Planning: Proceedings of the International*

*Islamic Conference held in Rabat,* December 1971. Vol. 2, part 4. Beirut, 1974.

_____. *Seminar on Voluntary Sterilization and Post-Conceptive Regulation* (January 30, 1974 to February 2, 1974). Kuala Lumpur: 1974.

_____. *Sterilization as a Method of Family Planning.* Publication No. 22. London: October 1972.

IRHPF (Institute of Rural Health and Family Planning), *A Brief Report on the Study of Persons Who Have Undergone Vasectomy in the Institute Area.* Gandhigram: (Mimeographed), n.d.

Islam, A.I.M.M. *A Cause for Vasectomy in Population Control Programme in East Pakistan.* Mimeographed. Rajshahi, East Pakistan: Family Planning Training-cum-Research Institute, 1966.

Iyer, H.P. and Selvaraj, S.R. *Demographic Particulars of Sterilised Persons in Cannanore District, 1965–1966.* District Report Series (F.P.). Paper No. 4. Kerala: Demographic Research Centre, Trivandrum, 1968.

Jain, A.K., and Sarma, D.V.H. *Some Explanatory Factors for Statewise Differential Use of Family Planning Methods in India.* New York: The Population Council, 1974 (mimeo).

Jain, S.C. *The Canvassar System: A Study of A Policy Pertaining to Delivery of Family Planning Services.* Draft: Research Proposal, 1969 (manuscript).

Jhaver, P.S. *Reversible Vasectomy: Progress Reports to the Rockefeller Foundation, May 1966 to January 1968.* Mimeographed. New York: The Rockefeller Foundation, 1968.

Kapil, K.K. and Saksena, D.N. *A Bibliography of Sterilisation and KAP Studies in India.* Bombay: Demographic Research and Training Center, 1968.

Kapoor, S.D. *Behavioral Effects of Male Sterilisation: A Research Model Employing Sensitive Behavioral Indices for Evaluation.* New Delhi: Social Research Division, Central Family Planning Institute, 1967.

_____ and Chandhoke, A.S. *Behavioral Characteristics of Camp and Non-Camp Vasectomized Clients: A Comparative Study.* New Delhi: Central Family Planning Institute (Mimeographed), 1968.

Kasirsky, G. *Vasectomy, Manhood, and Sex.* New York: Springer, 1972.

Katti, A.P. and Hasalkar, J.B. *A Follow-up Study of Sterilised Males in the Rural Areas of Belgaum District.* Vidyagiri, Mysore State, India: Demographic Research Center, Institute of Economic Research, 1970.

Kaufman, A.R. *Progress of Birth Control in Canada.* Kitchener, Ontario, Canada: Parents' Information Bureau, 1970.

Kessel, E. "Evaluation of Sterilization Programs." Evaluation Series Paper No. 7. Chapel Hill, N.C.: International Fertility Research Program, 1975.

Keyhan, R. *Family Planning: A World View and its Significance for Iran.* Tehran: Chape-Mahwan, 1969.

Konotey-Ahulu, F.I.D. *Medical Considerations for Legalizing Voluntary Sterilization: Sickle-Cell Disease As A Case in Point.* Law and Population Monograph,

No. 13. Medford, Mass.: Tufts University, Law and Population Programme, 1973.

Korea. National Family Planning Center. *Family Planning Monthly Report: January 1971.* Seoul: 1971.

Krishnakumar, S., *Ernakulam District Janapperuppa Pratirodha Ya jna (Crusade for Control of Population Growth): A Report on the Massive Vasectomy Camp at Ernakulam.* Cochin (Ernakulam District) (Mimeographed), 1971.

_____. *The Story of the Ernakulam Experiment in Family Planning.* Government of Kerala. (India), 1969.

_____. *The Story of the Ernakulam Experiment in Family Planning.* Cochin, Government of Kerala, 1971.

Kumar, A. *An Over-view of Sterilization Studies in India.* Bombay: International Institute for Population Studies, 1972.

Kumaran, N.O. and Khan, M.S.S. *Report on the Demographic Particulars of Sterilised Persons in Cannanore District for 1964-65.* Paper No. 40. Trivandrum (Kerala): Demographic Research Centre (Mimeographed), 1966.

Lader, Lawrence, ed. *Foolproof Birth Control: Male and Female Sterilization.* Boston: Beacon Press, 1972.

Lavergne, J.L., and E.E.E.L. "Opiniones sobre el crecimiento de nuestra población, conocimientos sobre la planificación de la familia y uso de anticonceptivos de un sector de la población masculina de la República de Panamá." (Attitudes Toward the Growth of Our Population, Knowledge for Family Planning and Use of Contraceptives in a Sector of the Male Population of the Republic of Panama). Asociación Panameña para el Planeamiento de la Familia (APLAFA). Panama City: 1971.

Loraine, J.A. *Sex and the Population Crisis: An Endocrinologist's View of the 20th Century.* London: Heinemann Medical, 1970.

Lyons, T.C. *Legislation-Regulation-Availability of Contraception, Sterilization, Abortion in Selected Countries.* Mimeographed. Washington D.C.: Population and Program Analysis Division, Population Service, 1968.

Mandke, M.B. *Communication and Motivation for Vasectomy.* Mimeographed. Bombay: Demographic Training and Research Centre, 1967.

Mannan, M.A. *Male Sterilization in Commilla (A Follow-up Study on 100 Vasectomy Clients in Comilla Kotwali Thana).* Kotbari. Comilla: Pakistan Academy for Rural Development, April, 1969.

Monsma, J.C., ed. *Religion and Birth Control: Twenty-one Medical Specialists Write in Plain Language about Control of Conception, Therapeutic Abortion, Sterilization, Natural Childbirth and Artificial Insemination.* Garden City, N.Y.: Doubleday, 1963.

Morcos, M. et al. *The Attitude of Christianity Towards Family Planning (a Social Study).* Population Studies, No. 26, November 1975.

Myaing, T.T. and Reynolds, J. *Esterilizacion Femenian en Costa Rica, 1959-*

*1969* (Female Sterilization in Costa Rica, 1959-1969). Universidad de Costa Rica, 1973.

Nair, G.S. and Nair, K.N.R. *Report on the Demographic Particulars of Sterilized Persons in Kozhi Kode District 1964-65.* Paper No. 37. Trivandrum: Demographic Research Centre, 1966.

Nair, K.R. and Pillai, N.K. *A Report on the Demographic Particulars of Sterilised Persons in Kottavam District,* 1964-65. Paper No. 35. Trivandrum: Demographic Research Centre, 1966.

Nair, P.S.G. and Ayyappan, K.S. *Demographic Particulars of Sterilised Persons in Trichur District, 1965-66.* District Report Series (Family Planning), Paper No. 1. Trivandrum: Demographic Research Centre (Mimeographed), 1967.

Nepal. Family Planning and Maternal Child Health Project, Research, Planning and Evaluation Unit. *Vasectomy Acceptors: Evaluation Report of February, March, April, May, June 1970 (Falgun, Chaitra, Baisakh, Jestha, Asnad, 2026-27).* 1970.

Nepal. Family Planning and Maternal Child Health Project, Research, Planning and Evaluation Unit. *Vasectomy Evaluation Report: July and August 1969 (Scrawan and Bhadra, 2026).* 1969.

Nortman, D. *Population and Family Planning Programs: A Factbook.* New York: Population Council, and Columbia University, July 1970.

_____. *Population and Family Planning Programs: A Factbook.* Reports on Population/Family Planning. New York: Population Council, June 1971.

_____ and Hofstatter, E. *Population and Family Planning Programs: A Factbook.* Publication No. 2. New York: Population Council, December 1974.

O'Neill, C.J. *The Demographic Implications of Contraception, Sterilization and Abortion in New Zealand.* Hamilton, N.Z.: University of Waikato, September 1975.

Pai, D.N. *India's Vasectomy Camps.* Mimeographed. Bombay: Maternal and Child Health Division, Municipal Corporation of Greater Bombay, 1969.

Pakistan (East). Family Planning Board. *Progress Report on Family Planning.* Dacca, June 1967.

Pakistan. National Research Institute of Family Planning. *Proceedings of the Fifth Biannual Seminar on Research and Family Planning.* Lahore, November 7-9, 1968. Karachi: 1969.

Pakistan. National Research Institute of Family Planning. *Proceedings of the Sixth Biannual Seminar on Research and Family Planning.* Karachi, April 23-26, 1969. Karachi: 1970.

Patel, V.M. *A Study of Effectiveness of Card System for Using Vasectomy Cases as Motivators and a Plan of Action for Gujarat State, 1970-71.* Mimeographed. Ahmedabad, India: State Family Planning Bureau, 1969.

Pilpel, H.F. *Know Your Rights About Voluntary Sterilization.* New York: Association for Voluntary Sterilization, 1971.

Piotrow, P.E., ed. *Voluntary Sterilization.* Draper World Population Fund Report, Monograph Series No. 3. Washington, D.C.: Population Crisis Committee, 1976.

Pohlman, E.W. *Incentives and Compensations in Birth Planning.* Monograph Series No. 11. Chapel Hill, N.C.: Carolina Population Center, 1971.

_____. *The Psychology of Birth Planning.* Cambridge, Mass.: Schenkman, 1969, pp. 405-409.

Poole, K. *Topical Investigation and Analysis of Intensive vs. Extensive Use of Resources Where Sterilization is the Primary Method of Contraception.* Research Triangle Park, N.C.: Research Triangle Institute, 1970.

Population Crisis Committee. *Mankind's Great Need: Population Research.* Washington, D.C., 1971.

Population Crisis Committee. *Voluntary Sterilization.* Draper World Population Fund Report, Monograph No. 3. Washington, D.C., Autumn-Winter 1976.

Potts, M. and Wood, C., eds. *New Concepts in Contraception: A Guide to Developments in Family Planning.* Baltimore: University Park Press, 1972.

Presser, H.B. *Sterilization and Fertility Decline in Puerto Rico.* Berkeley, Calif.: University of California, Institute of International Studies, International Population and Urban Research, Population Monograph Series, No. 13, 1973.

_____. *Voluntary Sterilization: A World View.* New York: Population Council, and Columbia University, July 1970.

Rajagopal, T.P. and Sukamaran, K.K. *Demographic Particulars of Sterilized Persons in Ernakulam District (1964-65 and 1965-66).* (Two Issues). Trivandrum: Demographic Research Centre, Government of Kerala, 1968.

Raman, M.V. *A Critique of Some of the Targets for IUCD and Sterilization.* Calcutta: Demography Unit, Indian Statistical Institute, 1966.

Rama Rao, G. *Impact of Long-Term Sterilisation Programme on Some Demographic Characteristics of the Population.* Bombay: International Institute for Population Studies, June 1972.

_____ and Yeole, B.B. *Impact of Long-Term Sterilization Programme on Some Demographic Characteristics of the Population.* Bombay: International Institute for Population Studies, 1972.

Rao, V.K.R.V. *The Indian Experiment in Family Planning: A Review and Suggestions for the Future.* Bombay: International Institute for Population Studies, 1974.

Rasheed, C. *A Pilot Vasectomy Program in a Rural Area of West Pakistan.* Lahore: West Pakistan Research and Evaluation Center, 1967.

Rastogi, S.R. *Demographic Rationality in Vasectomy Acceptance in Rural Communities.* Series C: Occasional Paper, No. 10. Lucknow: Lucknow

University, Demographic Research Centre, July 1975.

Repetto, R. "Temporal Aspects of Indian Development." Ph.D. thesis. Cambridge, Mass.: Harvard University, 1969.

Research and Marketing Services. *A Study on the Evaluation of the Effectiveness of the Tata Incentive Programme for Sterilisation: vol. 1, The Report.* Bombay, 1970.

Richart, R.M. and Prager, D.J. *Human Sterilization.* Springfield: Charles C. Thomas, 1972.

Rogers, E.M. and Shoemaker, F.F. *Communication of Innovations: A Cross-Cultural Approach.* New York: Free Press of Glencoe, 1971.

Ross, J.A. et al. *Findings from Family Planning Research.* Reports on Population/Family Planning Series. New York: Population Council, October 1972.

Russia, K.G. *Madras State Family Planning Program: Present Twin Emphasis on Sterilization and IUD.* Student paper written for the School of Public Health, University of North Carolina at Chapel Hill. Chapel Hill, N.C., Spring 1969.

Ryder, N.B. and Westoff, C.F. *Reproduction in the United States, 1965.* Princeton: Princeton University Press, 1971.

Sally, K.P. and Bhardwaj, K.S. *A Report on Demographic Particulars of Sterilized Persons in Alleppey District, 1964-65.* Paper No. 41. Trivandrum: Demographic Research Centre, 1966.

Sandhu, S.K. *Report on Follow-Up Study of Vasectomized Cases in Paharganj Area.* New Delhi: Central Family Planning Institute, 1969.

Sanwal, H. and Agarwala, S.N., eds. *Problems and Prospects of Family Planning in India.* Lucknow: Population Centre, 1975.

Sciarra, J.J. et al., eds. *Control of Male Fertility: Proceedings of a Workshop on Control of Male Fertility Held in San Francisco, California.* Hagerstown: Harper & Row, Medical Department, 1975.

Schima, M.E., et al., eds. *Advances in Voluntary Sterilization,* Proceedings of the Second International Conference. Princeton: Exerpta Medica, 1974.

Segal, S.J. and Tietze, C. *Contraceptive Technology: Current and Prospective Methods.* New York: Population Council, 1974.

Sengupta, A. *Behavior Patterns of Manual Workers Towards Fertility Control in a CAR Project.* Calcutta: Indian Statistical Institute, 1969.

_____. *Family Life and Fertility Control of Non-white Collar Workers in a Research Institute.* Calcutta: Indian Statistical Institute, 1969.

Sikes, O.J. and Greene, D.T. *Sterilization in Caswell County, North Carolina, 1957-1958.* Caswell County, N.C.: Department of Public Health, 1969.

Simmons, G.B. *The Indian Investment in Family Planning.* An Occasional Paper of the Population Council. New York: Population Council, 1971.

Simon Population Trust. *Vasectomy: Followup of a Thousand Cases.* Cambridge, 1969.

Singapore. Family Planning and Population Board, National Statistical Commission. *Report of the 1st National Survey on Family Planning in Singapore, 1973.* By Wan Fook Kee and Saw Swee-Hock. Singapore, September 1974.

Singh, K.M. *Family Planning Programme in Punjab State for 1968-1969: Policies and Other Relevant Information.* Punjab, India: Directorate of Health Services, 1970.

Soni, V. *The Ernakulam Camps.* New Delhi: Ford Foundation, 1971.

Spillane, W.H. and Ryser, P.E. *Male Fertility Survey: Fertility Knowledge, Attitudes and Practices of Married Men.* Cambridge, Mass.: Ballinger, 1975.

Srikantan, K.S. *Comparative Analysis of Family Planning Programs in the Context of Socio-Economic Infrastructure: States of India.* New York: The Population Council, 1974 (mimeo).

Stepan, J. and Kellog, G.J. *The World's Laws on Voluntary Sterilization for Family Planning Purposes.* Law and Population Monograph Series. No. 8. Medford, Mass.: Fletcher School of Law and Diplomacy, Tufts University, 1972.

Stolnitz, G.J. *Estimating the Birth Effects of India's Family Planning Targets: A Report on Statistical Methodology and Illustrative Projections, 1968-1978.* Washington, D.C.: USAID Consultant Report, 1968.

Sundaram, C. *A Follow-Up Study of Sterilised Male Industrial Workers in Bombay.* Publication Series No. 3. Bombay: Family Planning Association of India, 1969.

Thiery, M. *Anticoncepti* (Contraception). Leiden, Netherlands: Stafleu's Wetenschappelijke Uitgeversmaatschappi, NV, 1971.

Tietze, C. and Neumann, L., eds. *Surgical Sterilization of Men and Women: A Selected Bibliography.* Publication No. 11. New York: National Committee on Maternal Health, 1962.

Udry, J.R. *Sterilization as a Terminal Contraceptive Method.* Chapel Hill, N.C.: Department of Maternal and Child Health, School of Public Health, University of North Carolina at Chapel Hill, 1971 (Mimeographed).

United Nations, Department of Economic and Social Affairs, Commissioner For Technical Cooperation, Advisory Mission, *An Evaluation of the Family Planning Program for the Government of India,* 1972.

United Nations, Department of Economic and Social Affairs, Interagency Mission, *Population and Family Planning in Iran,* 1971.

U.S. Agency for International Development. Office of Population. *Family Planning Service Statistics.* Annual Report, 1974.

———. Office of Population. *Family Planning Service Statistics.* Washington, D.C.: U.S. Government Printing Office, January 1976.

U.S. Commission on Population Growth and the American Future, Report of the Commission. *Population and the American Future.* Washington, D.C.: U.S. Government Printing Office, 1972.

U.S. National Center for Health Statistics. *Relationship of Social and Demographic and Maternal Health Factors to Postpartum Sterilization: Findings from the 1972 National Natality Survey.* By Paul Placek. Washington, D.C.: 1975.

Vig, O.P. and Yeole, B.B. *Reduction in Birth Rate Due to Various Combinations of Sterilization, I.U.C.D. and Contraceptive Programme in India Through Use of Birth Order Statistics.* Bombay: International Institute for Population Studies, 1973.

Weisbord, R.G. *Genocide? Birth Control and the Black American.* New York: Two Continents Publishing Group, 1975.

Whelpton, P.K., Campbell, A.A., and Patterson, J.E. *Fertility and Family Planning in the United States.* Princeton: Princeton University Press, 1966.

Wood, C. *Vasectomy and Sterilization.* London: T. Smith, 1974.

Woodside, M. *Sterilization in North Carolina.* Chapel Hill, N.C.: The University of North Carolina Press, 1950.

Wortman, J. *Tubal Sterilization: Review of Methods.* Publication No. 7. Washington, D.C.: George Washington University, Department of Medical and Public Affairs, May 1976.

_____ and Piotrow, P.T. *Vasectomy—Old and New Techniques.* Population Report, Sterilization, Series D., No. 1. Washington, D.C.: George Washington University Medical Center, December 1973.

Wylie, E.M. *The New Birth Control: A Guide to Voluntary Sterilization.* New York: Grosset and Dunlap, 1972.

Yosuf, M. and Hameed, A.S. *Demographic Particulars of Sterilised Persons in Quilon District, 1965-66.* Trivandrum, India: Demographic Research Center, Bureau of Economics and Statistics, August 1967.

Ziegler, F.J. et al. *Vasectomy: Current Research in Male Sterilization.* New York: MSS Information Corporation, 1973.

## II. Periodical Articles

"APHA Recommended Program Guide for Voluntary Sterilization." *American Journal of Public Health* 62 (July 1972): 1265-67.

Adams, T.W. "Female Sterilization." *American Journal of Obstetrics and Gynecology* 89 (June 1, 1964): 395-401.

Adatia, M.D. and Adatia, S.M. "A Ten Year Survey of Sterilization Operations (in Women)." *Journal of Obstetrics and Gynecology of India* 16 (1966): 423-26.

Addison, P.H. "Sterilisation." *Lancet* 1 (May 20, 1972): 1115-16.

"After Sterilization, No Regrets." *Medical World News* 13 (March 17, 1972): 31.

Agarwala, S.N. "The Arithmetic of Sterilization in India." *Eugenics Quarterly* 13 (September 1966): 209-13.

——. "Sterilisation as a Population Control Device: Its Economics." *Economic Weekly* 16 (1964): 1091-94.

Ager, J.W. et al. "Vasectomy: Who Gets One and Why?" *American Journal of Public Health* 64, 7 (July 1974): 680-86.

Alderman, P.M. "Vasectomy for Voluntary Male Sterilisation." (Letter to the Editor) *Lancet* 2 (November 23, 1968): 1137-38.

Alexander, N.J. "Vasectomy: Long-Term Effects." *Science* 182, 4115 (November 30, 1973): 946-47.

Alvarado, C.R. de and Tietze, C. "Birth Control in Puerto Rico." *Human Fertility* 12 (1): 15-17; 24-25/1947.

Araica, H. "Algunas Estimaciones Sobre La Práctica Anticonceptiva en la República de Panama" (Some Estimations on Contraceptive Practice in the Republic of Panama). *Notas de Población* 3, 8 (August 1975): 89-96.

Arasteh, J.D. "Parenthood, Some Antecedents and Consequences: A Preliminary Survey of the Mental Health Literature." *Journal of General Psychology* 118 (June 1971): 179-202.

Altman, M. "Place of Vasectomy." *British Medical Journal* 1 (January 29, 1972): 311.

Apte, J.S. and Gandi, V.N. "A Follow-up Study of Vasectomy Cases." *Journal of Family Welfare* 17 (September 1970): 3-17.

Arthure, H. "Morbidity and Mortality of Abortions." *Lancet* 2 (August 7, 1971): 310-11.

"Asian Experts Call for Cost Benefit Studies." *International Planned Parenthood News,* No. 211 (September 1972).

*Association for Voluntary Sterilization News.* Published on irregular basis. New York.

Atkinson, S.M. and Chappell, S.M. "Vaginal Hysterectomy for Sterilization." *Obstetrics and Gynecology* 39 (May 1972): 759-66.

Auger, M., Bernard, P.E., and Dessureault, P. "Vasectomie et Vaso-vasotomie" (Vasectomy and vasovasotomy). *Union Medicale du Canada* 101 (January 1972): 115-17.

Back, K.W., Hill, R., and Stycos, J.M. "Population Control in Puerto Rico: The Formal and Informal Framework." *Law and Contemporary Problems* 25 (1960): 562-65.

Baird, C. "The Obstetrician and Society." *American Journal of Public Health* 60 (April 1970): 628-40.

Balswick, J.O. "Attitudes of Lower-Class Males Toward Taking a Male Birth Control Pill." *Family Coordinator* 21 (April 1972): 195-99.

Banerjee, S.N. "Family Planning Workers and Mass Vasectomy Camps." *Journal of Family Welfare* 22, 1 (September 1975): 22-31.

Banerji, T.P. "A Study of Male Sterilisation at Kanpur: Report on 202 Cases of Vasectomy." *Journal of the Indian Medical Association* 36 (June 16, 1961): 578-80.

Barglow, P. and Eisner, M. "An Evaluation of Ligation in Switzerland." *American Journal of Obstetrics and Gynecology* 95 (August 15, 1966): 1083-94.

————, Gunther, M.S., Johnson, M.A., Johnson, A., and Meltzer, H.S. "Hysterectomy and Tubal Ligation: A Psychiatric Comparison." *American Journal of Obstetrics and Gynecology* 25 (April 1965): 520-27.

Barglow, P. "Pseudocyesis and Psychiatric Sequelae of Sterilization." *Archives of General Psychiatry* 11, 6 (December 1964): 571-80.

Barnes, A.C. and Zuspan, F. "Patient Reaction to Puerperal Surgical Sterilization." *American Journal of Obstetrics and Gynecology* 75 (1958): 65.

Barnes, M.N. "One Thousand Vasectomies." *Family Planning* 22, 4 (January 1974): 81-86.

Barson, M. and Wood, C. "A Survey of the Role of the General Practitioner in Family Planning." *Medical Journal of Australia* 1 (May 20, 1972): 1069-71.

Bartova, D., Kolarova, O., Stanicek, J. et al. "Nekteré Psychologické a sexuologické Aspekty Sterilizace u Zen" (Some psychological and sexological aspects of sterilization in women). *Ceskoslovenska Gynekologie* 33 (April 1968): 267-69.

Bass, M.S. "Attitudes of Parents of Retarded Children Toward Voluntary Sterilization." *Eugenics Quarterly* 14 (March 1967): 45-53.

Batliwalla, A.S. "Vasectomy in India." *IPPF Medical Bulletin* 1 (1967): 1-2.

Batts, J.A., Jr. "Hospital-based Family Planning Program." *American Journal of Obstetrics and Gynecology* 110 (May 1, 1971): 49-53.

Baudry, F., Herzig, N., and Wiener, A. "Assessment of Patients Seeking Tubal Sterilization on Psychological Ground." *Journal of Obstetrics and Gynecology* 38, 3 (September 1971): 411-15.

Beazley, J.M. and Fraser, W.J. "Voluntary Sterilization." *Lancet* 2 (September 6, 1969): 531-33.

Beck, A.D. "The Effect of Vasectomy upon the Incidence and Morbidity of Post-prostatectomy Epididymitis." *Australian and New Zealand Journal of Surgery* 39 (February 1970): 286-89.

Beckles, F.N. "A Five-year Plan for Population Research and Family Planning Services: (3) Family Planning Services." *Family Planning Perspectives* 3 (October 1971): 49-64.

Bendel, R.B. "Female Sterilization." *Minnesota Medicine* 55 (March 1972): 235.

Benjamin, R. "Vasectomy as an Office Procedure." *Bulletin of St. Louis Park Medical Center* 14 (Winter 1970): 13-25.

Bergen, R.P. "Legal Consent for Vasectomy of a Mentally-retarded Minor." *Journal of the American Medical Association* 221 (July 17, 1972): 310.

Bernstein, A.H. "The Law and Sterilization." *Hospitals* 46 (March 1, 1972): 160-64.

Bhagwanani, S., Mirchandani, J., and Sikand, S. "Psychological Aspects of Sterilization in Female." *Journal of Obstetrics and Gynecology in India* 18 (1968): 279-81.

Bhandari, V. "Opinion Study of Rural Male Toward Vasectomy." *Family Planning News* 10 (November 1969): 16-18.

Bhardwaj, K.S. "Influence of IUCD & Sterilisation Programmes." *Indian Journal of Medical Science* 22 (1968): 454-56.

_____and Virmani, R. "Post-operative Reactions of Vasectomised Persons." *Punjab Medical Journal* 19 (1970): 439-41.

Bhashti, A.M.H. "Islamic Attitude Towards Abortion and Sterilization." *Birthright* (Lahore) 7, 1 (1972): 49-51.

Bhatnagar, N.K. "Vasectomy—A Study of Effects and Reactions." *Journal of Family Welfare* 11 (December 1964): 1-13.

Blacker, C.P. "Voluntary Sterilization." *British Medical Journal* 1 (February 21, 1970): 499.

_____. "Voluntary Sterilisation for Family Welfare." *Lancet* 1 (April 30, 1966): 971-74.

_____. "Voluntary Sterilization: Its Role in Human Betterment." *Eugenics Review* 56 (1964): 77-80.

_____. "Voluntary Sterilization: Transitions Throughout the World." *Eugenics Review* 54 (October 1962): 143-62.

_____and Peel, J.H. "Sterilisation of Women." *British Medical Journal* 1 (March 1, 1969): 566-67.

_____and Jackson, L.M. "Male Sterilisation." *British Medical Journal* 2 (July 9, 1966): 111.

Bloom, L.J. and Houston, B.K. "The Psychological Effects of Vasectomy for American Men." *The Journal of Genetic Psychology* 128 (1976): 173-82.

"The Boom in Vasectomies." *Emko Newsletter* 6 (December 1972): 6

Bopp, F. "Indications for Surgical Sterilization." *Obstetrics and Gynecology* 35 (1970): 760-64.

Bopp, J.R. and Hall, D.G. "Indications for Surgical Sterilization." *Obstetrics and Gynecology* 35 (May 1970): 760-64.

Borland, B.L. "Behavioural Factors in Non-coital Methods of Contraception: A Review." *Social Science and Medicine* 6 (February 1972): 163-78.

Bragonier, J.R. and Lowe, E.W. "The Experience of Two County Hospitals in Implementation of Therapeutic Abortion." *Clinical Obstetrics and Gynecology* 14 (December 1971): 1237-42.

Brat, T. et al. "La Stérilisation Féminine. Analyse Statistique 1961-1966." (Female Sterilization. Statistical Analysis, 1961-1966). *Bulletin de la Societé Royale Belge de Gynécologie et d'Obstétrique* 38 (1968): 97-107.

Brewer, H. "Reversibility Following Sterilization by Vasectomy." *Eugenics Review* 56 (1964): 147-50.

Buckle, A.E.R. and Loung, K.C. "Sterilization of the Female: A Positive

Approach to Family Limitation." *Journal of Biosocial Science* 3, 3 (July 1971): 289–300.

Buckley-Sharp, M.D. "Mortality of Abortion." *Lancet* 2 (August 28, 1971): 490-91.

Bumpass, L.L. and Presser, H.B. "Contraceptive Sterilization in the U.S.: 1965 and 1970." *Demography* 9, 4 (November 1972): 531-48.

Burch, T.K. and Shea, G.A. "Catholic Parish Priests and Birth Control: A Comparative Study of Opinion in Colombia, the United States, and the Netherlands." *Studies in Family Planning* 2 (June 1971): 121-36.

Burnight, R.G. et al. "Male Sterilization in Thailand: A Follow-up Study." *Journal of Biosocial Science* 7, 4 (October 1975): 377-91.

Campbell, A.A. "The Incidence of Operations that Prevent Contraception." *American Journal of Obstetrics and Gynecology* 89 (July 1964): 694-700.

Carlson, H.E. "Vasectomy of Election." *Southern Medical Journal* 63 (July 1970): 766-70.

Cates, W., Jr., Pedersen, V.H., and O'Brien, N.N. "Door-to-door Canvassing as a Means of Family Planning Patient Recruitment." *Yale Journal of Biology and Medicine* 42 (August 1969): 21-29.

Ceong, C.K. "A Baseline Survey on a Maximum Pill Dissemination Project in Ansung County." *Journal of Family Planning Studies* 2 (June 1975): 96-138.

Chakravarty, S. "Follow-Up Studies of Surgical Sterilisation in Women with Special Reference to Ovarian Changes." *Journal of Obstetrics and Gynaecology of India* 16 (1966): 418-22.

Charyk, W.R. "Potential Legal Difficulties with Voluntary Sterilization." *Medical Annals of the District of Columbia* 41 (July 1972): 459-60.

Chaset, N. "Male Sterilization." *Journal of Urology* 87 (March 1962): 512-17.

_____. "Vasectomy." *Medical Technique Quarterly* 18 (1971): 170-76.

Chez, R.A. "Mental Disability as a Basis for Contraception and Sterilization." *Social Biology* 18 (Supplement) (September 1971): 120-26.

Chitre, K.T., Sexena, R.N., and Ranganathan, H.N. "Motivation for Vasectomy." *Journal of Family Welfare* 11 (September 1964): 36-49.

Chopra, P. L. "Male Sterilisation: Its Aspects and Effects." *Journal of the Indian Medical Association* 45 (1965): 100.

Claman, A.D., Wakeford, J.R., Turner, J.M., and Hayden, B. "Impact on Hospital Practice of Liberalizing Abortions and Female Sterilizations." *Canadian Medical Association Journal* 105 (July 10, 1971): 35-41.

Clement, J.E. "A Program of Indigent Obstetric Care and Planned Parenthood in a Rural North Carolina County." *American Journal of Obstetrics and Gynecology* 108 (September 1, 1970): 63-67.

Coburn, J. "Sterilization Regulations: Debate Not Quelled by HEW Document." *Science* 183 (4128) (March 8, 1974): 935-39.

Cohen, M.R. "Hazards of Laparoscopy." *Arizona Medicine* 28 (November 1971): 830.

, Taylor, M.B., and Kass, M.B. "Interval Tubal Sterilization Via Laparoscopy." *American Journal of Obstetrics and Gynecology* 108 (October 1970): 458-61.

Cole, S.G. and Bryon, D. "Couples Served by the Fort Worth Vasectomy Clinic: An Evaluative Examination." As cited in *Family Planning Digest* 2, 2 (March 1973): 9.

 and Bryon, D. "A Review of Information Relevant to Vasectomy Counselors." *The Family Coordinator* 22, 2 (April 1973): 215-21.

"Control of Fertility by Sterilization." *Canadian Medical Association Journal* 104 (March 20, 1971): 527-28.

"Controlling Human Fertility." *Canadian Medical Association Journal* 102 (April 25, 1970): 871-72.

Corbett, H.V. "Sterilization." *Lancet* 1 (June 17, 1972): 1345.

Corfman, P.A. "A Five-year Plan for Population Research and Family Planning Services: (2) Population Research." *Family Planning Perspectives* 3 (October 1971): 41-48.

Corman, L. and Schaefer, J.B. "Population Growth and Family Planning." *Journal of Marriage and the Family* 35, 1 (February 1973): 89-92.

Cowgill, D.O. et al. "Sterilization: A Case of Extensive Practice in a Developing Nation." *Milbank Memorial Fund Quarterly* 49, 3, Part 1 (July 1971): 363-78.

Coyaji, B.J. "Report on 2,847 Sterilizations." *Journal of Obstetrics and Gynaecology of India* 14 (1964): 485-93.

Craft, I. "Vasectomy." *Lancet* 2 (September 23, 1972): 654.

and Diggory, P. "Problems in Male and Female Sterilization." *Lancet* 1 (May 6, 1972): 1011.

Craft, J.H. "The Effects of Sterilization as Shown by a Follow-up Study in South Dakota." *Journal of Heredity* 27 (October 1936): 379-87.

Curran, W.J. "A Vasectomy Case: The Meaning of 'Malpractice' and the 'Discovery Rule.'" *New England Journal of Medicine* 286 (March 2, 1972): 469.

Daily, E. and Nicholas, N. "Tubal Ligations on General Service Patients Seen by Peer-Level Family Planning Counselors in Thirty New York City Voluntary and Municipal Hospitals." *American Journal of Obstetrics and Gynecology* 123, 6 (1975): 656-58.

Dandekar, D. "After-effects of Vasectomy." *Artha Vijnana* 5 (September 1963): 212-24.

. "Sterilization Programme: Its Size and Effects on the Birth Rate." *Artha Vijnana* 1 (1959): 220-32.

. "Vasectomy Camps in Maharashtra." *Population Studies* 17 (November 1963): 147-54.

Darity, W.A. and Turner, C.B. "Research Findings Related to Sterilization: Attitudes of Black Americans." *American Journal of Orthopsychiatry* 44 (March 1974): 184-185.

Das, D. "Inter-state Variations in the Cost-Effectiveness of Family Planning

During 1969-1970." *Journal of Family Welfare* 18, 2 (December 1971): 55-69.

Das Gupta, S. "Vasectomy Operation for Control of Population." *Indian Journal of Public Health* 9 (1965): 82-84.

Datta, A.K. "Vasectomy in Family Planning." *Journal of the Indian Medical Association* 50 (January 16, 1968): 52-54.

_____ and Ghosh, S. "Failed Vasectomy." *Journal of the Indian Medical Association* 45 (1965): 186-87.

Davis, J.E. "Voluntary Male Sterilisation." *Lancet* 1 (March 1, 1969): 465.

_____ and Hulka, J.F. "Elective Vasectomy by American Urologists in 1967." *Fertility and Sterility* 21 (August 1970): 615-21.

_____ and Lubell, I. "Advances in Understanding the Effects of Vasectomy." *Mount Sinai Journal of Medicine* 42, 5 (September-October 1975): 391-97.

Dawn, C.S. "Late Effects of Sterilization." *Journal of Obstetrics and Gynecology* 16 (1966): 435-38.

_____ , Samanta, S., and Poddar, D.L. "Female Sterilisation as a Method of Population Control." *Journal of Obstetrics and Gynaecology of India* 18 (April 1968): 276-78.

De, A.K. and Basu, N.K. "Progress of Sterilization Operations in West Bengal." *Family Planning News* 10 (January 1969): 14-16.

Deisher, J.B. "Fertile Period After Vasectomy." *Science* 169 (1970): 816-17.

Delee, S.T. "Voluntary Sterilization." *International Surgery* 54 (October 1970): 304-11.

Deodhar, N.S. and Nadkarni, M.G. "Early Morbidity After Vasectomy—A Study of 137 Cases." *Indian Journal of Medical Sciences* 16 (May 1962): 391-96.

Diamond, E.F. "A Physician Views the Directives." *Hospital Progress* 53 (November 1972): 56-60.

Diggory, P. "The Place and Timing of Contraception and Sterilization." *Practitioner* 206 (March 1971): 409-11.

_____ . "Place and Timing of Contraception and Sterilization." *Proceedings of the Royal Society of Medicine* 64, 9 (September 1971): 955-58.

_____ and Craft, I. "Legal Problems Following Vasectomy." *Lancet* 2 (July 8, 1972): 87.

Dlhos, E. "Závery z konferencie venovanej problematike sterilizácie mužou a žien." (Conclusions from the Conference Devoted to the Problems of Sterilization of Males and Females). *Ceskoslovenska Gynekologie* 33 (April 1968): 301-302.

Doll, R. and Vessey, M.P. "Rare Adverse Effects of Systemic Contraceptives." In *British Medical Bulletin*, ed. G.I.M. Swyer. Vol. 26, No. 1. London: 1970.

Dubey, D.C. "Family Life Cycle Hypothesis and Its Importance in Explaining Fertility Behavior in India." *Journal of Family Welfare* 14 (1967): 42-52.

Dudley, H.A. "Reflections on Male Sterilisation Today." *Medical Journal of Australia* 2 (August 28, 1971): 490-93.

Dunbar, E. "Foolproof Birth Control." *Look*, pp. 45-48, March 9, 1971.

Ebbing, R.N. "Sterilisation by Hysterectomy." *Lancet* 2 (October 24, 1970): 879.

Edey, H. "Psychological Aspects of Vasectomy." *Medical Counterpoint* 4 (January 1972): 19-24.

———. "Sterilization." *New York Medicine* 26 (1970): 339-43.

———. "Voluntary Sterilization and the Medical Profession." *New York State Journal of Medicine* 71 (February 15, 1971): 483-84.

Edgerton, R.B. and Sabagh, G. "Sterilized Mental Defectives Look at Eugenic Sterilization." *Eugenics Quarterly* 9 (December 1962): 213-22.

Edwards, L.E. and Hakanson, E.Y. "Changing Status of Tubal Sterilization." *American Journal of Obstetrics and Gynecology* 115 (1973): 347-53.

Eisner, T., Van Tienhoven, A., and Rosenblatt, F. "Population Control, Sterilization, and Ignorance." *Science* 167 (January 23, 1970): 337.

Elahi, V.K. "A Family Planning Survey in Halifax, Nova Scotia." *Canadian Journal of Public Health* 64, 6 (November-December 1973): 515-20.

Eliot, J.W. "Fertility Control and Coercion." *Family Planning Perspectives* 5, 3 (Summer 1973): 132-87.

Ellison, R.M. "Psychiatric Complications Following Sterilization of Women." *The Medical Journal of Australia* 2 (October 17, 1964): 625-28.

Elstein, M. "Sterilization and Family Planning," *Practitioner* 205 (July 1970): 30-37.

Enke, S. "A Rejoinder to Comments on the Superior Effectiveness of Vasectomy-bonus Schemes." *Economic Development and Cultural Change* 9 (July 1961): 645-47.

Erling, C.B. "One GP's Personal and Professional Commitment." *Medical Opinion* 7 (March 1971): 58-59.

Fathalla, M.F. "Laparoscopic Sterilization in the Family Planning Program in Developing Communities." *Contraception* 6 (October 1972): 295-303.

Ferber, A.S. and Ferber, W.L. "Vasectomy." *Medical Aspects of Human Sexuality* 2 (June 1968): 29-35.

———, Tietze, C., and Lewit, S. "Men with Vasectomies: A Study of Medical, Sexual, and Psychosocial Changes." *Psychosomatic Medicine* 29 (July-August 1967): 354-66.

Ferguson, R.M. "The Status of Sterilization in the United States." *Journal of Family Welfare* 5 (December 1958): 45-46.

Fischer, H.K. "Emotional Problems Associated with Gynecologic Surgery." *Clinical Obstetrics and Gynecology* 5 (1962): 597-614.

Fitzgerald, J.A. "The Female Response to Male Vas Ligation." *Medical Insight* 4 (1972): 23-27.

Fleming, M. and Joyce, T.C. "Elective Sterilization of the Human Male." *Canadian Hospital* 45 (1968): 39-41.

Flowers, C.E. "Tubal Ligation and Abortion in the State of Alabama." *Journal of the Medical Association of the State of Alabama* 39 (April 1970): 945-47.

"Follow-up After Vasectomy." *Lancet* 1 (February 28, 1970): 483.

Foreman, J.R. "Vasectomy Clinic." *American Journal of Nursing* 73, 5 (May 1973): 819-21.

Fort, A.T. "Abortion and Sterilization: An Insight into Obstetrician-Gynecologists' Attitudes and Practices." *Social Biology* 18 (June 1971): 192-94.

Franda, M.F. "Mass Vasectomy Camps and Incentives in Indian Family Planning." *American University Field Service Reports* 16 (June 1972): 1-16.

Freund, M. and Davis, J.E. "A Follow-up Study of the Effects of Vasectomy on Sexual Behavior." *The Journal of Sex Research* 9, 3 (August 1973): 241-68.

_____ and Davis, J.E. "Disappearance Rate of Spermatozoa From the Ejaculate Following Vasectomy." *Fertility and Sterility* 20 (1969): 163-70.

Fried, J.J. "The Incision Decision." *Esquire* 77 (June 1972): 118.

Fujita, B.N. et al. "Voluntary Sterilization of the Male: A Survey of Elective Vasectomies Performed by Washington State Urologists." *Northwest Medicine* 70 (November 1971): 755-58.

Gaal, R.J. "The Position of Tubal Ligation in Family Planning." *Medical Journal of Australia* 2 (October 9, 1971): 772-74.

Gandotra, M.M. "Mass Vasectomy Camp—An Evaluation." *Demography India* 4, 1 (June 1975): 158-66.

Garrison, P.L. and Gamble, C.J. "Sexual Effects of Vasectomy." *Journal of the American Medical Association* 144 (September 23, 1950): 293-95.

Gesenius, H. "Freiwillige Sterilisierung ab 25. Lebensjahr Straffei Zum Alternativentwurf eines Strafgestzvuches von 1970" (Voluntary Sterilization Legal Beyond the Age of 25: On the Suggested Alternate Criminal Code of 1970). *Medizinische Klinik* 66 (December 1971): 1700-02.

Ghatikar, N.V. and Bhoopatkar, I. "Aftermaths of Puerperal Sterilisation." *Journal of Obstetrics and Gynaecology of India* 56 (1966): 572-78.

Ghazi, A.R. "A Pilot Vasectomy Programme in a Rural Area of West Pakistan." *Pakistan Journal of Family Planning* 2 (January 1968): 38-48.

Gilroy, A. "Family Planning on Tea Estates in Assam with Special Reference to IUD's and Sterilizations." *Journal of Family Welfare* 16 (June 1970): 3-8.

Gokhale, V.V. "Vasectomy Camps in Ahmdednagar District." *Journal of Family Welfare* 7 (September 1960): 9-11.

Goldsmith, A. et al. "Vasectomy in Columbia: A Pilot Study." *Journal of Biosocial Science* 5, 4 (October 1973): 497-505.

_____, Goldberg, R.J., and Echeverria, G. "Vasectomy in Latin America." International Planned Parenthood Federation, England, *IPPF Medical Bulletin* 7, 2 (April 1973): 1-2.

Gonzales, B. "Voluntary Sterilization." *American Journal of Nursing* 70 (December 1970): 2581-83.

Gopalakrishnan, S.V. "Fertility Patterns of the Sterilized and Contraceptive

Users in Kerala." *Journal of Family Welfare* 18, 4 (June 1972): 48-56.

Gopalan, C. and Nair, C.P.G. "A Study of 300 Vasectomized Cases in Kerala." *Family Planning News* 10 (May 1969): 7-8.

Gopalaswami, R.A. "Advantages of Vasectomy." Directorate General of Health Services, Ministry of Health, New Delhi. *Family Planning News* 3, 2 (1962): 34-35.

Gore, S.S. "Safeguards to be Adopted in Sterilization." *Journal of Family Welfare* 5 (December 1958): 5-12.

Gould, R.S. "Vasectomy." *Journal of the American Medical Association* 220 (June 11, 1972): 1495.

Greene, L.F. "Bilateral Partial Vasectomy for Elective Sterilization." *American Family Physician* 4 (August 1971): 73-80.

Greenhill, J.P. "World Trends of Therapeutic Abortion and Sterilization." *Clinical Obstetrics and Gynecology* 7 (March 1964): 37-42.

Grimwade, J. and Patterson, P. "Female Sterilisation Using the Laparoscope." *Medical Journal of Australia* 1 (February 12, 1972): 316-19.

Grindstaff, C.F. and Ebanks, G.E. "Male Sterilization as a Contraceptive Method in Canada: An Empirical Study." *Population Studies* 27, 3 (November 1973): 443-55.

_____ and Ebanks, G.E. "Protestant and Catholic Couples Who Have Chosen Vasectomy." *Sociological Analysis* 36, 1 (Spring 1975): 29-42.

_____ and Ebanks, G.E. "Vasectomy: Canada's Newest Method of Family Planning." *Canada's Mental Health* 21, 5 (September-October 1973): 3-5.

Grosswirth, M. "Who's Afraid of Vasectomy." *Saturday Review* 55 (June 10, 1972): 38.

Gudgeon, D. "Sterilisation or Abortion." *Lancet* 1 (June 12, 1972): 1240.

Gunn, A.D. "Male Sterilization: An Ultimate in Family Planning." *Nursing Times* 66 (May 14, 1970): 627.

Gustavus, S.O. and Hanley, J.R., Jr. "Correlates of Voluntary Childlessness in a Select Population." *Social Biology* 18 (1971): 277-84.

Guttmacher, A.F. "Puerperal Sterilization on the Private and Ward Services of a Large Metropolitan Hospital." *Fertility and Sterility* 8 (1957): 591-602.

"Gynaecological Illness After Sterilisation." *British Medical Journal* 1 (March 18, 1972): 748-49.

Haas, H.I. and Maehr, M.L. "Two Experiments on the Concept of Self and the Reaction of Others." *Journal of Personality and Social Psychology* 1 (1965): 100.

Hacket, R.E. and Waterhouse, K. "Vasectomy—Reviewed." *American Journal of Obstetrics and Gynecology* 116, 3 (June 1, 1973): 438-55.

Halder, B.N. "Follow-Up Study of 250 Vasectomy Cases in Madhya Pradesh." *Family Planning News* (October 1968).

_____ and Sivaraman, N. "A Follow-up Study of Vasectomy Cases in Orissa." *Family Planning News* 10 (March 1969): 11-17.

Hall, R.E. "Therapeutic Abortion, Sterilization, and Contraception." *American Journal of Obstetrics and Gynecology* 91 (February 15, 1965): 518-32.

Hammer, E.F. "An Investigation of Sexual Symbolism: A Study of H-T-P's of Eugenically Sterilized Subjects." *Journal of Projective Techniques* 17 (1953): 401-13.

Han, S.H. "A Calculation of the Couple Years Protection for the Korean Family Planning Program." *Journal of Family Planning Studies* 2 (June 1975): 24-29.

Hanley, H.G. "Vasectomy for Voluntary Male Sterilization." *Lancet* 2 (July 27, 1968): 207-09.

Haralambidis, G. and Spinnelli, A.N. "Vasectomy: An Evaluation." *Journal of Urology* 89 (April 1963): 591-94.

Hardin, G. "Parenthood: Right or Privilege?" *Science* 169 (July 31, 1970): 427.

Hauschild, T.B. "The Role of the Psychiatrist in Therapeutic Abortion and Sterilization." *U.S. Army, Europe: Medical Bulletin* 2 (November 1963): 322-26.

Hauser, E. "Die Sterilisation des Mannes zur Verhutung von Schwangerschaften." *Praxis* 44 (1955): 477-84, 500-06.

Haynes, D.M. and Wolfe, W.M. "Tubal Sterilization in an Indigent Population: Report of Fourteen Years' Experience." *American Journal of Obstetrics and Gynecology* 106 (April 1, 1970): 1044-53.

Haynes, M.A., Immerwahr, G.E., George, A., and Nayar, P.S.J. "A Study on the Effectiveness of Sterilizations in Reducing the Birth Rate." *Demography* 6 (February 1969): 1-12.

Hayt, E. "Legal Responsibility for Unsuccessful Sterilization." *Hospital Management* 109 (February 1970): 50-52.

────. "Legal Responsibility for Unsuccessful Sterilization." *Hospital Management* 109 (March 1970): 12-15.

Hellman, R. "Die Sterilisierung als Legitime Ärztliche Aufgabe" (Sterilization as a Legitimate Medical Task). *Medizinische Welt*, no. 1, pp. 41-47 (1970).

Henker, F.O. "Abortion and Sterilization From Psychiatric and Medicolegal Viewpoints." *Journal of the Arkansas Medical Society* 57 (February 1961): 368-73.

Hershey, N. "Abortion and Sterilization: Status of the Law in Mid-1970." *American Journal of Nursing* 70 (September 1970): 1926-27.

Hibbard, L.T. "Sexual Sterilization by Elective Hysterectomy." *American Journal of Obstetrics and Gynecology* 112 (April 15, 1972): 1076.

Hinderer, M. "Uber die Sterilization des Mannes und ihre Auswirkungen" (On the Sterilization of Men and its Effects). *Archiv der Neurologie und Psychiatric* 60 (1947): 145-76.

Hobbs, J.J. "Vasectomy in General Practice." *British Medical Journal* 1 (March 25, 1972): 802.

Hodson, J.M. "Vasectomy for Voluntary Sterilization." *Postgraduate Medicine* 52 (July 1972): 99-103.

Holden, C. "Sperm Banks Multiply as Vasectomies Gain Popularity." *Science* 176 (April 7, 1972): 32.

Holder, A.R. "Compulsory Sterilization." *Journal of the American Medical Association* 221 (July 10, 1972): 229-30.

————. "Vasectomies." *Journal of the American Medical Association* 217 (September 27, 1971): 1943-44.

Homesley, H.D. and Zelenik, J.S. "Is There a Best Time for Postpartum Vaginal Hysterectomy?" *American Journal of Obstetrics and Gynecology* 112 (April 1, 1972): 972-77.

Hooper, P.D. "A Problem In Vasectomy." *Lancet* 2 (October 30, 1971): 892.

Horn, H.J. "Der Leidensdruck asls Indikationskriterium. Bemerkungen zur 'Medikamentösen Kastration' " (Psychological Stress as an Indication Criterion. Remarks on "Medicamentous Castration"). *Nervenarzt* 42 (June 1971): 312-16.

Houghton, B. "Vasectomies Affect Women, Too." *American Journal of Nursing* 73, 5 (May 1973): 821.

Houseman, R.J. "Sterilisation of Young Wives." *British Medical Journal* 3 (July 17, 1971): 184.

Huda, N., Ratcliffe, J.W., and Croley, H.T. "A Study of Vasectomy Physicians in East Pakistan." *Pakistan Journal of Family Planning* 3 (July 1969): 60-74.

Huether, C.A. "Vasectomy Services, Inc." *ZPG National Reporter* 3 (March 1971): 10-11.

Hulka, J.F. "Teaching Laparoscopy: A Pilot Regional Program in North Carolina." *Contraception* 6 (August 1972): 151-62.

————and Davis, J.E. "Vasectomy and Reversible Vasocclusion." *Fertility and Sterility* 23, 9 (1972): 683-96.

Huntingford, P.J. "Sterilization from the Aspect of Family Planning." *Deutsches Medizinisches Journal* 22 (October 1971): 630-32.

Hurst, J.A. "Birth Control: The Views of Women." *Medical Journal of Australia* 2 (October 31, 1970): 835-38.

Husslein, H. "Familienplanung und Derzeitige Rechtssituation in Osterreich" (Family Planning and the Present Law Situation in Austria). *Weiner Klinische Wechenschrift* 83 (March 5, 1971): 141-44.

Hynie, J. "Indikace sterilizace u mužu" (Indications for Sterilization of Men). *Ceskoslovenska Gynekologie* 33 (April 1968): 295-96.

Islam, A.I.M.M. "Experience with Vasectomy in Rajshahi." *Pakistan Journal of Family Planning* 1 (July 1967): 57-66.

Jackson, L.M. "Sterilisation of Women." *Lancet* 2 (August 29, 1970): 463.

————. "Vasectomy." *Lancet* 1 (January 17, 1970): 140-41.

————. "Vasectomy in the United Kingdom." *Practitioner* 203 (1969): 320-23.

————. "Voluntary Sterilisation." *Family Planning* 16 (October 1967): 72-73.

_____. "Voluntary Sterilisation." *Lancet* 2 (September 27, 1969): 690.

_____. "Voluntary Sterilisation in the U.K." *Lancet* 2 (October 22, 1966): 906-07.

Jackson, P., Phillips, B., Prosser, E., Jones, H.O., Tindall, V.R., Crosby, D.L., Cooke, I.D., McGarry, J.M., and Rees, R.W. "A Male Sterilization Clinic." *British Medical Journal* 4 (October 31, 1970): 295-97.

Jaffe, F.S. "Toward the Reduction of Unwanted Pregnancy: An Assessment of Current Public and Private Programs." *Science* 174 (October 8, 1971): 119-27.

_____, Dryfoos, J.G., and Varky, G. "Who Needs Organized Family Planning Services? A Preliminary Projection, 1971-1975." *Family Planning Perspectives* 3 (July 1971): 22-32.

Jain, S.P. "The Indian Family Planning Programme—An Assessment of Past Performance." *Journal of Family Welfare* 21, 4 (1975): 10-27

Jain, P.K. and Sharma, B.B.L. "Socio-Demographic Evaluation of Mass Vasectomy Camps in Bihar." *Journal of Population Research* 1, 1 (July-December 1974): 51-58.

Janke, L.D. and Wiest, M. "Effects of Vasectomy on Psychosocial Adjustment and Medical Health in a Sample of Subscribers to the Kaiser Foundation Health Plan." Reed College. Privately Circulated Paper. Portland, Oregon, 1973.

Jhaver, P.S. "The Place of Surgery in the Family Planning Programme." *Journal of Family Welfare* 5 (June 1959): 46-48.

_____. "Reversibility of Sterilization Produced by Vas Occlusion." *Fertility and Sterility* 22 (April 1971): 263-69.

_____. "Surgery and Family Planning." *Times of India,* September 25, 1960.

Johnson, D.S. "Contraception and Sterilization." *New England Journal of Medicine* 285 (December 9, 1971): 1380.

_____. "Reversible Male Sterilization: Current Status and Future Directions, A Report." *Contraception* 5 (April 1972): 327-38.

Johnson, M.H. "Author's Reply." *Journal of Sex Research* 7 (1971): 73.

_____. "Social and Psychological Effects of Vasectomy." *American Journal of Psychiatry* 121 (November 1964): 482-86.

_____and Miller, C. "The Wives Reconsider Vasectomy." *Journal of Sex Research* 6 (February 1970): 36-40.

Jordan, J.A., Edwards, R.L., Pearson, J., and Maskery, P.J.K. "Laparoscopic Sterilisation and Follow-up Hysterosalpingogram." *Journal of Obstetrics and Gynecology of the British Commonwealth* 78 (May 1971): 460-66.

Kaij, L. and Malmiquist, A. "Prognosis after Sterilization in Connection with Parturition." *Acta Psychiatrica Scandinavica* 41 (1965): 204-17.

Kakar, D.N. "After-effects of Vasectomy on Sex Behaviour: An Exploratory Investigation." *Journal of Family Welfare* 17 (December 1970): 37-46.

_____. "Sexual Problems Related to Vasectomy: Suggested Guidance for

Future Research." *Journal of Family Welfare* 21, 3 (1975): 16-20.

Kalasur, S.B. "A Study of 280 Vasectomy Cases." *Family Planning News* 11 (April/May 1970): 14-15.

Kangas, L.W. "Integrated Incentives for Fertility Control." *Science* 169 (1970): 1278-83.

Kapil, K.K. "Study of Factors Leading to Drop-out Among Men Registered for Vasectomy Operation." *Journal of Family Welfare* 8 (March 1962): 28-38.

Kar, J.K. "Surgical Correction of Post-Vasectomy Sterility." *Journal of Family Welfare* 15, 3 (1969): 50-53.

Kepp, R. "Fragen aus der Praxis: Medicinische und Juristische Aspekte der Sterilization" (Questions from Medical Practice: Medical and Legal Aspects of Sterilization). *Deutsche Medizinische Wochenschrift* 96 (November 5, 1971): 1777-78.

Kestelman, P. "Mortality and Morbidity of Abortion." *Lancet* 2 (August 14, 1971): 368-69.

——. "Mortality of Abortion." *Lancet* 2 (September 11, 1971): 607.

Khati, T.D. "Sterilization in Gujarat." *Family Planning News* 9 (July 1968): 20.

Khorana, A.B. "Acceptor-Characteristics of Women Undergoing Tubectomy." *Journal of Family Welfare* 22, 3 (March 1976): 33-39.

Kildare-Donaldson, E. et al. "Tubal Ligations in Dominica." *West Indian Medical Journal* 21, 4 (1972): 236-39.

Kind, H. "Die Sterilisation des Mannes und ihre Auswirkung im Lichte einer Katamnestischen Untersuchung" (Sterilization of Men and its Effect in the Light of a Catamnestic Survey). *Praxis* 53 (May 14, 1964): 652-56.

—— and Petersen, P. "Fuhrt die Sterilisation zu Seelischen Fehlentwicklungen? Eine Erwiderung auf W. Mende: Forensisch-psychiatrische Fragen bei Sterilisation und Kastration" (Does Sterilization Lead to Psychological Disturbance? A rebuttal to W. Mende: Forensic-Psychiatric Questions Related to Sterilization and Castration). *Nervenarzt* 41 (June 1970): 287-88.

Kohli, K.L. "Factors Leading to Drop-Out Among Men Registered for Vasectomy." *Journal of Family Welfare* 21, 3 (March 1975): 30-37.

Kohli, K.L. "Motivational Factors and Socio-Economic Characteristics of Vasectomized Males." *Journal of Biosocial Science* 5, 2 (April 1973): 169-77.

Kothari, M.L. and Pardanani, D.S. "Temporary Sterilisation of the Male by Intravasal Contraceptive Device (VCD)." *Indian Journal of Surgery* 29 (July 1967): 357-63.

Koya, Y. "Sterilization in Japan." *Eugenics Quarterly* 8 (September 1961): 135-41.

——. "Sterilization in Japan." *Journal of Family Welfare* 8 (March 1962): 28-38.

Krishef, C.H. "State Laws on Marriage and Sterilization of the Mentally Retarded." *Mental Retardation* 10 (June 1972): 36-38.

Krishnakumar, S. "Ernakulam's Third Vasectomy Campaign Using the Camp

Approach." *Studies in Family Planning* 5, 2 (February 1974): 58-61.
_____. "Kerala's Pioneering Experiment in Massive Vasectomy Camps." *Studies in Family Planning* 3 (August 1972): 177-85.
_____. "Organization of Massive Vasectomy Camps—A Study of the Ernakulam Experiment." *Journal of the Indian Medical Association* 59 (October 16, 1972): 375-80.
Kroger, W.S. "Hypnotic Pseudo-orientation in Time as a Means of Determining the Psychological Effects of Surgical Sterilization in the Male and Female." *Fertility and Sterility* 14 (1963): 535-39.
Kumar, J. "A Comparison Between Current Indian Fertility and Late Nineteenth-Century Swedish and Finnish Fertility." *Population Studies* 25, 2 (July 1971): 269-82.
Kundu, M.S. "Vasectomy." *Indian Medical Journal* 60 (1966): 98.
Kwon, E.H., Kim, T.R., Park, H.J., Hong, J.W., Park, S.Y., Lee, Y.W., and Yum, B.J. "Characteristics, Circumstances, Knowledge, and Attitudes of Vasectomized Men in Urban Area." *Journal of Population Studies* 11 (November 1970): 5-51, 178-82.
Laidlaw, R.W. and Bass, M.S. "Voluntary Sterilization as It Relates to Mental Health." *American Journal of Psychiatry* 120 (June 1964): 1176-80.
Lakshmi, A.K.S. "An Application of the Generalised Distance Concept in a Family Planning Study in Kerala." *Journal of Family Welfare* 18 (December 1971): 32-36.
Lakshmi, P. "A Note on the Progress of Sterilisation in Madras State." *Journal of Family Welfare* 8 (March 1962): 12-17.
Lal, A. "Sterilization in Mainland China." *Maharashtra Medical Journal* 11 (1965): 1033-34.
Landis, J.T. "Attitudes of Individual California Physicians and Policies of State Medical Societies on Vasectomy for Birth Control." *Journal of Marriage and the Family* 28 (August 1966): 277-83.
_____ and Poffenberger, T. "Hesitations and Worries of 330 Couples Choosing Vasectomy for Birth Control." *Family Life Coordinator* 15 (October 1966): 143-47.
_____. "The Marital and Sexual Adjustment of 330 Couples Who Chose Vasectomy as a Form of Birth Control." *Journal of Marriage and the Family* 27 (February 1965): 57-58.
Lapham, R.J. "Family Planning and Fertility in Tunisia." *Demography* 7 (May 1970): 241-53.
_____. "Family Planning in Tunisia and Morocco: A Summary and Evaluation of the Recent Record." *Studies in Family Planning* 2 (May 1971): 101-110.
Lapinski, A. and Wieszcyzycki, W. "Contemporary Trends in Sterilization of Women." *Ginekologia Polska* 41, 3 (1970): 219-25.
Larson, S.L. "Laparoscopic Sterilization." *Minnesota Medicine* 55 (April 1972): 369-71.

Laube, W. "Rekanalisierung nach Vasketomie mit Schwangerschaftsfolge und Haftpflichtbegehren" (Recanalization Following Vasectomy Resulting in Pregnancy and Liability Claim). *Helvetia Chirurgica Acta* 38 (December 1971): 481-83.

Laufe, L.E. and Kreutner, A.K. "Vaginal Hysterectomy: A Modality for Therapeutic Abortion and Sterilization." *American Journal of Obstetrics and Gynecology* 110 (August 15, 1971): 1096-99.

Leader, A.J. "The Houston Story: A Vasectomy Service in a Family Planning Clinic." *Family Planning Perspectives* 3 (July 1971): 46-49.

Lear, H. "Psychosocial Characteristics of Patients Requesting Vasectomy." *Journal of Urology* 108 (November 1972): 767-69.

———. "Vasectomy—A Note of Concern." *Journal of the American Medical Association* 219 (February 28, 1972): 1206-07.

Lecomte, J. and Marcoux, A. "Contraception and Fertility in Morocco and Tunisia." *Studies in Family Planning* 7, 7 (July 1976): 182-87.

Lee, H.Y. et al. "Effects of Vasectomy on Medical and Psychosocial Aspects." *Journal of Population Studies* 11 (1970): 145-77.

———. "Studies on Vasectomy: (3) Clinical Studies on the Influence of Vasectomy." *Korean Journal of Urology* 7 (1966): 11-29.

———. "Studies on Vasovasostomy: (5) Effects of Early Ambulation on Success Rate and Report of 85 Vasovasostomies." *Journal of the Korean Medical Association* 13 (1970): 897-903.

———. "Summary of Studies on Vasectomy." *New Medical Journal of Korea* 13 (1970): 507-519.

Lee, L.T. "Law and Family Planning." *Studies in Family Planning* 2 (April 1971): 81-98.

Leeton, J. "Population Control in Australia Today: Contraception, Sterilization and Abortion." *Medical Journal of Australia* 2 (October 25, 1975): 682-86.

Lefebvre, Y. et al. "Clinical Experience with the Dalkon Shield Intrauterine Device." *British Medical Journal* 5872 (July 28, 1973): 143-45.

"Legality of Sterilisation." *British Medical Journal* 1 (March 21, 1970): 704-05.

Lewit, S. "Sterilization Associated with Induced Abortion: JPSA Findings." *Family Planning Perspectives* 5, 3 (Summer 1973): 177-82.

Liebman, H.G. and Lehfeldt, H. "Population Control in India." *Journal of Sex Research* 8 (August 1972): 189-93.

———. "La Stérilisation Chirurgicale de la Femme dans un Milieu Canadien-Français" (Surgical Sterilization of Women in a French-Canadian Setting). *Union Médicale du Canada* 102, 2 (February 1973): 357-60.

Lippitt, T., Ranganathan, K.V., and Hulka, J.F. "Tubal Ligation as Part of Family Planning in India." *American Journal of Obstetrics and Gynecology* 105 (October 1, 1969): 434-39.

Lipson, G. and Wolman, D. "Polling Americans on Birth Control and Population." *Family Planning Perspectives* 4 (January 1972): 39-42.

Livingstone, E.S. "Vasectomy: A Review of 3200 Operations." *Canadian Medical Association Journal* 105 (November 20, 1971): 1065.

Lu, T. and Chun, D. "Long Term Follow-up Study of 1055 Cases of Post-partum Tubal Ligation." *Journal of Obstetrics and Gynecology of the British Commonwealth* 74 (1967): 875-80.

Mabray, C.R., Malinak, L.R., and Flowers, C.E. "Tubal Sterilization: Morbidity on a Charity Hospital Service." *Obstetrics and Gynecology* 36 (August 1970): 204-207.

MacCorquodale, D.W. et al. "How Doctors in Bolivia and the Philippines View Sterilization." *Studies in Family Planning* 6, 12 (December 1975): 426-28.

McEwan, J. "Control of Fertility: The General Practitioner's Role." *Proceedings of the Royal Society of Medicine* 64 (September 1971): 949-52.

_____ et al. "Hospital Family Planning: A Vasectomy Service." *Contraception* 9, 2 (February 1974): 177-92.

McIntyre, R.J. "The Fertility Response to Abortion Reform in Eastern Europe: Demographic and Economic Implications." *American Economist* 16 (Fall 1972): 45-63.

MacKay, M. and Edey, H. "The Law Concerning Voluntary Sterilization as it Affects Doctors." *Journal of Urology 103* (April 1970): 482-84.

Madrigal, V. et al. "Male Sterilization in El Salvador: A Preliminary Report." *Journal of Reproductive Medicine* 14, 4 (April 1975): 167-70.

Maehr, M.L., Mensing, J., and Nafzger, S. "Concept of Self and Reaction of Others." *Sociometry* 25 (December 1962): 353.

Mathur, B.L. and Srivastava, G.P.L. "Some Aspects of the Bihar Mass Vasectomy Camps." *The Journal of Family Welfare* 20, 3 (March 1974): 73-83.

Mauldin, W.P. "Family Planning Programs and Fertility Declines in Developing Countries." *Family Planning Perspectives* 7, 1 (January-February 1975): 32-38.

Maxwell, I. "Sexual Sterilization: Legal Position of a Doctor." *Nova Scotia Medical Bulletin* 49 (1970): 18.

Measham, A.R., Hatcher, R.A., and Arnold, C.B. "Physicians and Contraception: A Study of Perceptions and Practices in an Urban Southeastern United States Community." *Southern Medical Journal* 64 (April 1971): 499-503.

Mehta, D.C. et al. "Demographic Characteristics of Tubectomy Acceptors in Kaira District." *Journal of Family Welfare* 22, 1 (September 1975): 32-40.

Mehta, P.F. et al. "Effectiveness of Female Sterilization in Greater Bombay: Some Vital Issues for Reconsideration for the National Programme." *Demography India* 4, 1 (1975): 146-57.

Melody, G.F. "Depressive Reactions Following Hysterectomy." *American Journal of Obstetrics and Gynecology* 83 (1962): 410-13.

Mencher, J.P. "Family Planning in India: The Role of Class Values." *Family Planning Perspectives* 2 (March 1970): 35-39.

Mende, W. "Forensische-psychiatriche Fragen bei Sterilization und Kastration."

(Forensic-psychiatric Problems in Sterilization and Castration). *Nervenarzt* 40 (October 1969): 463-66.

Middleman, R.R. "Services for Males in A Family Planning Program." *American Journal of Public Health* 62, 11 (November 1972): 1451-53.

Misra, B.D. "Family Planning: Differential Performance of States." *Economical and Political Weekly* 8 (1973): 1769-79.

Momose, T.O. et al. "Side Effects Following Male Sterilization." *Japanese Journal of Fertility and Sterility* 9 (1964): 111-15.

"The Mood of the Nation." *The Gallup Opinion Index,* Report No. 64, pp. 20-21, 1970.

Moore, D.W. "Sequelae of Tubal Ligation, Medical and Psychological." *American Journal of Obstetrics and Gynecology* 101 (June 1, 1968): 350-51.

Moore, J.L. and Vickery, T.E. "Voluntary Sterilization Law Recommended Forms." *Journal of the Medical Association of Georgia* 59 (September 1970): 374-77.

Morcos, M. et al. "The Attitude of Christianity Towards Family Planning (A Social Study)." *Population Studies* 26 (November 1975): 1-61.

"More than 100,000 Persons a Year Are Reported Seeking Sterilization as Method of Contraception." *New York Times,* p. 17, March 22, 1973.

Morgan, R.E. "Vasectomy." *Pennsylvania Medicine* 75 (November 1972): 38-40.

Mukherjee, B. "Role of Vasectomy in Family Planning." *Indian Medical Journal* 60 (1966): 169-70.

Muldoon, M.J. "Gynaecological Illness After Sterilisation." *British Medical Journal* 1 (January 8, 1972): 84-85.

Mullen, P., Reynolds, R., Cignetti, P., and Dornan, D. "Vasectomy Education Program: Implications From Survey Data." *The Family Coordinator* 22, 3 (July 1973): 331-38.

Muller, C.F. "The Cost of Contraceptive Sterilization." *Family Planning Perspectives* 6, 1 (Winter 1974): 39-41.

_____and Jaffe, F.S. "Financing Fertility—Related Health Services in the United States, 1972-1973: A Preliminary Projection." *Family Planning Perspectives* 4 (January 1972): 6-19.

Munroe, G.S. and Jones, G.W. "Mobile Units in Family Planning." *Reports on Population and Family Planning* 10 (October 1971): 1-32.

Murty, S.D.V.R. "The Place of IUCD, Sterilisation and Contraception in the Family Planning Programme in India." *Journal of Family Welfare* 12 (December 1965): 15-21.

Nag, M. "Attitudes Towards Vasectomy in West Bengal." *Population Review* 10 (January 1966): 61-64.

Nag, M., Shokeir, M.H., Board, F.A. et al. "Is Sterilization the Answer?" *Science* 168 (1970): 62.

Nagaraj, B.B. and Shirwadker, P.S. "A Study of Sterilised Cases in South Kanara

District." *Journal of Family Welfare* 20, 1 (September 1973): 22-25.

Nair, P.S.G. and George, N.C. "Correlates of Inter-District Variation in the Progress of Family Planning in Kerala." *Journal of Family Welfare* 18, 3 (March 1972): 37-49.

Nash, J.L. and Rich, J.D. "The Sexual Aftereffects of Vasectomy." *Fertility and Sterility* 23 (October 10, 1972): 715-18.

Newman, S.H. and Kelty, M.F. "Support for Psychologists in the Population and Family Planning Areas." *American Psychologist* 27 (January 1972): 31-36.

Nichols, E.E. "Current Practices in Female Sterilization in the United States: Incidence and Methods." *American Journal of Obstetrics and Gynecology* 101, 3 (June 1, 1968): 345-48.

Noble, N.S. "Policies and Practices in Iowa Hospitals Relating to Human Sterilization." *Fertility and Sterility* 6 (July-August 1955): 375-80.

Norman, F.W., ed. "Vasectomy." *California GP* 14 (1963): 15-25.

Norris, A.S. "An Examination of the Effects of Tubal Ligation: Their Implications for Prediction." *American Journal of Obstetrics and Gynecology* 90 (1964): 431.

Nortman, D.L. "Status of National Family Planning Programmes of Developing Countries in Relation to Demographic Targets." *Population Studies* 26, 1 (March 1972): 5-18.

O'Conor, V.J. "Sexual Effects of Vasectomy." *Journal of the American Medical Association* 144 (December 1950): 1502.

Okraku, Ishmael O. "Fishing and Fertility: A Study of a Nova Scotia Fishing Village." *Social Biology* 22, 4 (Winter 1975): 326-37.

Orleans, L.A. "China's Experience in Population Control: The Elusive Model." *World Development* 3 (July-August 1975): 497-525.

Pallister, P.D. and Perry, R.M. "Reflections on Marriage for the Retarded: The Case for Voluntary Sterilization." *Hospital and Community Psychiatry* 24, 3 (March 1973): 172-74.

Palmer, J. "Festivals with a Purpose." *War on Hunger* 6 (January 1972): 6-9.

Paniagua, M.E., Tayback, M., Janer, J.L., and Vazquez, J.L. "Medical and Psychological Sequelae of Surgical Sterilization of Women." *American Journal of Obstetrics and Gynecology* 90, 4 (October 15, 1964): 421-30.

Pare, C.M. and Raven, H. "Follow-up of Patients Referred for Termination of Pregnancy." *Lancet* 1 (March 28, 1970): 635-38.

Pathak, U.N. "Postpartum Sterilisation." *West Indian Medical Journal* 20 (March 1971): 17-24.

Paul, J. "Population 'Quality' and 'Fitness for Parenthood' in the Light of State Eugenic Sterilization Experiences, 1907-1966." *Population Studies* 21 (November 1967): 295-99.

———. "The Psychiatrist as Public Administrator: Case in Point—State Sterilization Laws." *American Journal of Orthopsychiatry* 38 (January 1968): 76-82.

———. "The Return of Punitive Sterilization Proposals." *Law and Society Review* 3 (August 1968): 77-106.

Peberdy, M. "Family Planning as Social Medicine." *Lancet* 1 (June 22, 1968): 1363-65.

Pec, J. and Kohlicek, J. "Sterilizácia u muža urobená za terapeutickým účelom a jej prípadné nasledky." (Sterilization in Men Carried Out for Therapeutical Reasons and its Possible Consequences). *Ceskoslovenska Gynekologie* 33 (April 1968): 297-300.

Peck, S.L. "Voluntary Female Sterilization: Attitudes and Legislation." *Hastings Center Report* 4, 3 (June 1974): 8-10.

Peel, J. "The Health of Women." *British Medical Journal* 3 (July 31, 1971): 267-71.

Petersen, P. "Die Freiwillige Sterilisation als Mittel der Familien-planung" (Voluntary Sterilization as a Family Planning Measure). *Fortschritte der Neurologie, Psychiatrie und Ihrer Grenzgebiete* 38 (January 1970): 33-52.

Phadke, A.M. "The Fate of Spermatozoa After Vasectomy." *The Journal of Family Welfare* 19, 2 (December 1972): 36-39.

———. "Sterilization as a Method of Family Limitation." *Maharashtra Medical Journal* 11 (1964): 237-44.

———. "Vasectomy: Sterilisation of the Male." *Journal of the Indian Medical Association* 37 (1961): 241-46.

Phadke, G.M. and Phadke, A.T. "Experiences in the Reanastomosis of the Vas Deferens." *Journal of Urology* 97 (1967): 888-90.

Phillips, N. "The Prevalence of Surgical Sterilization in a Suburban Population." *Demography* 8 (May 1971): 261-70.

Phoenix, C.H. "Sexual Behavior in Rhesus Monkeys After Vasectomy." *Science* 179, 4072 (February 2, 1973): 493-94.

Pillai, K.M. "Decision-making in Contraceptive Behaviour: A Systems Approach." *Demography India* 3, 2 (December 1974): 397-408.

Pilpel, H. "Family Planning and the Law." *Social Biology* 18 (September 1971): 127-33.

Poffenberger, S.B. and Sheth, D.L. "Reactions of Urban Employees to Vasectomy Operations." *Journal of Family Welfare* 10 (December 1963): 7-23.

———and Poffenberger, T. "Interview Report of Fifty-six Sterilization Cases Performed at a Rural 'Camp.'" *Journal of Family Welfare* 9 (September 1962): 1-7.

Poffenberger, T. "Age of Wives and Number of Living Children of a Sample of Men Who had the Vasectomy in Meerut District, U.P." *Journal of Family Welfare* 13 (June 1967): 48-51.

———. "Two Thousand Voluntary Vasectomies Performed in California: Background Factors and Comments." *Marriage and Family Living* 25 (November 1963): 469-74.

———and Patel, H.G. "The Effect of Local Beliefs on Attitudes Toward

Vasectomy in Two Indian Villages in Gujarat State." *Population Review* 8 (July 1964): 37-44.

_____ and Poffenberger, S.B. "A Comparison of Factors Influencing Choice of Vasectomy in India and the U.S.." *Indian Journal of Social Work* 25 (January 1965): 339-51.

_____. "Vasectomy as a Preferred Method of Birth Control: A Preliminary Investigation." *Marriage and Family Living* 25 (August 1963): 326-30.

Pond, D.A. "Psychological Aspects of Sterilization." *Family Planning* 19 (January 1971): 109-12.

Popenoe, P. "Eugenic Sterilization in California: (18) Effect of Vasectomy on the Sexual Life." *Journal of Abnormal and Social Psychology* 14 (October-December 1929): 251-68.

"Population Control, Morality, and the Doctor." *Scott Medical Journal* 17 (June 1972): 201-02.

Population Council. "India: UN Mission Evaluation of the Family Planning Program." *Studies in Family Planning* 56 (1970): 4-18.

Porter, C.W., Jr. and Hulka, J.F. "Female Sterilization in Current Clinical Practice." *Family Planning Perspectives* 6, 1 (Winter 1974): 30-38.

Potts, D.M. "Liberalization of Abortions and Female Sterilization." *Canadian Medical Association Journal* 105 (November 1971): 901.

Potts, I.F. "Medico-legal Implications of Vasectomy." *British Journal of Urology* 42 (December 1970): 737-38.

Potts, M. "Control of Human Fertility." *Carnets de L'Enfance/Assignment Children* (UNICEF) 18 (1972): 19-28.

Poulson, A.M. Jr. "Analysis of Female Sterilization Techinques." *Obstetrics and Gynecology* 42 (July 1973): 131-35.

Prasad, M.R.N. "Limiting Male Fertility by Selectively Depriving the Epididymis of Androgen." *Research in Reproduction* 5, 3 (May 1973): 3.

"Pregnancy Termination: The Impact of New Laws: An Invitational Symposium." *Journal of Reproductive Medicine* 6 (June 1971): 274-301.

Presser, H.B. "Puerto Rico: The Role of Sterilization in Controlling Fertility." *Studies in Family Planning* 45 (September 1969): 8-12.

_____. "The Role of Sterilization in Controlling Puerto Rican Fertility." *Population Studies* 23 (November 1969): 343-61.

_____. "Voluntary Sterilization: A World View." *Reports on Population/Family Planning* 5 (July 1970): 1-36.

_____. "Voluntary Sterilization—A World View." *Participant Journal* 7, 4 (October 1972): 30-33.

_____ and Bumpass, L.L. "The Acceptability of Contraceptive Sterilization Among U.S. Couples: 1970." *Family Planning Perspectives* 4 (October 1972): 18-26.

"Preventive Medicine?" *Family Planning Perspectives* 4 (January 1972): 5.

"Public Voices Approval of Sterilization Cases." *Washington Post,* p. A6, April 13, 1966.

Quddus, A.H.G. "The Unofficial Vasectomy Agent in East Pakistan." *News and Views on Family Planning in East Pakistan* pp. 26-35, Autumn 1969.

———, Ratcliffe, J.W., and Croley, H.T. "A Follow-up Study of Vasectomy Clients in East Pakistan." *Pakistan Journal of Family Planning* 3 (July 1969): 38-48.

———. "The Unofficial Vasectomy Agent of East Pakistan." *Pakistan Journal of Family Planning* 3 (January 1969): 17-26.

Raju, B.S. "Cost-Benefit Analysis of the Family Planning Programme in Andhra Pradesh (1963-74)." *Journal of Family Welfare* 22, 3 (March 1976): 10-20.

Ram, B. "A Demographic Evaluation of the Family Planning Programme in India." *Journal of Family Welfare* 18, 2 (December 1971): 37-54.

Rao, H.K., Saha, S.K., and Sadasivaiah, K. "A Follow-Up of Tubectomy Operations: Pilot Study at Vanivilas Hospital, Bangalore, Regional Health Office (Southern Region)." *Family Planning News,* November 1968.

Rao, G.G.P. "A Glance at Psychological and Other Aspects of Family Planning." *Indian Medical Journal* 63 (1969): 95-96.

Rathore, H.S. "After Effects of Vasectomy and Its Social Acceptance." *The Journal of Family Welfare* 19, 2 (December 1972): 20-25.

Rattan, W.C. "The Case for Voluntary Sterilization." *Wisconsin Medical Journal* 69 (August 1970): 20-21.

Reddy, S.V.R. et al. "Retrospective Study of 800 Families Tubectomised-Vasectomised Under Family Planning Programme." *Indian Pediatrics* 12 (September 1975): 899-902.

Reed, S.D. "New Voluntary Sterilization Law." *Eugenics Quarterly* 9 (September 1962): 166-67.

Reed, T.H. "Practice of Vasectomy Increasing." *Northwest Medicine* 71 (January 1972): 13.

"Regaining Fertility: and Vasectomy Complications Aplenty. Tough Road." *Medical World News* 13 (November 3, 1972): 17-18.

Regan, N.A. "Vasectomy." *British Medical Journal* 4 (October 23, 1971): 233.

Reiger, H.J. "Fragen aus der Parxis: Friewillige Sterilisienung" (Questions from Medical Practice: Voluntary Sterilization). *Deutsche Medicinische Wechenschrift* 97 (August 25, 1972): 1267-68.

Reimann-Huniziker, R. and Reimann-Huniziker, G. "Our Experiences with Over 1,000 Vasectomies During the Last 20 Years." *Zeitschrift fur Präventivmedizin* 7 (1962): 537.

——— and Reimann-Hunziker, F.J. "Twenty Years Experience with Vasectomized Patients." *Journal of Sex Research* 2 (July 1966): 99-110.

———, Reimann-Hunziker, G., and Friesewinkel, H. "Klinische Erfahrungen mit dem IBM-Computer 1401 über die freiwillige Sterilisation des Ehemannes auf Grund einer 25 jährigen Erfahrung." (Clinical Studies with the IBM 1401 Computer on Voluntary Sterilization of the Husband Based on 25 Years of Experience). *Praxis* 55 (September 8, 1966): 1013-14.

Rem-Picci, M. "Controllo delle Nascite in India" (Birth Control in India).

*Minerva Medicine* 31 (1972): 10-19.

Repetto, R. "India: A Case Study of the Madras Vasectomy Program." *Studies in Family Planning* 31 (1968): 8-16.

Roach, C.J., Krolack, J.D., Powell, J.L., Llorers, A.S., and Deubles, K.F. "Vaginal Hysterectomy for Sterilization." *American Journal of Obstetrics and Gynecology* 114 (November 1, 1972): 670-73.

Roberto, E.L. "Vasectomy Responses." *Family Planning Perspectives* 5 (Winter 1973): 5-6.

Roberts, H.J. "Thrombophlebitis after Vasectomy." *New England Journal of Medicine* 284 (June 10, 1971): 1330.

Rochar, R.W. "Regional Variation in Sterility, United States: 1970." *Advances in Planned Parenthood* 11, 1 (1976): 1-11.

Rodgers, D.A. and Ziegler, F.J. "Changes in Sexual Behavior Consequent to Use of Non-coital Procedures of Contraception." *Psychosomatic Medicine* 30 (September-October 1968): 495-505.

Rodgers, D.A., Ziegler, F.J., Prentiss, R.J., and Martin, P.L. "Comparisons of Nine Contraceptive Procedures by Couples Changing to Vasectomy or Ovulation Suppression Medication." *The Journal of Sex Research*, 1 (1965): 87-96.

_____, Ziegler, F.J., Altrocchi, J., and Levy, N. "A Longitudinal Study of the Psycho-social Effects of Vasectomy." *Journal of Marriage and the Family* 27 (February 1965): 59-64.

_____, Ziegler, F.J., and Levy, N. "Prevailing Cultural Attitudes about Vasectomy: A Possible Explanation of Postoperative Psychological Response." *Psychosomatic Medicine* 29 (July-August 1967): 367-75.

_____ and Ziegler, F.J. "Social Role Theory, the Marital Relationship, and Use of Ovulation Suppressors." *Journal of Marriage and the Family* 30 (1968): 584-91.

_____, Ziegler F.J., Rohr, P., and Prentiss, R.J. "Sociopsychological Characteristics of Patients Obtaining Vasectomies from Urologists." *Marriage and Family Living* 25 (August 1963): 331-35.

Rodriguez, F. and Phillips, C.M. "Vasectomy: Review of 579 Operations." *Journal of the Florida Medical Association* 60 (November 1973): 25-26.

Roe, A. "Vasectomy: Research Proposal." *Science* 168 (June 26, 1970): 1523-25.

Roe, R.E., Lares, R.K., Jr., and Work, B.A., Jr. "Female Sterilization: (1) The Vaginal Approach." *American Journal of Obstetrics and Gynecology* 112 (April 15, 1972): 1031-36.

Rogers, D.R. "Vasectomy." *Alaska Medicine* 12 (1970): 60.

Rogers, E.M. "Incentives in the Diffusion of Family Planning Innovations." *Studies in Family Planning* 2, 12 (1971): 241-48.

Rogers, W.C. "Beating the Drum for Vasectomy." *Family Planning Perspectives* 4, 4 (1972): 56-58.

Rosenfield, A.G., Hemachudha, C., Asavasena, W., and Varakamin, S. "Thailand: Family Planning Activities, 1968-1970." *Studies in Family Planning* 2 (September 1971): 181-92.

———and Varakamin, S. "The Postpartum Approach to Family Planning: Experiences in Thailand, 1966-1971." *American Journal of Obstetrics and Gynecology* 113 (May 1972): 1-13.

Rosoff, J.I. "Sterilization: The Montgomery Case—and Its Aftermath." *The Hastings Center Report* 3, 4 (September 1973): 6.

Ross, J.A., Germain, A., Forrest, J.E., and Van Ginneken, J. "Findings From Family Planning Research." *Reports on Population/Family Planning* 12 (October 1972). 1-47.

Ryder, N.B. "Contraceptive Failure in the U.S.." *Family Planning Perspectives.* 5, 3 (1973): 133-42.

Sabagh, G. and Edgerton, R.B. "Sterilized Mental Defectives Look at Eugenic Sterilization." *Eugenics Quarterly* 9 (December 1962): 213-22.

Sackler, A.M. "Vasectomy: Long-Term Effects." *Science* 182, 4115 (November 30, 1973): 947.

Sacks, S. and LaCroix, G. "Gynecologic Sequelae of Postpartum Tubal Ligation." *American Journal of Obstetrics and Gynecology* 19 (1962): 22.

Sadashivaiah, K. "A Retrospective Study of the Delivery Ratio and Post-Partum Sterilisation in Mission Hospitals in India." *Journal of Family Welfare* 22, 3 (March 1976): 21-32.

———and Rao, M.S.S. "Family Planning Project of the Christian Medical Association of India: Bangalore, Facts and Figures, 1970." *Journal of the Christian Medical Association of India* 46 (October 1971): 567-78.

Saha, H. "An Evaluation of Family Planning Programme in a Rural Area in West Bengal." *Journal of Family Welfare* 18, 1 (September 1971): 10-15.

Sahay, S.S. "A Study of 350 Vasectomy Cases." *Family Planning News* 10 (March 1969): 18.

Saigal, M.D. "Tubectomy Operations in Kaira District." *Family Planning News* 4, 3 (1963): 58-60.

Saksena, D.N. "Follow-Up Study of Rural Vasectomy Acceptors in Uttar Pradesh." *Studies in Family Planning* 5, 2 (February 1974): 50-53.

———. "Vasectomy: Field Experience of a District Hospital in Bihar." *Journal of Family Welfare* 18, 2 (December 1971): 9-19.

Sandhu, S.K. and Bhardwajk, S. "Follow-up Study of Vasectomized Cases in Mehrauli Block." *Family Planning News* 9 (1968): 17-20.

Sarma, R.S.S. "Demographic Effects of a Large-scale Sterilization Policy." *Artha Vijnana* 5, 1 (March 1963): 17-23.

Satish, C. and Hanumanulu, V.V. "Study of Demographic and Socioeconomic Characteristics of the Sterilised Cases at the Intensive Sterilization Drive (September-October 1972)." *Parivar Kalyan,* pp. 31-34, Special Number, 1973.

Savage, P.M., Jr. "An Economic and Efficient Vasectomy Program." *HSMHA Health Reports* 86, 8 (August 1971): 682-83.

_____. "Vasectomy and Psychosexual Damage." *Health Service Reports* 87, 9 (November 1972): 803-04.

Sawhney, Y.L. and Langoo, P.N. "A Study of Male Sterilization in Jammu and Kashmir." *Family Planning News* 10 (January 1969): 2-5.

Saxena, R.N., Chitre, K.T.O., and Lobo, J.A. "Follow-up of Vasectomy." *Journal of Family Welfare* 11 (March 1965): 1-12.

Saxena, D.M. "Vasectomy: What Are the Qualitative Gains?" *International Journal of Health Association* 16 (1973): 188-98.

Schirren, C. "Vasektomie" (Vasectomy). *Zeitschrift fur Haut- und Geschlechts-Krankheiten* 46 (May 1, 1971): 317-18.

Schmidt, S.S. "Vasectomy." *Journal of the American Medical Association* 216 (April 19, 1971): 522.

Schneider, H.E. "Aussagen und Ergebnisse nach Tubensterilisation" (A Retrospective Study on the Results of Sterilization by Tubal Ligation). *Geburtschilfe und Frauenheilkunde* 32 (April 1972): 290-97.

_____. "Mögliche Folgen nach Freiwilliger Sterilisation der Frau: Präoperative Beurteilung" (Possible Consequences of Voluntary Sterilization in Women). *Munchener Medizinische Wochenschrift* 113 (September 3, 1971): 1185-88.

_____. "Statistische und Soziologische Aspekte nach Sterilisation-operationen" (Statistical and Sociological Aspects After Sterilization Surgery). *Geburstshilfe Frauenheilkd* 30 (December 1970): 1064-70.

Schramm, W. "Communication in Family Planning." *Reports on Population/Family Planning* 7 (April 1971): 1-43.

Schulman, J. "Major Surgery for Abortion and Sterilization." Editorial, *American Journal of Obstetrics and Gynecology* 40 (1972): 738.

Schwyhart, W. and Kutner, S.J. "Reanalysis of Female Reactions to Contraceptive Sterilization." *The Journal of Nervous and Mental Disease* 156, 5 (1975): 354-70.

Scott, L.S. "Sterilisation of Women." *Lancet* 2 (August 22, 1970): 417.

_____. "Voluntary Vasectomy." *Scottish Medical Journal* 17 (June 1972): 203-09.

Scrimshaw, S.C. and Pasquariella, B. "Obstacles to Sterilization in One Community." *Family Planning Perspectives* 2 (October 1970): 40-42.

Seal, K.C. and Bhatnagar, N.K. "Cost-Effectiveness of Family Planning Programme—Variation by Methods and by States." *Journal of Family Welfare* 20, 1 (September 1973): 56-70.

Segal, S.J. "Contraceptive Technology: Current and Prospective Methods." *Milbank Memorial Fund Quarterly* 49 (October 1971): 145-70.

"Sexual Sterilization for Non-medical Reasons." *Canadian Medical Association Journal* 102 (January 31, 1970): 211.

Sharma, B.P. "Observation Upon Patients Following Vasectomy in Nepal." *Southern Medical Journal* 63 (July 1970): 771-72.

Sharp, H.C. "The Severing of the Vas Deferentia and the Relation to the Neuro-psychopathic Constitution." *New York Medical Journal* 75 (March 8, 1902): 411-14.

Shearman, R.P. "Recent Advances in Contraceptive Technology." *Medical Journal of Australia* 2 (October 9, 1971): 767-72.

Shepard, M.K. "Female Contraceptive Sterilization." *Obstetrical and Gynecological Survey* 29, 11 (November 1974): 739-87.

Sheth, S.S. and Batliwala, P. "Vaginal Sterilisation as Conception Control." *Journal of Obstetrics and Gynaecology of India* 18 (April 1968): 274-76.

Shinozaki, N. "Mutual Connection and Diffusion of Contraception, Abortion, and Sterilization." *Archives of the Population Association of Japan* 4 (1963): 63-80.

Shugarr, G. "Role as Population Curb Ruled Out for Sterilization." *Obstetrics-Gynecology News* 6, 3 (February 1, 1971): 1.

Shulman, J.J. "Contraceptive Provision in the Immediate Postpartum Period." *Obstetrics and Gynecology* 40 (September 1972): 403-08.

Shulman, S., Zappi, E., Ahmed, U., and Davis, J.E. "Immunologic Consequences of Vasectomy." *Contraception* 5 (April 1972): 269-78.

Siegler, A.M. "A Review of Tubal Sterilization." *Journal of Obstetrics, Gynecology and Neonatal Nursing* 1 (July-August 1972): 23-28.

Silver, M.A. "Birth Control and the Private Physician." *Family Planning Perspectives* 4 (April 1972): 42-46.

Sim, M. et al. "Psychiatric Aspects of Female Sterilization." *British Medical Journal* 5873 (July 28, 1973): 220-22.

Simcock, B.W. "The Position of Tubal Ligation in Family Planning." *Medical Journal of Australia* 2 (December 11, 1971): 1258.

Simlote, P.N. and Chittora, M.P. "Vasectomy in Bhilwara District." *Family Planning News* 11 (June-July 1967): 5.

Singapore, National Statistical Commission. "Statistics Related to Family Planning in Singapore, 1966-1974." *Singapore Statistical Bulletin* 4, 2 (December 1975): 99-102.

Sinha, S.N., Jain, P.C., and Prasad, B.G. "Socio-medical Study of Urban Sterilized Males in Lucknow: (1) Socio-demographic Data and Pre-operative Phase Reactions." *Journal of the Indian Medical Association* 53 (July 16, 1969): 68-77.

_____. "Socio-medical Study of Urban Sterilized Males in Lucknow: (2) Postoperative Effects and Reactions." *Journal of the Indian Medical Association* 53 (August 1, 1969): 134-41.

Sobrero, A.J. and Kohli, K.L. "Two Years' Experience of an Outpatient Vasectomy Service." *American Journal of Public Health* 65, 10 (October 1975): 1091-94.

_____ and Kohli, K.L. "Vasectomized Men: Follow-Up Results at One Year." *Studies in Family Planning* 5, 2 (February 1974): 54-57.

"Some Effects of Vasectomy Need More Study." *Journal of the American*

*Medical Association* 220 (June 12, 1972): 1419-20.

Southwick, S.J. "Psychological Side Effects of Vasectomy." *New York Times,* p. 33, January 14, 1972.

Speidel, J.J. and Spreche, J.T. "A Family Planning Strategy Based on Irreversible Means of Fertility Control." *Population Index* 38 (July-September 1972): 287-88.

Srinivasan, K. and Kachirayan, E. "Vasectomy Follow-up Study: Findings and Implications." *Bulletin of the Institute of Rural Health and Family Planning, Gandhigram* 3 (July 1968): 13-23.

Srivastav, V.C. "Demographic and Socio-Economic Characteristics of Females Sterilised in Camps." *Journal of Family Welfare* 19, 4 (June 1973): 52-56.

Steptoe, P.C. "Recent Advances in Surgical Methods of Control of Fertility and Infertility." *British Medical Bulletin* 26, 1 (1970): 60-64.

"Sterilization: Simpler Methods Boost Public Acceptance." *Family Planning Digest* 1 (May 1972): 4-7.

"Sterilisation Camp at Coondapoor." *Planned Parenthood (India)* 19 (April 1972): 4.

"Sterilizations and IUCD Insertions in the States and Union Territories." *Family Planning News* 8 (August 1967): 19-24.

"Sterilizations and IUCD Insertions in the States and Union Territories." *Family Planning News* 9 (July 1968): 15-19.

"Sterilisation in Man." *British Medical Journal* 66 (June 25, 1966): 1553-54.

"Sterilization Status Report." *Hospital Practice* 3 (May 1968): 16-20.

Stycos, J.M. "Female Sterilization in Puerto Rico." *Eugenics Quarterly* 1 (1954): 3-9.

Sundaram, C. "A Follow-Up Study of Sterilised Male Industrial Workers in Bombay." *Journal of Family Welfare* 16, 1 (September 1969): 48-56.

"Surgery in Planned Parenthood." *IPPF Medical Bulletin* 6 (June 1972): 4.

Tauber, A.S. "A Long-term Experience with Vasectomy." *The Journal of Reproductive Medicine* 10, 4 (April 1973): 147-49.

Thakor, V.H. and Patel, V.M. "The Gujarat State Massive Vasectomy Campaign." *Studies in Family Planning* 3, 8 (August 1972): 186-92.

Thiyagarajan, B. and Narayanaswami, S.S. "A Statistical Study of the Vasectomised Persons at Government General Hospital, Madras, During 1967-1968." *Journal of Family Welfare* 17 (March 1971): 46-51.

Thompson, B. and Aitken-Swan, J. "Pregnancy Outcome and Fertility Control in Aberdeen." *British Journal of Preventive and Social Medicine* 27 (August 1973): 137-45.

Thompson, B. and Baird, D. "Follow-up of 186 Sterilised Women." *Lancet* 1 (May 11, 1965): 1023-27.

_____ and Illsley, R. "Sterilisation: Social and Psychological Aspects." *IPPF Medical Bulletin* 6 (February 1972): 1-3.

_____ and Wheeless, C.R. "Outpatient Sterilization by Laparoscopy: A Report of 666 Patients." *Obstetrics and Gynecology* 38 (December 1971): 912-15.

Thompson, D.S. et al. "Postpregnant Vasectomies." *American Journal of Public Health* 65, 7 (July 1975): 735-37.

Thomsen, K. "Über die Möglichkeiten der temporären Sterilisation der Frau" (Possibilities of Temporary Sterilization of the Female). *Archiv für Gynackologie* 219, 1-4 (November 18, 1975): 43-44.

Tietze, C. "Induced Abortion and Sterilization as Methods of Fertility Control." *Journal of Chronic Disease* 18 (November 1965): 1161-74.

Tietze, C. "The Current Status of Fertility Control." *Law and Contemporary Problems* 25 (1960): 426-44.

"Tiny Gold Values to Control Fertility." *Life*, p. 54, July 28, 1972.

Todd, I.A.D. "Vasectomy." *Canadian Nurse* 67 (August 1971): 20-23.

Trehan, P.L. "Population Control by Sterilization in Underdeveloped Countries." *Journal of Family Welfare* 5 (December 1958): 55-56.

Truesdale, C.W. "Assessment of Vasectomy as Means of Voluntary Sterilization." *Lancet* 85 (1965): 155-56.

"Tubal Ligation in Population Control." *British Medical Journal* 1 (March 28, 1970): 770-71.

Turner, G. and Hooper, N. "Sterilization and Thrombo-embolism." *Journal of Obstetrics and Gynecology of the British Commonwealth* 78 (August 1971): 737-40.

Tyler, E.T. "How Soon Will We Have the 'Ideal' Contraceptive?" *Journal of the American Medical Association* 219 (March 6, 1972): 1333.

Tyson, J.E.A. and Washburn, H.H. "Canadian County-Sponsored Family Planning: (3) A Second Survey." *Obstetrics and Gynecology* 35 (March 1970): 377-80.

Uehling, D.T. and Wear, J.B. "Patient Attitudes Towards Vasectomy." *Fertility and Sterility* 23 (November 1972): 838-40.

Uppal, S. "A Study of Women Who Have Undergone Tubal Ligation." *Journal of Family Welfare* 20, 2 (December 1973): 74-88.

Urquhart-Hay, D. "Voluntary Sterilisation in the Male." *New Zealand Medical Journal* 71 (April 1970): 230-32.

Van Tienhoven, A., Eisner, T., and Rosenblatt, F. "Education and the Population Explosion." *BioScience* 21 (January 1971): 16-21.

Varma, R.N. and Boparai, M.S. "Vasectomy in the Army." *Indian Journal of Medical Research* 59 (April 4, 1971): 655-59.

"Vasectomy." *Lancet* 2 (November 18, 1972): 1074-75.

"Vasectomy Complications Aplenty." *Medical World News* 13 (November 3, 1972): 19.

"Vasectomy in Britain." *IPPF Medical Bulletin* 4 (April 1970): 40.

"Vasectomy on the National Health Service." *British Medical Journal* 1 (May 9, 1970): 312-13.

"Vasectomy Report." *Journal of the American Medical Association* 222 (October 2, 1972): 14-15.

"A Vasectomy that Is Reversible." *Business Week,* p. 72 September 4, 1971.

Vasquez Calzada, J.L. "La Esterilización Femenina en Puerto Rico" (Female Sterilization in Puerto Rico). *Revista de Ciencias Sociales* 17 (September 1973): 281-308.

Vaughn, D. and Sparer, G. "Ethnic Group and Welfare Status of Women Sterilized in Federally Funded Family Planning Program, 1972." *Family Planning Perspectives* 6, 4 (Fall 1974): 224-29.

_____. "Demographic Characteristics of Persons Sterilized in OEO Planning Services in 1972." A Working Paper, 1973.

Venkatachary, N.K. "A Model to Estimate Births Averted Due to IUCD's and Sterilizations." *Demography* 8 (November 1971): 491-505.

Verghese, S.I. "Tubectomy Camps: A Case Study." *Journal of Family Welfare* 17 (June 1971): 75-86.

Vokaer, R. "Le Côntrole de la Nalité: Avenir des Différentes Méthodes Contraceptives et Abortives" (Birth control: Future of the Different Contraceptive and Abortion Methods). *Gynecologie et Obstetrique* 70 (January-February 1971): 15-44.

"Voluntary Male Sterilization." *Journal of the American Medical Association* 204 (1968): 821-22.

"Voluntary Male Sterilization." *Medical Journal of Australia* 1 (February 27, 1971): 455-56.

"Voluntary Sterilization." *American Journal of Public Health* 63, 7 (1973): 573-75.

"Voluntary Sterilization." *Consumer Reports,* pp. 384-86, June 1971.

"Voluntary Sterilization in the Male." *British Medical Journal* 2 (June 1, 1968): 508.

Wadhwa, R.K. and McKenzie, R. "Complications of Band-aid Surgery for Sterilization." *Journal of the American Medical Association* 222 (December 18, 1972): 1558.

Wadia, A.B. "Notes on the Schemes for Sterilization in Madras State." *Journal of Family Welfare* 5 (December 1958): 38-44.

Wallace, D.N. and Riddle, P. "Vasectomy." *British Medical Journal* 4 (October 9, 1971): 100-102.

Walton, H.C.M. "Male Sterilisation." *British Medical Journal* 4 (December 19, 1970): 748.

Wan, F. "Sexual Sterilisation in Singapore: Some Epidemiological Aspects and Demographic Impact." *Annals of the Academy of Medicine Singapore* 3, 4 (1974): 324-30.

_____ and Sundarason, R. "Vasectomy in Singapore." *Annals of the Academy of Medicine Singapore* 3, 4 (1974): 353-56.

Westoff, C.F. "The Modernization of U.S. Contraceptive Practice." *Family Planning Perspectives* 4 (July 1972): 9-12.

———. "Trends in Contraceptive Practice: 1965-1973." *Family Planning Perspectives* 8, 2 (March-April 1976): 54-57.

Wheeless, C.R. "Laparoscopic Sterilization: Review of 3600 Cases." *Obstetrics and Gynecology* 42, 5 (November 1973): 751-58.

———. "Outpatient Tubal Sterilization." *Obstetrics and Gynecology* 36 (August 1970): 208-211.

———. "The Status of Outpatient Tubal Sterilization by Laparoscopy Improved Technics and Review of 1000 Cases." *Obstetrics and Gynecology* 39 (April 1972): 635-36.

Whitehouse, D.B. "Sterilisation of Young Wives." *British Medical Journal* 2 (June 19, 1971): 707.

Wiest, W.M. and Janke, L.D. "A Methodological Critique of Research on Psychological Effects of Vasectomy." *Psychosomatic Medicine* 36 (1974): 438-49.

Wig, N.N., Singh, S., Sahasi, G., and Issac, P. "Psychiatric Symptoms Following Vasectomy." *Indian Journal of Psychiatry* 12 (1970): 169-76.

Williams, P.P. and Bendel R.P. "Laparoscopic Sterilization." *Minnesota Medicine* 54 (November 1971): 887-88.

Winn, H. "Contraception." *Clinical Obstetrics and Gynecology* 13 (September 1970): 701-12.

Wolf, R.C. "Can New Laws Solve the Legal and Psychiatric Problems of Voluntary Sterilization?" *Journal of Urology* 93 (1965): 402-06.

Wolfers, D. and Wolfers, H. "Vasectomania." *Family Planning Perspectives* 5, 4 (Fall 1973): 196-98.

Wolfers, H. "Psychological Aspects of Vasectomy." *British Medical Journal* 4 (October 31, 1970): 297-300.

———, Subbiah, N., and Ariffin, B.M. "Psychological Aspects of Vasectomy in Malaysia." *Social Biology* 20, 3 (September 1973): 315-22.

"Women Give View on Sterilization." *New York Times,* p. 25, September 1, 1968.

Wood, H.C., Jr. (Letter to the Editor). *Journal of Sex Research* 7 (1971): 72-73.

Wood, H.C., Jr. "Vasectomy: How to Meet and Survive a Wave of Demand." *Medical Opinion* 7 (March 1971): 56-61.

Wood, W., Thomson, J.L., and Dowers, D.M. "Abortion or Contraception?" *British Medical Journal* 3 (August 21, 1971): 476-77.

Worth, G., Watson, W.R., Han, D.W., Finnigan, O.D., and Keeny, S.M. "Korea-Taiwan 1970: Report on the National Family Planning Programs." *Studies in Family Planning* 2 (March 1971): 57-69.

Wortman, J.S., Sciarra, J.J., and Markland, C. "Control of Male Fertility: Report of a Workshop." *Contraception* 10, 5 (November 1974): 561-68.

Wright, M.R. "Psychological Aspects of Vasectomy Counseling." *Family*

*Coordinator* 21 (July 1972): 259-65.

Yeates, W.K. "Voluntary Sterilisation." *Lancet* 2 (September 20, 1969): 641.

"Young Californians Opt for Permanent Method." *Family Planning Digest* 1 (January 1972): 6.

Young, D. "Vasectomy for Contraception." *British Medical Journal* 4 (November 11, 1967): 354-55.

Yuzpe, A.A., Allen, H., and Collins, J.A. "Tubal Sterilization: Methodology, Post-operative Management and Follow-up of 2,934 Cases." *Canadian Medical Association Journal* 107 (July 1972): 115-17.

Ziegler, F.J. "Vasectomy and Adverse Psychological Reactions." *Annals of Internal Medicine* 73 (November 1970): 853.

_____ and Kreigsman, S.A. "Vasectomy and Psychological Functioning." *Humanist* 25 (January-February 1965): 16-18.

_____ and Rodgers, D.A. "Vasectomy Ovulation Suppressors, and Sexual Behavior." *Journal of Sex Research* 4 (August 1968): 169-93.

_____, Rodgers, D.A., and Kriegsman, S.A. "Effect of Vasectomy on Psychological Functioning." *Psychosomatic Medicine* 28 (January-February 1966): 50-63.

_____, Rodgers, D.A., and Prentiss, R.J. "Psychosocial Response to Vasectomy." *Archives of General Psychiatry* 21 (July 1969): 46-54.

## Conference Papers

Ackner, B. "Emotional Aspects of Hysterectomy. A Follow-Up Study of Fifty Patients Under the Age of 40." In *Advances in Psychosomatic Medicine,* edited by A. Jores and H. Freyberger. Symposium of the Fourth European Conference on Psychosomatic Research. New York: Robert Brunner, Inc., 1961.

Agarwala, S.N. "Family Planning Performance in India." In *All India Seminar on Family Planning Problems in India* (February 20-22, 1972), pp. 27-50. Bombay: International Institute for Population Studies (Mimeographed), 1972.

Aguero, O. and Cardenas-Conde, L. "Tubal Ligation in Caracas, Venezuela." In *Human Sterilization,* edited by R.M. Richart and D.J. Prager, pp. 18-22. A Conference held in Cherry Hill, N.J. in 1969, sponsored by the International Institute for the Study of Human Reproduction, College of Physicians and Surgeons of Columbia University. Springfield, IL: Charles C. Thomas, 1972.

Alfaro, C. "Workshop K1: Motivation and Education in Voluntary Sterilization Programs." In *Advances in Voluntary Sterilization,* Proceedings of the Second International Conference, Geneva, 1973, edited by M.E. Schima, I. Lubell, J.E. Davis, and E. Connell, pp. 314-21. Princeton, N.J.: Excerpta, Medica, American Elsevier Publishing Co., Inc., 1974.

Anklesaria, S.B. "Statistical Review of 5900 Female Sterilizations at the Civil Hospital, Chinai Maternity Hospital (Vadilal Sarabhai Hospital) and Lallubhai Gordhandas Hospital, Ahmedabad, with a Prospective Follow-up of 1936 Patients for One to Five Years." In *Proceedings of the International Seminar on Maternal Mortality, Family Planning and Biology of Reproduction*. Bombay, March 3-8, 1969, edited by B.N. Purandare and C.L. Jhaveri, pp. 181-94. Bombay, 1970.

Australian and New Zealand Journal of Obstetrics and Gynaecology. "Clinical Proceedings of the First International Planned Parenthood Federation S.E. Asia and Oceania Regional Medical and Scientific Congress, Sydney, Australia, August 14-18, 1972." Melbourne, Australia, 1972.

Barnes, H.B. "Psycho-Social Aspects." In *Advances in Voluntary Sterilization*, Proceedings of the Second International Conference, Geneva, 1973, edited by M.E. Schima, I. Lubell, J.E. Davis, and E. Connell, pp. 289-90. Princeton, N.J.: Excerpta Medica, American Elsevier Publishing Co., Inc., 1974.

Barnes, J. "Medicolegal Aspects (Sterilisation)." In *Contraception Today: A Medical Text Based on the Proceedings of the FPA Medical Training Conferences in York, Bristol and London 1970*, edited by A.J. Smith, pp. 113-15. London: Family Planning Association, 1971.

Bernard, R. "Voluntary Sterilization Program Statistics—Collection and Evaluation." In *Advances in Voluntary Sterilization*, Proceedings of the Second International Conference, Geneva, 1973, edited by M.E. Schima, I. Lubell, J.E. Davis, and E. Connell, pp. 297-304. Princeton, N.J.: Excerpta Medica, American Elsevier Publishing Co., Inc., 1974.

Bhatla, P.C., ed. *Proceedings of the International Conference on Family Planning*, New Delhi, March 12-16, 1972. New Delhi: Indian Medical Association, 1972.

Blandy, J. "Male Sterilization." In *Contraception Today: A Medical Text Based on the Proceedings of the FPA Medical Training Conferences in York, Bristol and London 1970*, edited by A.J. Smith, pp. 101-07. London: Family Planning Association, 1971.

Bumpass, L. "The Increasing Acceptance of Sterilization in the U.S." In *Advances in Voluntary Sterilization*, Proceedings of the Second International Conference, Geneva, 1973, edited by M.E. Schima, I. Lubell, J.E. Davis, and E. Connell, pp. 104-11. Princeton, N.J.: Excerpta Medica, American Elsevier Publishing Co., Inc., 1974.

Burnight, R.G. "Current Practice of Sterilization in Thailand." In *Advances in Voluntary Sterilization*, Proceedings of the Second International Conference, Geneva, 1973, edited by M.E. Schima, I. Lubell, J.E. Davis, and E. Connell, pp. 367-73. Princeton, N.J.: Excerpta Medica, American Elsevier Publishing Co., Inc., 1974.

Chez, R.A. "The Use of Learning Aids in Human Sterilization Programs." In *Human Sterilization*, edited by R.M. Richart and D.J. Prager, pp. 48-52. A conference held in Cherry Hill, N.J. in 1969, sponsored by the International

Institute for the Study of Human Reproduction, College of Physicians and
Surgeons of Columbia University. Springfield, IL: Charles C. Thomas, 1972.
_____. "Male Sterilization in East Pakistan." In *Human Sterilization,* edited by
R.M. Richart and D.J. Prager, pp. 23-37. A conference held in Cherry Hill,
N.J. in 1969, sponsored by the International Institute for the Study of
Human Reproduction, College of Physicians and Surgeons of Columbia
University. Springfield, IL: Charles C. Thomas, 1972.
Conroy, F.D. and Wojcicki, H.M. "Functional Complications of Sterilization by
Vasectomy." Paper read at Annual Meeting of the American Urological
Association, Western Section, Coronado, California, February 1964.
Curt, J.N. "Evidence Relating to Acceptability of Sterilization in Puerto Rico."
In *Advances in Voluntary Sterilization,* Proceedings of the Second Inter-
national Conference, Geneva, 1973, edited by M.E. Schima, I. Lubell, J.E.
Davis, and E. Connell, pp. 112-23. Princeton, N.J.: Excerpta Medica,
American Elsevier Publishing Co., Inc., 1974.
Cutler, J.C. "The Role of the Voluntary Organization in Encouraging Use of
Voluntary Sterilization in Family Planning and Population Programs." In
*Advances in Voluntary Sterilization*, Proceedings of the Second Interna-
tional Conference, Geneva, 1973, edited by M.E. Schima, I. Lubell, J.E.
Davis, and E. Connell, pp. 187-93. Princeton, N.J.: Excerpta Medica,
American Elsevier Publishing, Co., Inc., 1974.
Deys, C.M. "Cultural Aspects of Male Sterilization." In *Abstracts of the First
International Planned Parenthood Federation, Southeast Asia and Oceania
Regional Medical and Scientific Congress.* Sydney, Australia, August 14-18,
1972, p. 50. Sydney: Family Planning Association of Australia, 1972.
Dourlen-Rollier, A.M. "Workshop E: The Legal Aspects of Voluntary Steriliza-
tion." In *Advances in Voluntary Sterilization,* Proceedings of the Second
International Conference, Geneva, 1973, edited by M.E. Schima, I. Lubell,
J.E. Davis, and E. Connell, pp. 273-76. Princeton, N.J.: Excerpta Medica,
American Elsevier Publishing Co., Inc., 1974.
Dubey, D.C. and Bardhan, A. "Role of Social Interaction and Incentives in
Social Change: A Case of Mass Acceptance of Vasectomy." Paper prepared
for 9th International Congress of Anthropological and Ethnological Sciences,
Chicago, August-September 1973.
Echeverria, C. Goldsmith, A., Goldberg, R., and Cadavid, C. "Vasectomy—The
Columbian Experience." Paper presented at the Second International
Conference on Voluntary Sterilization, February 25–March 1, 1973, Geneva.
Edey, H. "Workshop F: Psychologic and Psychiatric Aspects of Voluntary
Sterilization." In *Advances in Voluntary Sterilization,* Proceedings of the
Second International Conference, Geneva, 1973, edited by M.E. Schima,
I. Lubell, J.E. Davis, and E. Connell, pp. 277-82. Princeton, N.J.: Excerpta
Medica, American Elsevier Publishing Co., Inc., 1974.
Ghorbani, F.S. "Major Problems Concerning Motivation and Education in

Voluntary Sterilization Programs." In *Advances in Voluntary Sterilization,* Proceedings of the Second International Conference, Geneva, 1973, edited by M.E. Schima, I. Lubell, J.E. Davis, and E. Connell, pp. 332-33. Princeton, N.J.: Excerpta Medica, American Elsevier Publishing Co., Inc., 1974.

Gillespie, D.G. and Spillane, W.H. "Knowledge and Approval of Vasectomy in the U.S.: Implications for Educational Programs." In *Advances in Voluntary Sterilization,* Proceedings of the Second International Conference, Geneva, 1973, edited by M.E. Schima, I. Lubell, J.E. Davis, and E. Connell, pp. 338-45. Princeton N.J.: Excerpta Medica, American Elsevier Publishing Co., Inc., 1974.

——and Spillane, W.H. "Vasectomy in the United States, 1971." Paper presented at Session of Maternal and Child Health, Annual Meeting of the American Public Health Association, Atlantic City, N.J., November 12-16, 1972.

Goldberg, R. and Goldsmith, A. "Male Sterilization in Latin America: Some Considerations Prior to Program Implementation." Paper presented at the Second International Conference on Voluntary Sterilization, February 25-March 1, 1973, Geneva.

Goldsmith, A., Goldberg, R., and Echeverria, G. "An In-depth Study of Vasectomized Men in Latin America—A Preliminary Report." Paper presented at Fourth Annual Meeting of the International Family Planning Research Association, Las Vegas, October 23-25, 1972.

Gutierrez Najar, A.J. "Culdoscopy as an Aid to Family Planning." In *Workshop on Female Sterilization: Prognosis for Simplified Outpatient Procedures,* edited by G.W. Duncan, R.D. Falb, and J.J. Speidel, pp. 41-49. New York: Academic Press, 1972.

Hannah, W.J. "The Role of Surgical Procedures in Family Planning." In *Proceedings of a Symposium for Clergy and Physicians Counselling in Family Planning.* Toronto, April 20, 1966, pp. 63-66. Toronto: Council for Social Services, The Anglican Church of Canada, 1968.

Hulka, J.F., Soderstrom, R.M., Corson, S.L., and Brooks, P.G. "Complications Committee of the American Association of Gynecological Laparoscopists—First Annual Report." Report from Las Vegas Meeting of the American Association of Gynecological Laparoscopists, November 13-14, 1972.

Islam, M. "A Follow-up Study of Vasectomy." In *Proceedings of the Sixth Biannual Seminar on Research in Family Planning,* Karachi, West Pakistan, April 23-25, 1969, pp. 91-99. Karachi: National Research Institute of Family Planning, 1969.

Jackson, P. "Assessment for Sterilization." In *Contraception Today: A Medical Text Based on the Proceedings of the FPA Medical Training Conferences in York, Bristol and London 1970,* edited by A.J. Smith, pp. 120-23. London: Family Planning Association, 1971.

Karp, R. "Workshop K2: Motivation and Education in Voluntary Sterilization Programs." In *Advances in Voluntary Sterilization,* Proceedings of the

Second International Conference, Geneva, 1973, edited by M.E. Schima, I. Lubell, J.E. Davis, and E. Connell, pp. 322-26. Princeton, N.J.: Excerpta Medica, American Elsevier Publishing Co., Inc., 1974.

Katagiri, T. "Sterilization and Other Family Planning Methods in the People's Republic of China." In *Advances in Voluntary Sterilization,* Proceedings of the Second International Conference, Geneva, 1973, edited by M.E. Schima, I. Lubell, J.E. Davis, and E. Connell, pp. 124-32. Princeton, N.J.: Excerpta Medica, American Elsevier Publishing Co., Inc., 1974.

Kessel, E. "Evaluation of a Sterilization Program." In *Advances in Voluntary Sterilization,* Proceedings of the Second International Conference, Geneva, 1973, edited by M.E. Schima, I. Lubell, J.E. Davis, and E. Connell, pp. 200-11. Princeton N.J.: Excerpta Medica, American Elsevier Publishing Co., Inc., 1974.

Lee, H.Y. "The Korean Vasectomy Program." In *Human Sterilization,* edited by R.M. Richart and D.J. Prager, pp. 38-47. A Conference held in Cherry Hill, N.J., in 1969, sponsored by the International Institute for the Study of Human Reproduction, College of Physicians and Surgeons of Columbia University. Springfield, IL: Charles C. Thomas, 1972.

_____. "A Modified Operative Technique for Vasectomy." In *Human Sterilization,* edited by R.M. Richart and D.J. Prager, pp. 71-75. A conference held in Cherry Hill, N.J., in 1969, sponsored by the International Institute for the Study of Human Reproduction, College of Physicians and Surgeons of Columbia University. Springfield, IL: Charles C. Thomas, 1972.

Lower, B.R. "Critical Assessment of Sterilization Procedures." In *Workshop on Female Sterilization: Prognosis for Simplified Outpatient Procedures,* edited by G.W. Duncan, R.D. Falb, and J.J. Speidel, pp. 151-58. New York: Academic Press, 1972.

Mannan, M.A. "Male Sterilization in Comilla: A Follow-up Study of 100 Vasectomy Clients in Comilla Kotkwali Thana." In *Proceedings of the Sixth Biannual Seminar on Research in Family Planning,* Karachi, West Pakistan, April 23-26, 1969, pp. 100-17. Karachi: National Institute of Family Planning, 1969.

Mati, J.K.G. et al. "Present Attitudes Towards Female Sterilization and Projected Attitudes in the Next Generation of Kenyan Women." In *Advances in Voluntary Sterilization,* Proceedings of the Second International Conference, Geneva, 1973, edited by M.E. Schima, I. Lubell, J.E. Davis, and E. Connell, pp. 352-58. Princeton, N.J.: Excerpta Medica, American Elsevier Publishing Co., Inc., 1974.

McIntyre, R.J. "Pronatalist Policies in European Socialist Countries." Paper Presented at General Conference of the International Union for the Scientific Study of Population, Liege, Belgium, August 30, 1973.

Morgan, R.E., Jr. et al. "Workshop H: How to Establish a Voluntary Organization and Its Role in Voluntary Sterilization." In *Advances in Voluntary*

*Sterilization,* Proceedings of the Second International Conference, Geneva, 1973, edited by M.E. Schima, I. Lubell, J.E. Davis, and E. Connell, pp. 292-96. Princeton, N.J.: Excerpta Medica, American Elsevier Publishing Co., Inc., 1974.

Murty, D.V.R. "Estimated Reductions in Birth Rate Resulting from Different Combinations of Sterilisation and Contraception Programmes in India." Paper presented at the United States World Population Conference, Belgrade, 1965.

Okediji, F.O. "Workshop G: The Acceptability of Voluntary Sterilization: Sociological, Political and Religious Aspects." In *Advances in Voluntary Sterilization,* Proceedings of the Second International Conference, Geneva, 1973, edited by M.E. Schima, I. Lubell, J.E. Davis, and E. Connell, pp. 283-88. Princeton N.J.: Excerpta Medica, American Elsevier Publishing Co., Inc., 1974.

Pai, D.N. "Keynote Address: Voluntary Sterilization as a Component of a Family Planning Program." In *Advances in Voluntary Sterilization,* Proceedings of the Second International Conference, Geneva, 1973, edited by M.E. Schima, I. Lubell, J.E. Davis, and E. Connell, pp. 12-20. Princeton, N.J.: Excerpta Medica, American Elsevier Publishing Co., Inc., 1974.

———. "Indian Vasectomy Camps." In *Human Sterilization,* edited by R.M. Richart and D.J. Prager, pp. 5-11. A conference held in Cherry Hill, N.J. in 1969, sponsored by the International Institute for the Study of Human Reproduction, College of Physicians and Surgeons of Columbia University. Springfield, IL: Charles C. Thomas, 1972.

———. "Vasectomy in Greater Bombay." In *Proceedings of the International Seminar on Maternal Mortality, Family Planning and Biology of Reproduction, Bombay, 3-8 March 1969,* edited by B.N. Purandure, and C.L. Jhaveri, pp. 207-26. Bombay, 1970.

Parker, J.B., Hallock, H.L., and Longstaff, J.P. "Sequelae of Sterilization of Self or Marital Partner." Paper read at Meeting of the American Psychiatric Association, New York, May 1965.

Phadke, G.M. "Place of Sterilization (Especially of the Male) in Population Control in Underdeveloped Countries." In *Proceedings of the Seventh Conference of the International Planned Parenthood Federation,* Singapore, February 10-18, 1963, edited by G.W. Cadbury, et al. Amsterdam: Excerpta Medica Foundation, 1964.

———. "Sterilization of Men." In *Proceedings of the Fourth All India Conference of Family Planning,* Hyderabad, pp. 62-69, 1961.

———. "Vasectomy." In *Report of the Sixth International Conference on Planned Parenthood,* held at Delhi, 1959, pp. 342-45. Bombay: Family Planning Association of India, 1959.

Poffenberger, T. and Wells, H.B. "Research Designs for Evaluating After Effects of Vasectomy." Paper presented at Seminar on Sterilization.

Gokhale Institute of Politics and Economics, Poona, India, November 1965.

Pond, D., Jackson, P., Steptoe, P.C., and Barnes, J. "Panel Discussion (Sterilization)." In *Contraception Today: A Medical Text Based on the Proceedings of the FPA Medical Training Conferences in York, Bristol and London 1970,* edited by A.J. Smith, pp. 124-31. London: Family Planning Association, 1971.

Potts, M. "Current Status of Sterilization in the World—Prevalence, Incidence, Who and Where." In *Advances in Voluntary Sterilization,* Proceedings of the Second International Conference, Geneva, 1973, edited by M.E. Schima, I. Lubell, J.E. Davis, and E. Connell, pp. 97-103. Princeton, N.J.: Excerpta Medica, American Elsevier Publishing Co., Inc., 1974.

Purandare, B.N. "Development and Implementation of a Sterilization Program: India as an Example." In *Advances in Voluntary Sterilization,* Proceedings of the Second International Conference, Geneva, 1973 edited by M.E. Schima, I. Lubell, J.E. Davis, and E. Connell, pp. 218-28. Princeton, N.J.: Excerpta Medica, American Elsevier Publishing Co., Inc., 1974.

_____. "Evaluation of Operative Methods for Female Sterilization." In *Proceedings of the International Seminar on Maternal Mortality, Family Planning and Biology of Reproduction,* Bombay, March 3-8, 1969, edited by B.N. Purandare, and D.L. Jhaveri, pp. 265-69. Bombay, 1970.

Ragab, M. "Workshop L: Staffing Patterns for Voluntary Sterilization Programs: Needs, Training, and Utilization." In *Advances in Voluntary Sterilization,* Proceedings of the Second International Conference, Geneva, 1973, edited by M.E. Schima, I. Lubell, J.E. Davis, and E. Connell, pp. 327-31. Princeton, N.J.: Excerpta Medica, American Elsevier Publishing Co., Inc., 1974.

Ram, R. "Workshop J: The Organization and Administration of Voluntary Sterilization Service Programs." In *Advances in Voluntary Sterilization,* Proceedings of the Second International Conference, Geneva, 1973, edited by M.E. Schima, I. Lubell, J.E. Davis, and E. Connell, pp. 305-08. Princeton, N.J.: Excerpta Medica, American Elsevier Publishing Co., Inc., 1974.

Ratcliffe, J.W., Quddus, A.H.G., and Croley, H.T. "Factors Related to Vasectomy in East Pakistan." In *Proceedings of the Fifth Biannual Seminar on Research in Family Planning,* Lahore, East Pakistan, November 7-9, 1968, pp. 103-28. Karachi, West Pakistan: National Research Institute of Family Planning, 1969.

Ravenholt, R.T. "Overview of the Office of Population, AID, on Sterilization." In *Workshop on Female Sterilization: Prognosis for Simplified Outpatient Procedures,* edited by G.W. Duncan, R.D. Falb, and J.J. Speidel, pp. 1-2. New York: Academic Press, 1972.

Ravenholt, R.T. "World Epidemiology and Potential Fertility Impact of Voluntary Sterilization Services." Unpublished paper presented to the Third International Conference on Voluntary Sterilization, Tunis. February 2, 1976.

Rodgers, D.A. and Ziegler, F.J. "Changes in Sexual Behavior Consequent to

Use of Non-coital Procedures of Contraception." Paper presented at Symposium on Research in Birth Control and Changing Sex Behavior, Annual Meeting of the American Association for the Advancement of Science, New York, December 29, 1967.

_____ and Ziegler, F.J. "Effects of Surgical Contraception on Sexual Behavior." In *Advances in Voluntary Sterilization,* Proceedings of the Second International Conference, Geneva, 1973, edited by M.E. Schima, I. Lubell, J.E. Davis, and E. Connell, pp. 161-66. Princeton, N.J.: Excerpta Medica, American Elsevier Publishing Co., Inc., 1974.

Rosenfield, A.G. and Muangman, D. "Sterilization Procedures: Their Role in National Family Planning Programs." In *Advances in Voluntary Sterilization,* Proceedings of the Second International Conference, Geneva, 1973, edited by M.E. Schima, I. Lubell, J.E. Davis, and E. Connell, pp. 374-82. Princeton, N.J.: Excerpta Medica, American Elsevier Publishing Co., Inc., 1974.

Sciarra, J.J. "Research and Development Programs to Achieve Practical Outpatient Sterilization." In *Workshop on Female Sterilization:Prognosis for Simplified Outpatient Procedures,* edited by G.W. Duncan, R.D. Falb, and J.J. Speidel, pp. 159-63. New York: Academic Press, 1972.

Scrimshaw, S.C. "The Demand for Female Sterilization in Spanish Harlem: Experiences of Puerto Ricans in New York City." Paper presented at 69th Annual Meeting of the American Anthropological Association, San Diego, California, November 4, 1970.

Sharma, A.K. "Surgical Aspect of Family Planning (Males)." In *Advances in Voluntary Sterilization,* Proceedings of the Second International Conference, Geneva, 1973, edited by M.E. Schima, I. Lubell, J.E. Davis, and E. Connell, pp. 383-88. Princeton, N.J.: Excerpta Medica, American Elsevier Publishing Co., Inc., 1974.

Siddiqi, K.A. and Husain, I. "Some Characteristics of Vasectomy Clients in Karachi District." In *Proceedings of the Sixth Biannual Seminar on Research in Family Planning,* Karachi, West Pakistan, April 23-26, 1969, pp. 82-90. Karachi: National Research Institute of Family Planning, 1969.

Simmons, G.B. "The Economics of Voluntary Sterilization for the Parent and for the Nation." In *Advances in Voluntary Sterilization,* Proceedings of the Second International Conference, Geneva, 1973, edited by M.E. Schima, I. Lubell, J.E. Davis, and E. Connell, p. 154. Princeton, N.J.: Excerpta Medica, American Elsevier Publishing Co., Inc., 1974.

Sinha, S.N. "An Exploratory Study of One Hundred Urban Sterilized Males in Lucknow." Paper presented in the Seminar on Sterilization, Gokhale Institute of Politics and Economics, Poona, 1965 (Mimeographed).

Sobrero, A.J. and Edey, H. "A Vasectomy Service Within a Planned Parenthood Clinic." In *Advances in Planned Parenthood,* Vol. 6, edited by A.J. Sobrero and R. Harvey, pp. 130-32. Proceedings of the American Association of Planned Parenthood, 19th Annual Meeting, 1971. Amsterdam: Excerpta

Medica, 1971.

Soonawalla, R. "Vaginal Techniques of Surgical Sterilization." In *Abstracts of the First International Planned Parenthood Federation, Southeast Asia and Oceania Regional Medical and Scientific Congress,* Sydney, Australia, August 14-18, 1972, p. 49. Sydney: Family Planning Association of Australia, 1972.

Southam, A.L. "Summary and Directions for the Future." In *Human Sterilization,* edited by R.M. Richart and D.J. Prager, pp. 379-85. A conference held in Cherry Hill, N.J. in 1969, sponsored by the International Institute for Study of Human Reproduction, College of Physicians and Surgeons of Columbia University. Springfield, IL: Charles C. Thomas, 1972.

Speidel, J.J. "Male Sterilization and Its Contribution to Solution of Population Problems." Paper presented at a Symposium on the Role of the Urologist in Population Stabilization, Montreal, October 23, 1972. Mimeographed.

_____. "Research and Development Programs to Achieve Practical Outpatient Sterilization." In *Workshop on Female Sterilization: Prognosis for Simplified Outpatient Procedures,* edited by G.W. Duncan, R.D. Falb, and J.J. Speidel, pp. 159-63. New York: Academic Press, 1972.

_____. "The Role of Female Sterilization in Family Planning Programs." In *Workshop on Female Sterilization: Prognosis for Simplified Outpatient Procedures,* edited by G.W. Duncan et al., pp. 89-104. New York: Academic Press, 1972.

_____, Perry, M.I., and Duncan, G.W. "An Overview of Research on New Sterilization Technology." In *Advances in Voluntary Sterilization,* Proceedings of the Second International Conference, Geneva, 1973, edited by M.E. Schima, I. Lubell, J.E. Davis, and E. Connell, pp. 194-99. Princeton, N.J.: Excerpta Medica, American Elsevier Publishing Co., Inc., 1974.

_____ and Sprehe, J.T. "Irreversible Means of Fertility Control, a Neglected Family Planning Strategy." Paper presented at Meeting of the Population Association of America, Toronto, April 13-15, 1972. Mimeographed.

Tamayo, F. "Planning and Implementation of A Voluntary Sterilization Service." In *Advances in Voluntary Sterilization,* Proceedings of the Second International Conference, Geneva, 1973, edited by M.E. Schima, I. Lubell, J.E. Davis, and E. Connell, pp. 213-17. Princeton, N.J.: Excerpta Medica, American Elsevier Publishing Co., Inc., 1974.

Thiery, M., Cliquet, R.L., Wauters, M., and Maele, C.V. "A Prospective Investigation of Voluntary Sterilization." In *Advances in Voluntary Sterilization,* Proceedings of the Second International Conference, Geneva, 1973, edited by M.E. Schima, I. Lubell, J.E. Davis, and E. Connell, pp. 167-84. Princeton N.J.: Excerpta Medica, American Elsevier Publishing Co., Inc., 1974.

Veatch, R.M. "Sterilization: Its Socio-Cultural and Ethical Determinants." In *Advances in Voluntary Sterilization,* Proceedings of the Second International Conference, Geneva, 1973, edited by M.E. Schima, I. Lubell, J.E. Davis, and E. Connell, pp. 138-50. Princeton, N.J.: Excerpta Medica, American Elsevier Publishing Co., Inc., 1974.

Viel, B. "Development and Evaluation of Voluntary Sterilization Service Programs." In *Advances in Voluntary Sterilization,* Proceedings of the Second International Conference, Geneva, 1973, edited by M.E. Schima, I. Lubell, J.E. Davis, and E. Connell, pp. 309-11. Princeton, N.J.: Excerpta Medica, American Elsevier Publishing Co., Inc., 1974.

Wedderburn, C.C. "Factors Influencing a National Policy on Sterilization." In *Advances in Voluntary Sterilization,* Proceedings of the Second International Conference, Geneva, 1973, edited by M.E. Schima, I. Lubell, J.E. Davis, and E. Connell, pp. 133-37. Princeton, N.J.: Excerpta Medica, American Elsevier Publishing Co., Inc., 1974.

Ziegler, F.J., Rogers, D.A., and Kriegsman, S.A. "Effect of Vasectomy on Psychological Functioning." Paper presented at the annual Meeting of the American Psychosomatic Society. Philadelphia, May 1965.

## Chapters from Books and Articles in Books

Berquo, E. and Oya, D.R. "A Esterilizacao em Sao Paulo" (On Sterilization in Sao Paulo). In *Diferenciais de Fertilidade* (Differential Fertility), edited by E.S. Berquo et al., Vol. 1, pp. 75-91. Sao Paulo, Centro Brasiliero, de Analise e Planejamento (CEBRAP), 1971.

Dubey, D.C. and Bardhan, A. "Mass Acceptance of Vasectomy: The Role of Social Interaction and Incentives in Social Change." In *Population and Social Organization,* edited by M. Nag, pp. 295-305. The Hague: Mouton Publishers, 1975.

Ekblad, M. "The Prognosis After Sterilization on Social-Psychiatric Grounds, A Follow-Up Study of 225 Women." In *Acta Psychiatric Scandinavica,* Supplementum 161, Vol. 37, 1961.

Erickson, M.H. "The Psychological Significance of Vasectomy." In *Therapeutic Abortion,* edited by H. Rosen, pp. 57-86. New York: Julian Press, 1954.

Evans, T.M. "Sterilization of Women." In *Human Reproduction: Conception and Contraception,* edited by E.S.E. Hafez and T.N. Evans, pp. 383-404. New York: Harper & Row, 1973.

Ferber, W.L.F. "Male Sterilization." In *Manual of Family Planning and Contraceptive Practice,* edited by M.S. Calderone, pp. 246-49. Baltimore: Williams and Wilkins Company, 1970.

Gabriel, M.P., Jr., "The INC Sterilization Project: The Church that Really Cares." In *Voluntary Sterilization,* edited by P.T. Piotrow, pp. 9-11. Draper World Population Fund Report—Monograph No. 3. Washington, D.C.: Population Crisis Committee, 1976.

Grindstaff, C.F. and Ebanks, G.E. "Vasectomy as a Birth Control Method." In *Critical Issues in Canadian Society,* edited by C.L. Boydell, C.F. Grindstaff, and P.C. Whitehead, pp. 25-32. New York and Toronto: Holt, Rinehart & Winston, 1971.

———. "Male Sterilization in Canada." In *Social Process and Institution,* edited by J.E. Gallagher and R.D. Lambert, pp. 396-414. New York and Toronto: Holt, Rinehart, & Winston, 1971.

Gulhati, K. "Compulsory Sterilization: A New Dimension in India's Population Policy." In *Voluntary Sterilization,* edited by P.T. Piotrow, pp. 26-29. Draper World Population Fund Report—Monograph No. 3. Washington, D.C.: Population Crisis Committee, 1976.

Guttmacher, A.F. "The Place of Sterilization." In *The Population Crisis and the Use of Water Resources,* edited by S. Mudd, pp. 268-73. Bloomington: Indiana University Press, 1964.

Hulka, J.F. and Davis, J.E. "Sterilization of Men." In *Human Reproduction: Conception and Contraception,* edited by E.S.E. Hafez and T.N. Evans, pp. 427-46. New York: Harper & Row, 1973.

——— and Omran, K.F. "New Methods of Female Sterilization." In *New Concepts in Contraception,* edited by M. Potts and C. Wood, pp. 57-67. Baltimore: University Park Press, 1972.

India, Gandhigram. Institute of Rural Health and Family Planning, Research Division. "Vasectomy Follow-up Study." In *Summary of Projects Undertaken up to 31 March 1969,* pp. 9-11, 1969.

John-Stevas, N. "Human Sterilization." In *Life, Death and the Law: Law and Christian Morals in England and the United States,* by N. John-Stevas, pp. 160-97. Bloomington: Indiana University Press, 1964. (Issued separately as *Sterilization and Public Policy.* Washington, D.C.: Family Life Bureau, National Catholic Welfare Conference, 1965).

Kapil, K.K. "A Bibliography of Sterilization Studies in India, 1952-1968." In Newsletter No. 26 of the *International Institute for Population Studies,* pp. 3-18. Bombay, 1968.

Khandwala, S.D. "Vasectomy." In *Family Planning and Foetal Salvage,* edited by B.M. Purandare and N.A. Purandare, pp. 98-106. Bombay: Department of Obstetrics and Gynecology, K.E.M. Hospital, n.d.

Kleinman, R.L. "Sterilisation." In *IPPF Medical Handbook,* pp. 66-70. London: International Planned Parenthood Federation, 1968.

Krishnakumar, S. "Massive Vasectomy Camps—An Innovative Project in Ernakulam District." In *Family Planning in India: Policy and Administration,* edited by V. Jagannadhan, pp. 191-213. New Delhi: Indian Institute of Public Administration, 1973.

Kumar, A. "An Addendum to a Bibliography of Sterilization Studies in India, 1969-1970." In *Newsletter no. 39 of the International Institute for Population Studies,* pp. 4-7. Bombay, 1972.

Kunitz, S.J. and Slocumb, J.C. "The Use of Surgery to Avoid Childbearing Among Navajo and Hopi Inidans." In *Anthropological Studies of Human Fertility,* edited by B.A. Kaplan, pp. 9-21. Detroit: Wayne State University Press, 1976.

Long, W.N. "Black Attitudes Regarding Contraception, Abortion, and Sterilization." In *Abortion Techniques and Services,* edited by Sarah Lewit, pp.
151-60. Amsterdam: Excerpta Medica, 1972.

Lubell, I. and Frischer, R. "Sterilization Demand Exceeds Facilities." In
*Voluntary Sterilization,* edited by P.T. Piotrow, pp. 3-5. Draper World
Population Fund Report—Monograph No. 3. Washington, D.C.: Population
Crisis Committee, 1976.

Omran, K. et al. "Female Sterilization: A Review of the Middle East Experience."
In *Female Sterilization:* Series No. 29. Chapel Hill, N.C.: International
Fertility Research Program, 1975.

Osathanondh, V. " 'Minilap,' a Simple Technique for Female Sterilization." In
*Voluntary Sterilization,* edited by P.T. Piotrow, pp. 5-8. Draper World
Population Fund Report—Monograph No. 3. Washington, D.C.: Population
Crisis Committee, 1976.

Overstreet, E.W. "Female Sterilization." In *Manual of Family Planning and
Contraceptive Practice,* edited by M.S. Calderone, pp. 404-16. Baltimore:
Williams and Wilkins Company, 1970.

———. "Legal Aspects." In *Manual of Family Planning and Contraceptive
Practice,* edited by M.S. Calderone, pp. 398-404. Baltimore: Williams and
Wilkins Company, 1970.

———. "Permanent Contraception: Sterilization General Considerations." In
*Manual of Family Planning and Contraceptive Practice,* edited by M.S.
Calderone, pp. 389-97. Baltimore: Williams and Wilkins Company, 1970.

Parker, J.B. "Psychiatric Aspects of Sterilization." In *Psychological Aspects
of Sterilization,* edited by H.S. Abram, pp. 105-13. *International Psychiatry
Clinics,* vol. 4. Boston: Little, Brown and Company, 1967.

Paul, J. "Eugenic Sterilization Legislation in the United States." In *American
Philosophical Society Yearbook,* pp. 379-83. 1967.

Potts, M. "Bureaucratic Barriers to Sterilization." In *Voluntary Sterilization,*
edited by P.T. Piotrow, pp. 22-25. Draper World Population Fund Report—
Monograph No. 3. Washington, D.C.: Population Crisis Committee, 1976.

Presser, H.B. and Bumpass, L.L. "Demographic and Social Aspects of Contraceptive Sterilization in the United States: 1965-1970." In *Demographic
and Social Aspects of Population Growth,* edited by C.F. Westoff and R.
Parke, Jr., Vol. 1 of the Commission on Population Growth and the American Future, Research Reports. Washington D.C.: U.S. Government
Printing Office, 1972.

Rodgers, D.A. and Ziegler, F.J. "Psychological Reactions to Surgical Contraception." In *Psychological Perspectives on Population,* edited by J.T. Fawcett.
New York: Basic Books, May, 1973.

Schmidt, S.S. "Male Sterilization." In *Manual of Family Planning and Contraceptive Practice,* edited by M.S. Calderone, pp. 417-21. Baltimore: Williams
and Wilkins Company, 1970.

Setchell, B.P. "Bibliography on Vasectomy and Its Reversal in Man and Animals."
In *Bibliography on Reproduction,* V. 16, pp. 149-56, 277-87. Cambridge,
England: Research Information Service, LTD., August 1970.

Steptoe, P.C. "Female Sterilization." In *Contraception Today,* edited by A.J.
Smith, pp. 108-12. London: Family Planning Association, 1971.

Tietze, C. "Induced Abortion and Sterilization as Methods of Fertility Control."
In *Public Health and Population Change: Current Research Issues,* edited
by M.C. Sheps and J.C. Ridley, pp. 400-16. Pittsburgh: University of
Pittsburgh, 1965.

Viel, B. and Sanhueza, H. "Sterilization in Catholic Latin America." In
*Voluntary Sterilization,* edited by P.T. Piotrow, pp. 19-22. Draper World
Population Fund Report—Monograph No. 3. Washington, D.C.: Population
Crisis Committee, 1976.

# Indexes

# Author Index

271

# Subject Index

# About the Contributors

**Charles B. Arnold**, professor of public administration, New York University, utilizes a background in public health administration, epidemiology, and preventive medicine in his research on contraception, abortion, and sterilization. His interests include the psychosocial aspects of family planning and fertility regulation, unwanted pregnancies, and sex education, and he has published extensively.

**Nancy J. Cliff** worked at the Institute for Survey Research at Temple University from 1968 to 1974, and was involved in a variety of fertility research projects. She obtained the J.D. in 1977 and is currently engaged in the private practice of law in Miami, Florida.

**Henry P. David** received the Ph.D. in clinical psychology from Columbia University in 1951. He is director of the Transnational Family Research Institute, Bethesda, Maryland; associate clinical professor of psychology, Department of Psychiatry, University of Maryland Medical School, Baltimore; and author or editor of numerous scientific publications on fertility behavior, abortion, population psychology, and mental health.

**Herbert L. Friedman** received the Ph.D. from the University of London. His major areas of research are in communications and cross-cultural and psychosocial aspects of family planning. Former scientific director of the Transnational Family Research Institute in Geneva, he is presently attached to the Psychology Department of Claybury Hospital in Essex, England.

**Duff G. Gillespie** is chief of the Research Division, Office of Population, Agency for International Development. Dr. Gillespie's most recent publications have been concerned with the impact of family planning programs (with Louise Okada, "The Impact of Family Planning Programs on Unplanned Pregnancies," *Family Planning Perspectives,* July/August, 1977); and innovative family planning delivery systems for the developing world (with Dr. R.T. Ravenholt, *People*, Vol. 4, No. 1, 1977). His interest is in operations research, focusing on the cost-effectiveness of family planning programs.

**Leonard LoSciuto** is director of the Institute for Survey Research, Temple University. He is currently directing a number of large-scale projects in the area of population and fertility. His work includes a study of physicians' attitudes toward abortion, a methodological study of measures of unwanted childbearing, and a study of fertility-related decision-making.

**Warren B. Miller** is director of the Laboratory of Behavior and Population and Principal Research Scientist, American Institutes for Research. He is also a research consultant of the American Public Health Association. For a number of years, he has been engaged in research on the psychological aspects of pregnancy planning, unwanted pregnancy, teenage fertility, and childbearing, and has published extensively in these areas.

**Moni Nag** is senior associate at the Center for Policy Studies, The Population Council, New York and adjunct professor of anthropology at Columbia University, New York. At the time of writing this article he was the chief of Social Demography Section of the International Institute for the Study of Human Reproduction, Columbia University. He received the Ph.D. in anthropology from Yale University and worked for over a decade on the Anthropological Survey of India.

**Dorothy L. Nortman** of The Population Council, New York, has a major current interest in the design and application of computer models to assess the demographic impact of family planning practice and, conversely, the family planning practice requirements to meet state demographic goals. As the author of the Population Council's annual publication, *Population and Family Planning Programs: A Factbook,* Mrs. Nortman developed concepts and categories for monitoring and evaluating family planning service statistics on an international basis.

**Edward W. Pohlman** is the director of the Birth Planning Research Program at the University of the Pacific. He received the Ph.D. in psychology from Ohio State, and published *The Psychology of Birth Planning* in 1969, and other books and monographs on the topic subsequently. In 1972, he began a longitudinal study of psychological effects of vasectomy, started with a three-year grant from the Center for Population Research of the National Institute of Child Health and Human Development.

**Harriet B. Presser** is professor of sociology at the University of Maryland, College Park. She received the Ph.D. from the University of California, Berkeley, and has previously taught at the University of Sussex (England), Rutgers University, and Columbia University. She was also employed at The Population Council. Dr. Presser has published a book and a number of major reports on contraceptive sterilization.

**David A. Rodgers** is head of the section of psychology, Department of Psychiatry, Cleveland Clinic Foundation. A graduate of the University of Chicago, Dr. Rodgers has held faculty appointments at the University of California in Berkeley and at the University of California in San Diego. Among many

CAMBRIA COUNTY LIBRARY
JOHNSTOWN, PA. 15901

scientific and professional offices that he has held, he has served as acting chairman of the National Institutes of Health Population Research Study Section and on the Council of Representatives of the American Psychological Association. He has published numerous research and professional articles.

**Everett M. Rogers** is professor at the Institute for Communication Research, Stanford University. He is author of *Communication of Innovations* and *Communication Strategies for Family Planning*. Rogers' current research is concerned with interpersonal networks in the diffusion of family planning methods in Korean villages, and with family planning communication to low-income women in California.

**Paul E. Ryser** is vice-president for research and evaluation with Richard Katon and Associates, Inc., and adjunct associate professor of medical sociology at the Graduate School of Public Health, University of Pittsburgh. His current research interests are in the field of male fertility and the evaluation of health care facilities.

**George B. Simmons** is an associate professor of population planning and a lecturer in economics at the University of Michigan. He was formerly the director of the Economic Demography Training Program also at the University of Michigan. His research has been concerned with the economics of population policy in developing countries, particularly in India. He is currently working on an interdisciplinary study of the implementation of family planning programs in India and on the use of new techniques for the evaluation of family planning programs.

**William H. Spillane** combined training and experience in population, sociology, and public health to concentrate his research on male family planning attitudes and practices, with special attention to vasectomy. He is now director of the Division of Scientific and Program Information, National Institute on Drug Abuse.

**Helen Wolfers** is a psychology graduate of Melbourne University, Australia. She has been engaged in research into psychological effects of male and female sterilization during the past eight years, both in developing and developed countries. She is co-author with her husband of the controversial book, *Vasectomy and Vasectomania.*

## About the Editors

**Sidney H. Newman,** a psychologist, is a behavioral scientist administrator, Center for Population Research, National Institute of Child Health and Human Development. His background and experience is in the conduct and administration of research programs, including research and training grant programs. He is interested in stimulating and furthering behavioral-social population research on significant problems, such as contraceptive sterilization.

**Zanvel E. Klein** was a clinical psychologist in the Department of Psychiatry, Pritzker School of Medicine, University of Chicago when he co-edited this book. As a counselor with the Midwest Population Center he became interested in contraceptive sterilization. He has done research on sources of information about vasectomy, attitudes of clients, and factors that distinguish "continuers," "discontinuers," and those who never seriously considered vasectomy.

NO LONGER PROPERTY
OF CAMBRIA CO LIBRARY

301.321
B419

c-1

PJo

Behavioral-social aspects of
contraceptive sterilization / edited
by Sidney H. Newman, Zanvel E. Klein.
-- Lexington, Mass. : Lexington Books,
[c1978].
vii, 286 p. : ill. ; 24 cm.
Outgrowth of a workshop sponsored by
the National Institute of Child Health
and Human Development.
Bibliography: p. 217-268.
Includes indexes.

CAMBRIA COUNTY LIBRARY
Johnstown, Pa. 15901

FINES PER DAY: 5¢
Adults 5¢, Children 2¢
10¢
8

JOCCxc SEE NEXT CRD